Oh Joy Sex Toy

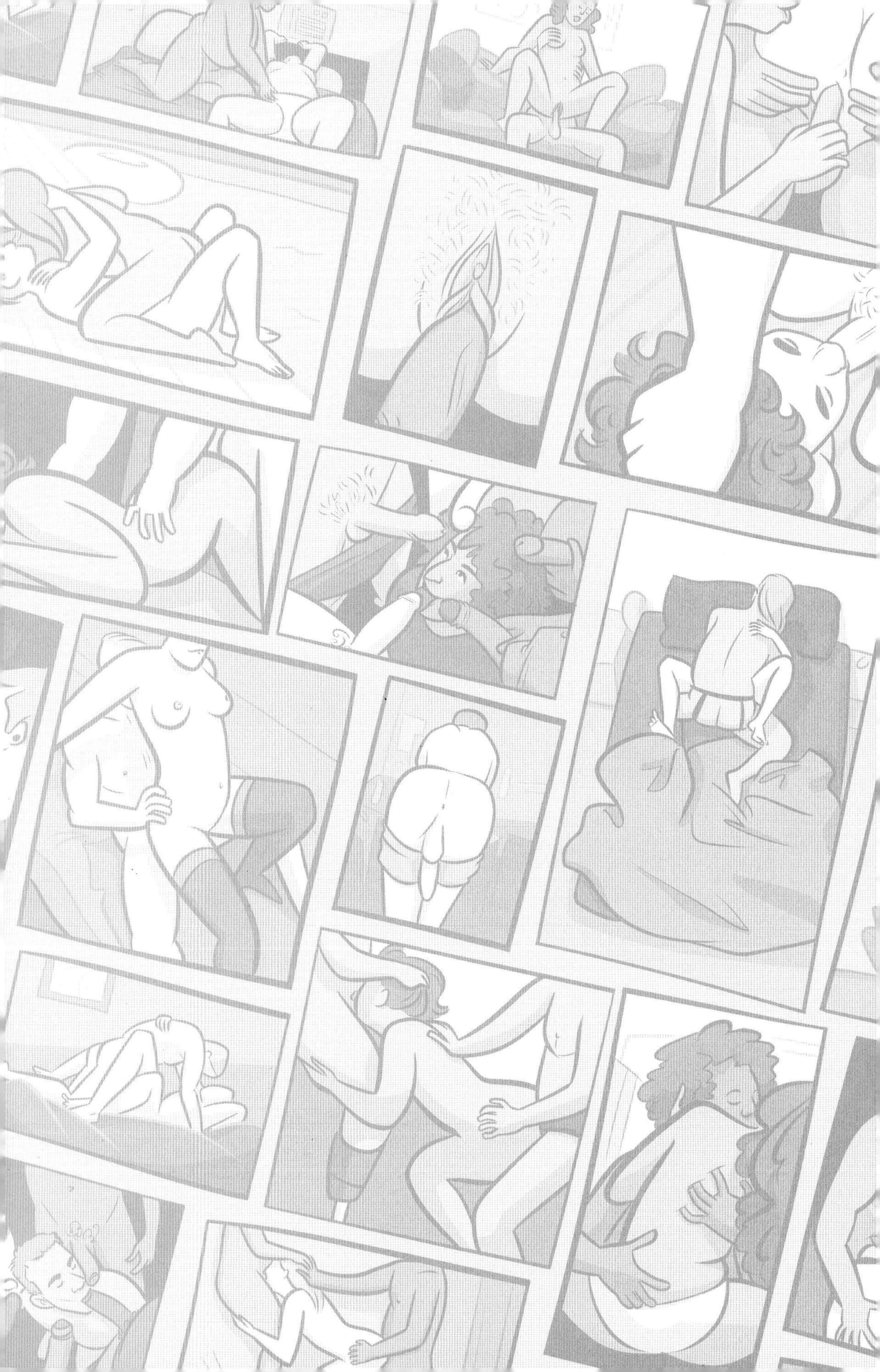

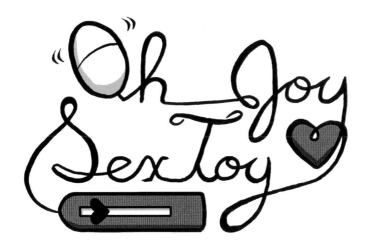

created by
ERIKA MOEN
&
MATTHEW NOLAN

Published by Erika Moen Comics & Illustration, LLC
Helioscope Studio
333 SW 5th Ave, Suite 500
Portland, OR 97204
Matthew Nolan, creator
Erika Moen, creator

Published by Limerence Press
Limerence Press is an imprint of Oni Press, Inc.
Joe Nozemack, publisher
James Lucas Jones, editor in chief
Andrew McIntire, v.p. of marketing & sales
Rachel Reed, publicity coordinator
Troy Look, director of design & production
Hilary Thompson, graphic designer
Jared Jones, digital art technician
Ari Yarwood, managing editor
Charlie Chu, senior editor
Robin Herrera, editor
Bess Pallares, editorial assistant
Brad Rooks, director of logistics
Jung Lee, logistics assistant

Edited by: Allyson Haller
Editorial Assists by: Ari Yarwood
Design by: Matthew Nolan, Erika Moen, Allyson Haller

OhJoySexToy.com
twitter.com/ErikaMoen
facebook.com/ErikaMoenComics
erikamoen.com

LimerencePress.com
twitter.com/limerencepress
limerencepress.tumblr.com

First edition: November 2016
Direct Market ISBN: 978-1-62010-361-6

PRINTED IN SINGAPORE.

Library of Congress Control Number: 2016940277
1 2 3 4 5 6 7 8 9 10

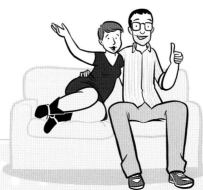

Table of Contents

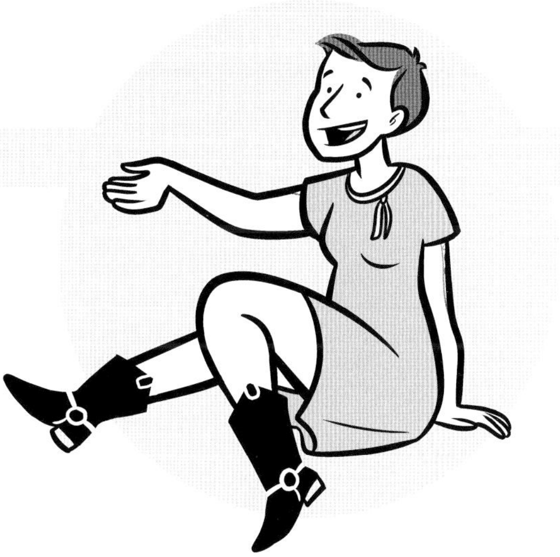

Introduction

GOOD THINGS COME IN THREES!!!

Dearest perverts*!

Salutations, smarty pants! Greetings Ladies, Gentlemen, and everyone betwixt and beyond…It is with immense pleasure (literally!) that I introduce to you… (drum roll please)...

Oh Joy Sex Toy, Volume 3!

The newest collection of comic sex toy reviews, erotic guest illustrations, and positively delightful sex geekery from celebrated artist-spouse duo Erika Moen and Matthew Nolan. Trust me, I'm just as excited as you are.

THE 'RULE OF THREE' suggests that things which come in threes are generally funnier, more satisfying, and more effective than any other numbers of things. (Examples range from *The Three Stooges* to *Star Wars*.) Well, this third volume is no exception to that rule, if only because it now means there exists a triad -- a jolly pink threesome, if you will -- to gayly display in your library, bedside table, or reading basket in your bathroom that everyone has but no one talks about.

I am particularly proud to introduce this third volume of *Oh Joy Sex Toy* because many of the strips in this book are about my favorite subject: P-O-R-N!

Aside from the salacious illustrations by guest artists, Volume 3 addresses the realities of porn production as told by voices from inside the industry. Like true sex geeks, Erika and Matthew go right to the source, interviewing actual professionals and featuring us in guest appearances as experts in our field, from pole dancing to porno. They even compensate us for our time. Loads of respect, right there!

The porn-curious will rejoice with Danny Wylde's DIY sex tape production tips, a review of Cocky Boys' gay porn website, and bear solemn witness as Erika weighs the pros and cons of whether she herself would choose to do porn and dip her toes in the jizz biz. ("Jizz biz!" You know I had to.) Speaking of "jiz"… Full disclosure: You'll see me again in a few pages when Erika and Matthew take a trip to San Francisco to watch Shine Louise Houston and her crew film

queer porn at the CrashPad! Erika also reviews my book, *Coming Out Like a Porn Star*, in which 57 porn professionals share their stories. From production angles to personal anecdotes, *Oh Joy Sex Toy*, Volume 3 just might be the porniest volume yet!

You know, I really could go on and on and on about porn…but there's much more to be said of this book. I laughed, I cried, and I got horny! There's three things *Oh Joy Sex Toy* does particularly well in Volume 3, so let's get right down to it.

THREE WAYS

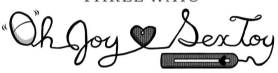

DOES WHAT IT DOES BEST

1

SEX TOYS!

Oh Joy Sex Toy takes a stab, a poke, a suck, and a slurp on some of the most sensational toys on the market. They go to bone town with newsmakers like the infamous Womanizer and the buzzworthy K-Goal, and get busy with popular toys like the Rechargeable Magic Wand Vibrator and esteemed dildo makers. They even let us peek into their bedroom—it's significant to see which toys make the cut for the coveted placement on a toy reviewer's nightstand.

Seeing toys (in-action!) in comics is wonderfully fun, but the real pleasure is how they're reviewed. Erika, Matt, and cartoon 'masturbateers' share what works for them and, importantly, what doesn't-work-for-them-but-might-work-for-someone-else. If you've ever visited a sex-positive toy store, you'll recognize this tone. It's a way of talking about a toy's function that is non-judgmental, respectful, and genuinely helpful. It's this honest and shame-free depiction of sexual exploration that makes learning about sex products and new information so palatable.

*"Pervert' is one of my favorite reclaimed sex-positive words. Whose idea of sexy are you calling 'abnormal' or 'inappropriate', huh!? Pick up a book (or three, ahem) and expand your horizons. The landscape of human sexuality is a wondrous world!

2 SEX EDUCATION!

I have a confession. While sex toy reviews are the comic's bread and butter, my favorite *Oh Joy Sex Toy* panels are actually the sex education specials. These drawings share the wondrous qualities of the toy reviews, but address important and hard to find information about some of the most central sexual health subjects.

In Volume 3, *Oh Joy Sex Toy* rolls up its sleeves, applies a generous amount of lube, and goes elbow deep in sex geekdom. What exactly happens in your brain during orgasm? How does society construct myths around sexual identity? What does it mean to be sex-positive? The wonders of the human body never cease! Learn about the foreskin, menstrual sponges, HPV, UTIs, asexuality, vaginismus, and… amazingly…HOMOLOGOUS GENITALS! You will not think about fleshy bits the same way ever again. Mind. Blown.

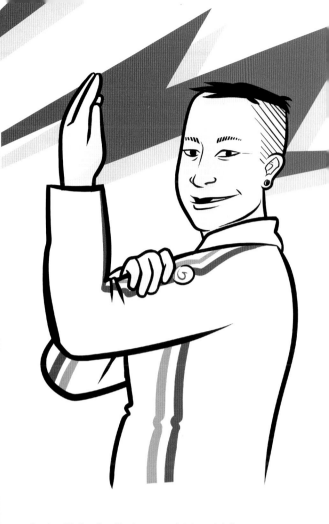

3 SEX SMART!

Oh Joy Sex Toy delivers some of the most truthful depictions of sexuality, bodies, and desires in sex-themed media. It is diverse, self-aware, and its creators grow as they build upon their experiences as sexual beings, and working artists. There's a transparency about their work that is disarmingly genuine and humble.

Sex can be a lot of things for different people: joyful, natural, traumatic, complex, messy, difficult, a job, intimate, and really fucking fun! All these places can gain from education. Erika and Matthew bare themselves on the pages, but also learn from their community and include us in the journey as key characters. It cannot be overstated that seeing bodies that are "outside the box" of what society deems is sexy -- or even "appropriate" -- is an important reality. We are sexy and to see our differences celebrated in *Oh Joy Sex Toy* illustrates that we all are capable and deserving of a happy, healthy sexuality.

So, let *Oh Joy Sex Toy* be your shining pink beacon to a world of sex-positivity. It's informative, hilarious, and completely one-of-a-kind. It's a page-turning series full of bite-sized sex education packaged in delightfully cute drawings with lots of cheeky puns that may make you simultaneously chuckle and groan. It will give you feels, wind you up, and spark your curiosity. The most "sexpert" among us will learn something new. It will probably blow your mind. And if all that isn't enough, just wait for an extra special bonus. Don't worry, I won't spoil the surprise. Sex is best left to be discovered. You know, like two people connecting. With four other people. And aliens… (Let your freak flag fly!)

-Jiz Lee
NSFW Legend
Jizlee.com

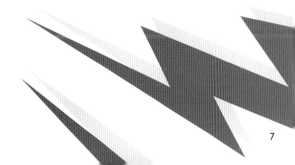

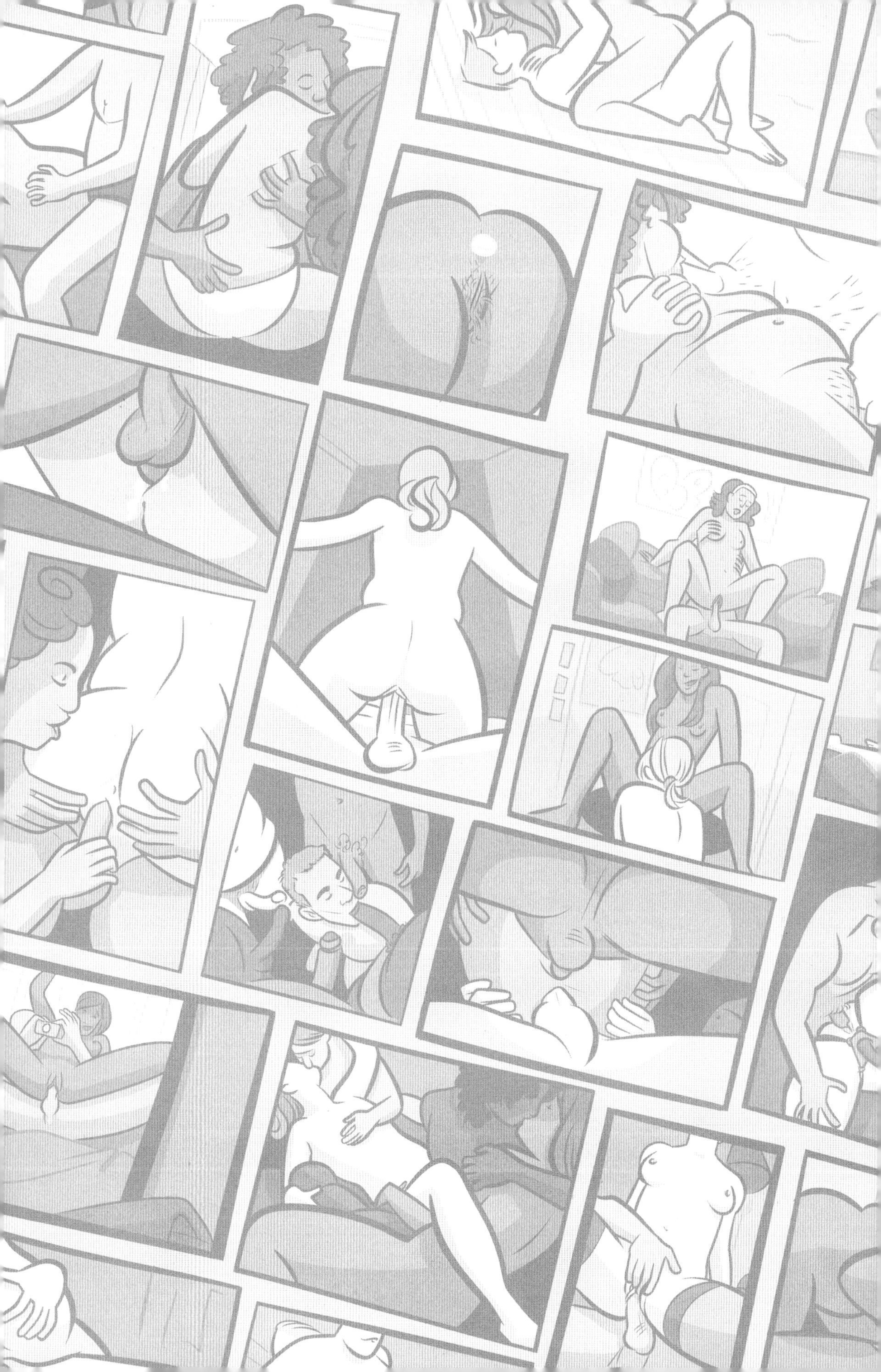

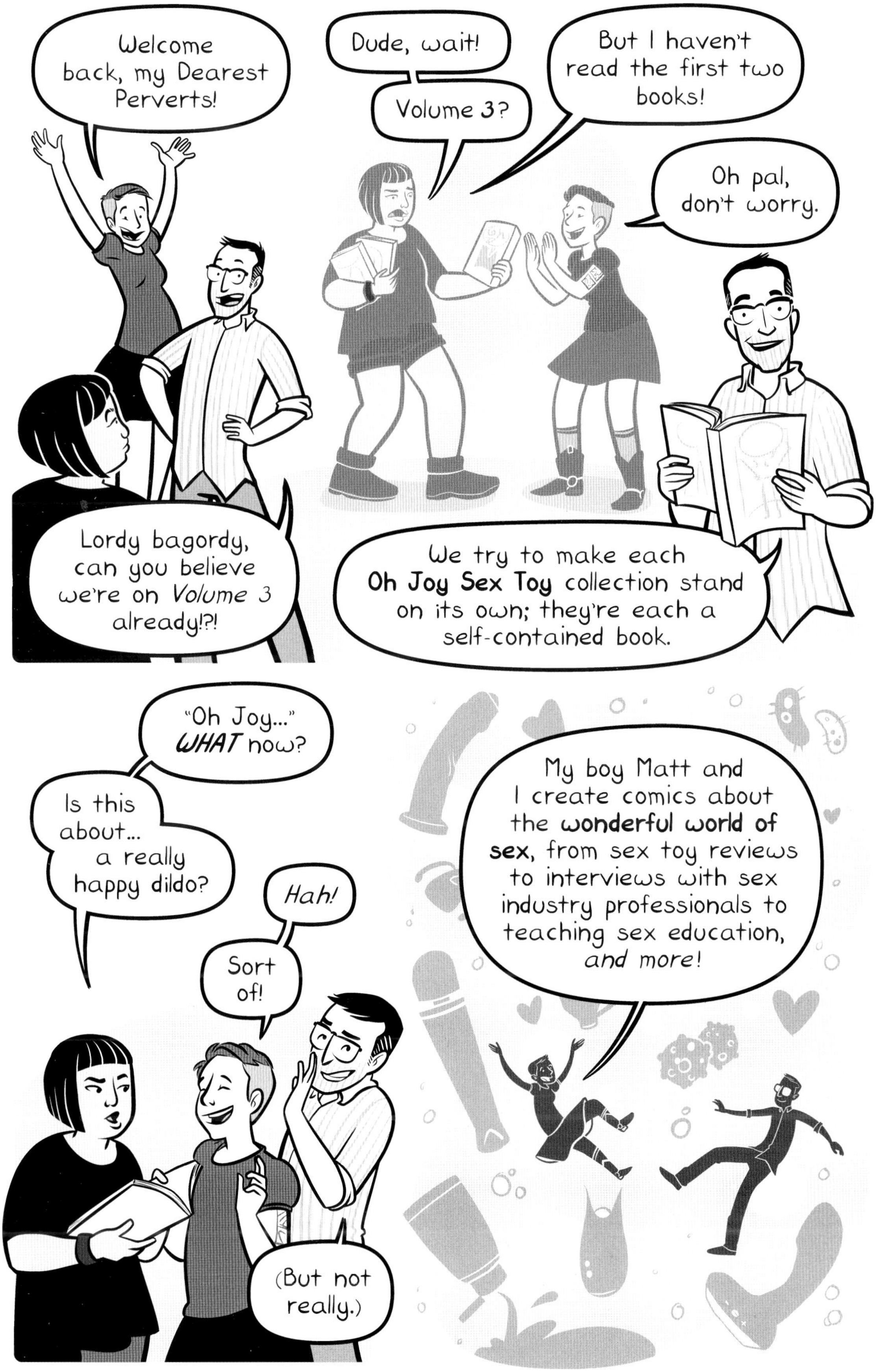
Welcome back, my Dearest Perverts!
Dude, wait!
Volume 3?
But I haven't read the first two books!
Oh pal, don't worry.
Lordy bagordy, can you believe we're on *Volume 3* already!?!
We try to make each **Oh Joy Sex Toy** collection stand on its own; they're each a self-contained book.
"Oh Joy..." *WHAT* now?
Is this about... a really happy dildo?
Hah!
Sort of!
(But not really.)
My boy Matt and I create comics about the **wonderful world of sex**, from sex toy reviews to interviews with sex industry professionals to teaching sex education, *and more*!

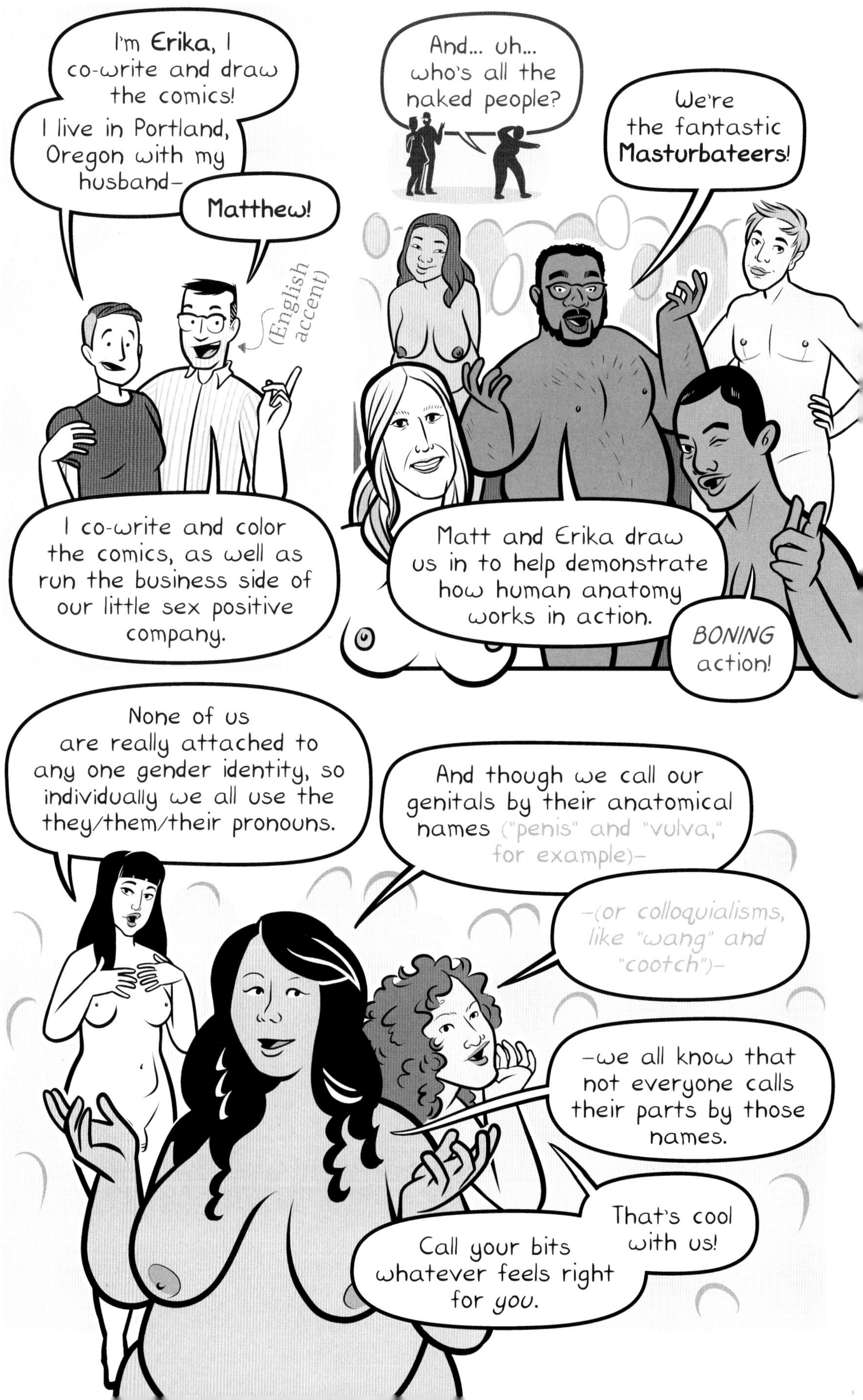

I'm Erika, I co-write and draw the comics! I live in Portland, Oregon with my husband–
Matthew!
(English accent)
I co-write and color the comics, as well as run the business side of our little sex positive company.
And... uh... who's all the naked people?
We're the fantastic Masturbateers!
Matt and Erika draw us in to help demonstrate how human anatomy works in action.
BONING action!
None of us are really attached to any one gender identity, so individually we all use the they/them/their pronouns.
And though we call our genitals by their anatomical names ("penis" and "vulva," for example)–
–(or colloquialisms, like "wang" and "cootch")–
–we all know that not everyone calls their parts by those names.
That's cool with us!
Call your bits whatever feels right for you.

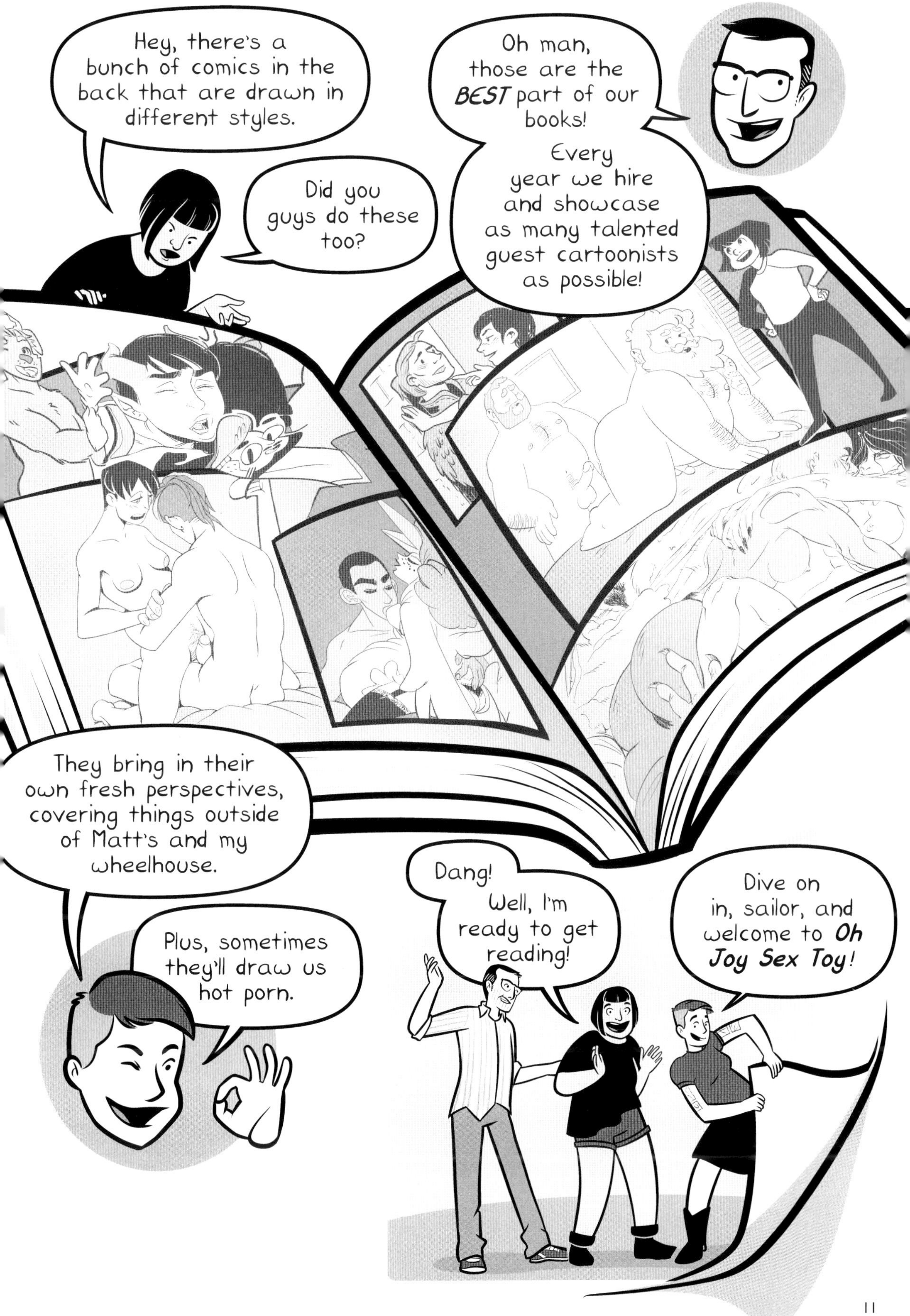
Hey, there's a bunch of comics in the back that are drawn in different styles.
Did you guys do these too?
Oh man, those are the BEST part of our books!
Every year we hire and showcase as many talented guest cartoonists as possible!
They bring in their own fresh perspectives, covering things outside of Matt's and my wheelhouse.
Plus, sometimes they'll draw us hot porn.
Dang!
Well, I'm ready to get reading!
Dive on in, sailor, and welcome to Oh Joy Sex Toy!

WE VIBE
WE VIBE

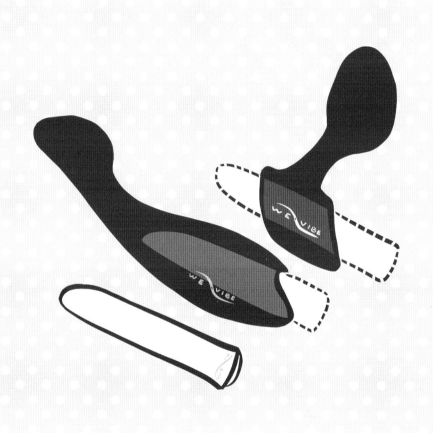

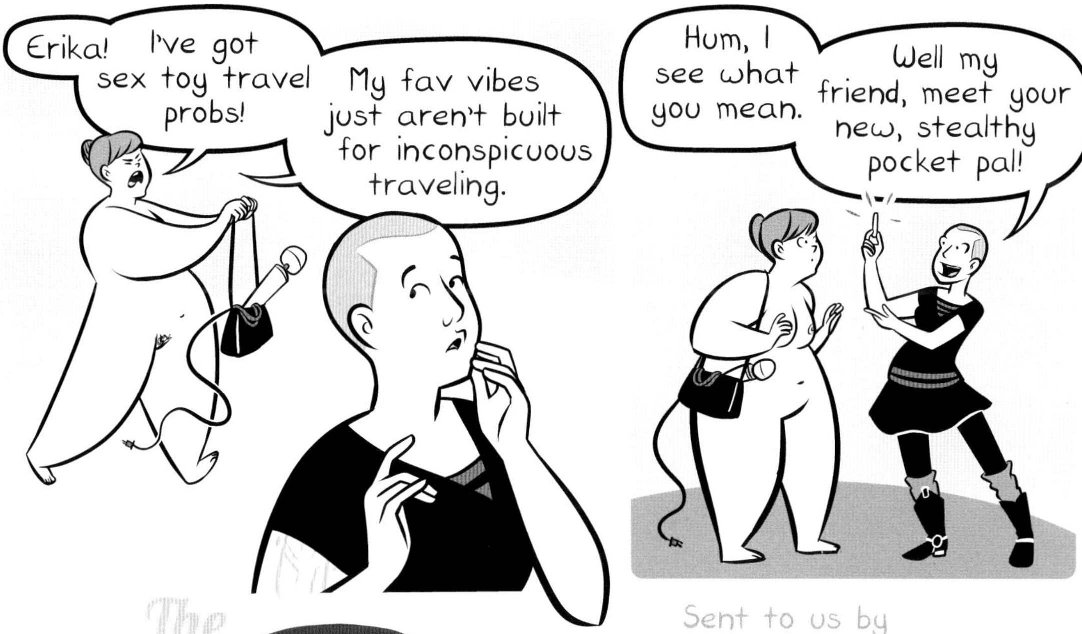

Erika! I've got sex toy travel probs!
My fav vibes just aren't built for inconspicuous traveling.
Hum, I see what you mean.
Well my friend, meet your new, stealthy pocket pal!

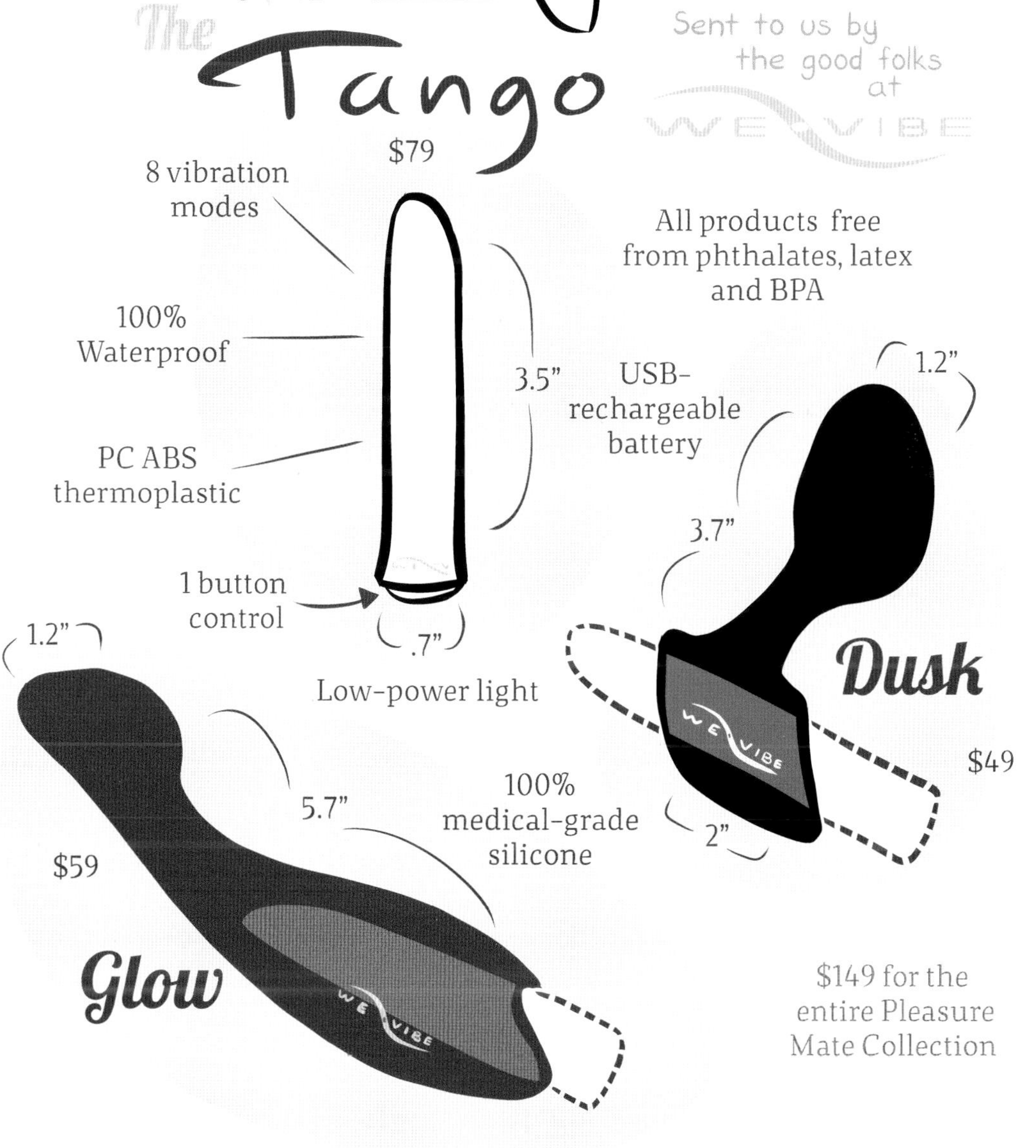

The Tango
Sent to us by the good folks at WE-VIBE
$79
8 vibration modes
100% Waterproof
PC ABS thermoplastic
1 button control
3.5"
.7"
Low-power light
All products free from phthalates, latex and BPA
USB-rechargeable battery
1.2"
3.7"
Dusk
$49
2"
1.2"
5.7"
100% medical-grade silicone
$59
Glow
$149 for the entire Pleasure Mate Collection

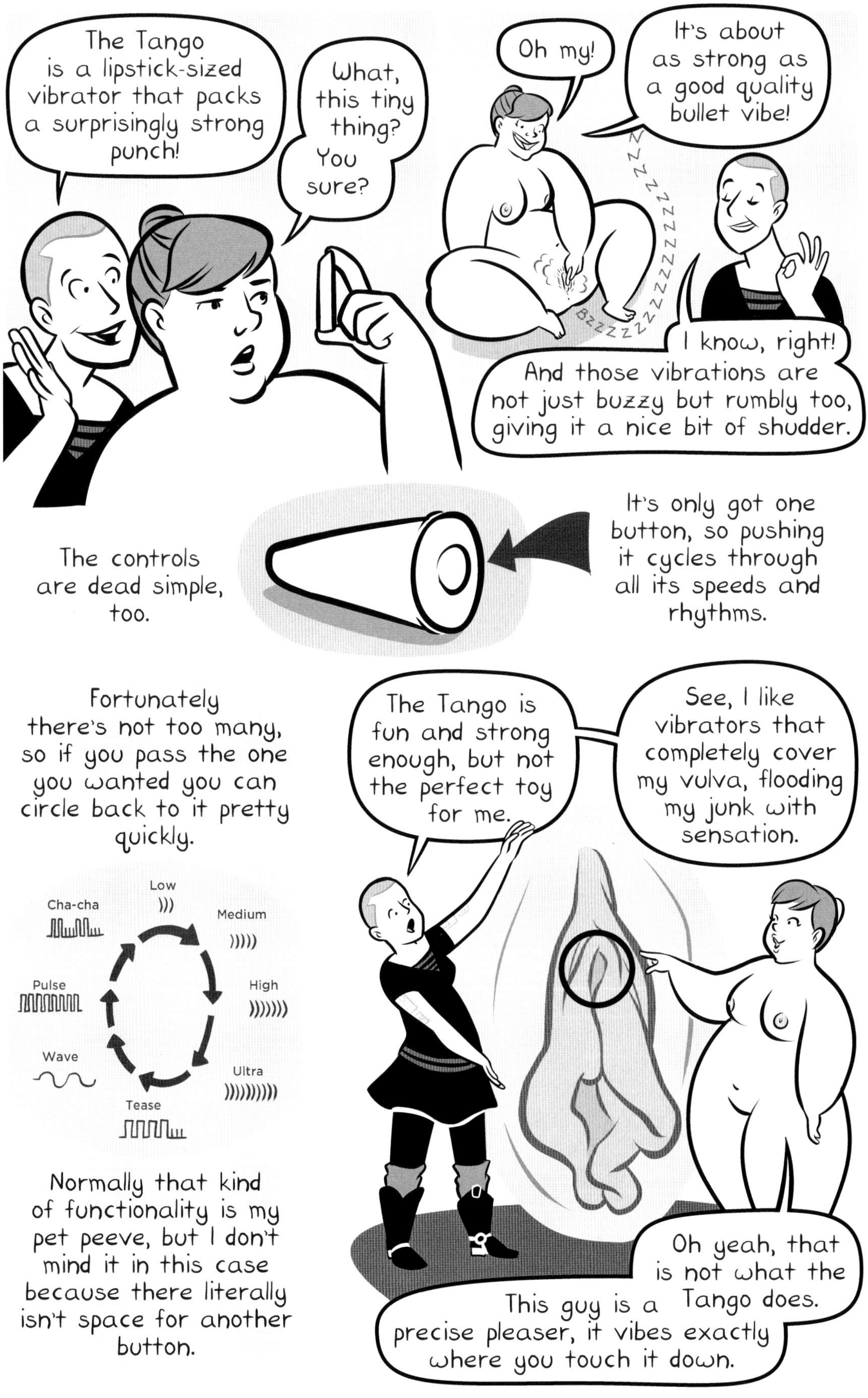
The Tango is a lipstick-sized vibrator that packs a surprisingly strong punch!
What, this tiny thing? You sure?
Oh my!
It's about as strong as a good quality bullet vibe!
I know, right! And those vibrations are not just buzzy but rumbly too, giving it a nice bit of shudder.
The controls are dead simple, too.
It's only got one button, so pushing it cycles through all its speeds and rhythms.
Fortunately there's not too many, so if you pass the one you wanted you can circle back to it pretty quickly.
Low
Medium
High
Ultra
Tease
Wave
Pulse
Cha-cha
Normally that kind of functionality is my pet peeve, but I don't mind it in this case because there literally isn't space for another button.
The Tango is fun and strong enough, but not the perfect toy for me.
See, I like vibrators that completely cover my vulva, flooding my junk with sensation.
Oh yeah, that is not what the Tango does.
This guy is a precise pleaser, it vibes exactly where you touch it down.

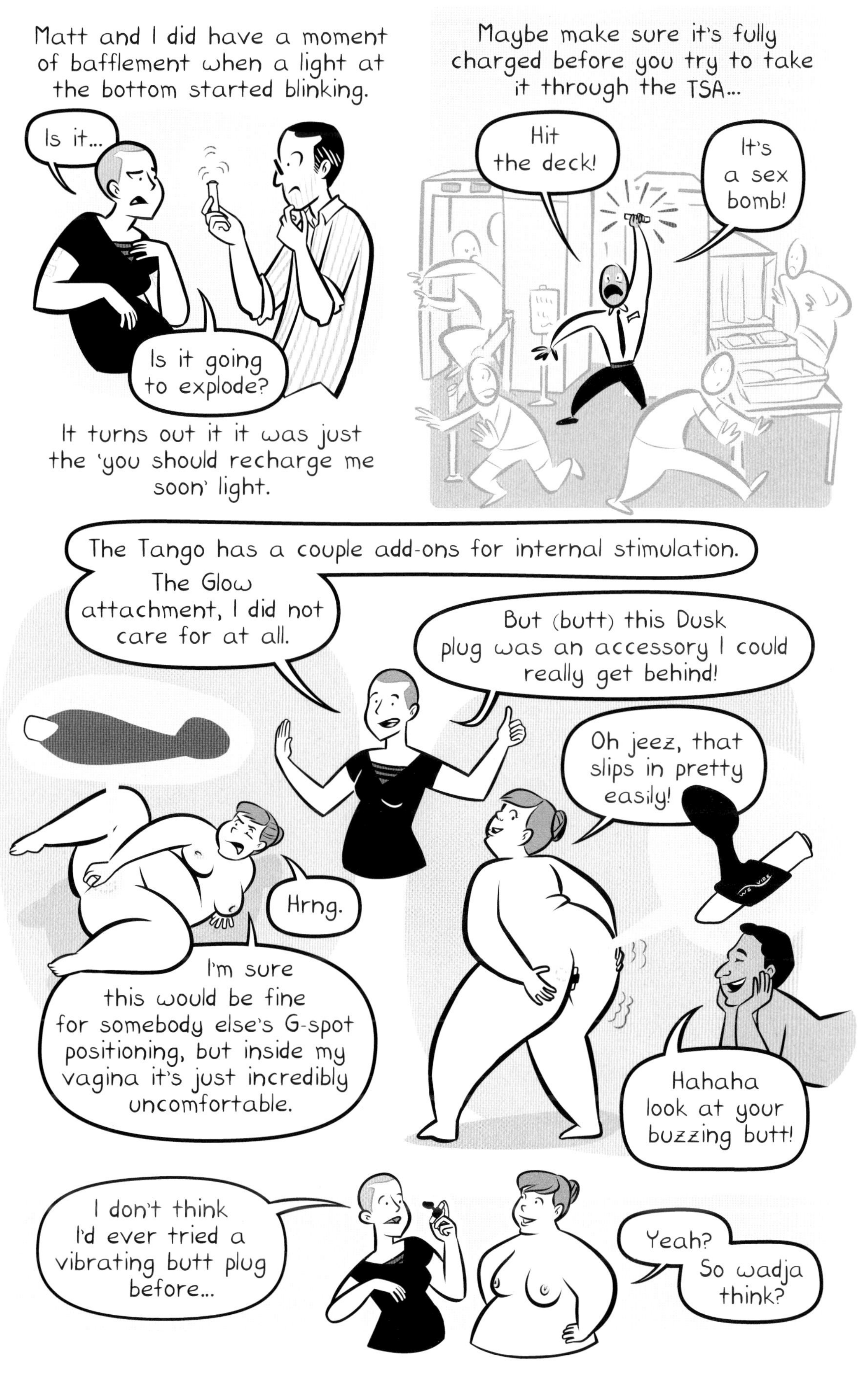
Matt and I did have a moment of bafflement when a light at the bottom started blinking.
Is it...
Is it going to explode?
It turns out it it was just the 'you should recharge me soon' light.
Maybe make sure it's fully charged before you try to take it through the TSA...
Hit the deck!
It's a sex bomb!
The Tango has a couple add-ons for internal stimulation.
The Glow attachment, I did not care for at all.
But (butt) this Dusk plug was an accessory I could really get behind!
Hrng.
I'm sure this would be fine for somebody else's G-spot positioning, but inside my vagina it's just incredibly uncomfortable.
Oh jeez, that slips in pretty easily!
Hahaha look at your buzzing butt!
I don't think I'd ever tried a vibrating butt plug before...
Yeah? So wadja think?

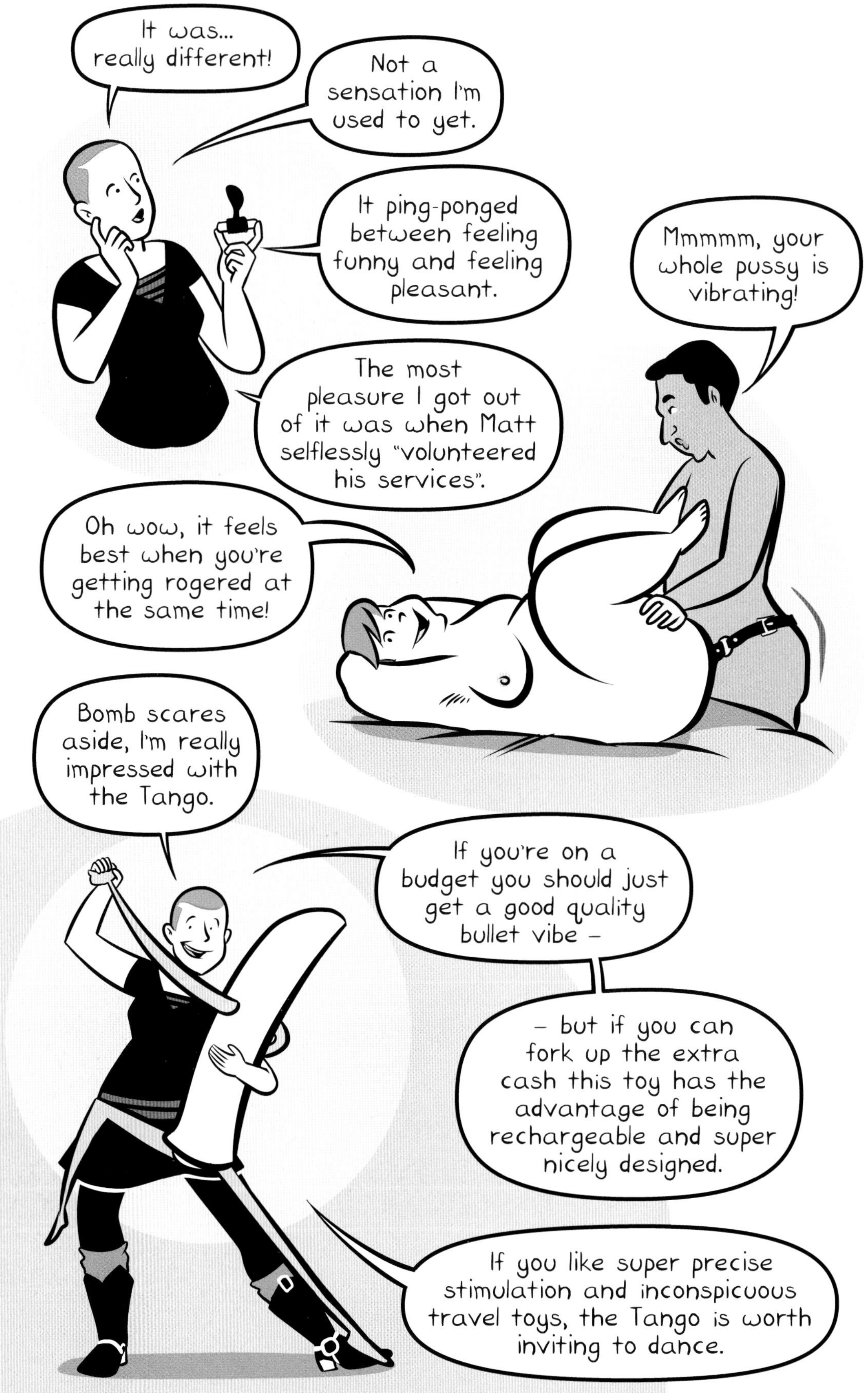
It was... really different!
Not a sensation I'm used to yet.
It ping-ponged between feeling funny and feeling pleasant.
The most pleasure I got out of it was when Matt selflessly "volunteered his services".
Mmmmm, your whole pussy is vibrating!
Oh wow, it feels best when you're getting rogered at the same time!
Bomb scares aside, I'm really impressed with the Tango.
If you're on a budget you should just get a good quality bullet vibe –
– but if you can fork up the extra cash this toy has the advantage of being rechargeable and super nicely designed.
If you like super precise stimulation and inconspicuous travel toys, the Tango is worth inviting to dance.

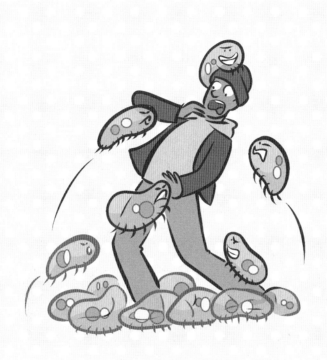

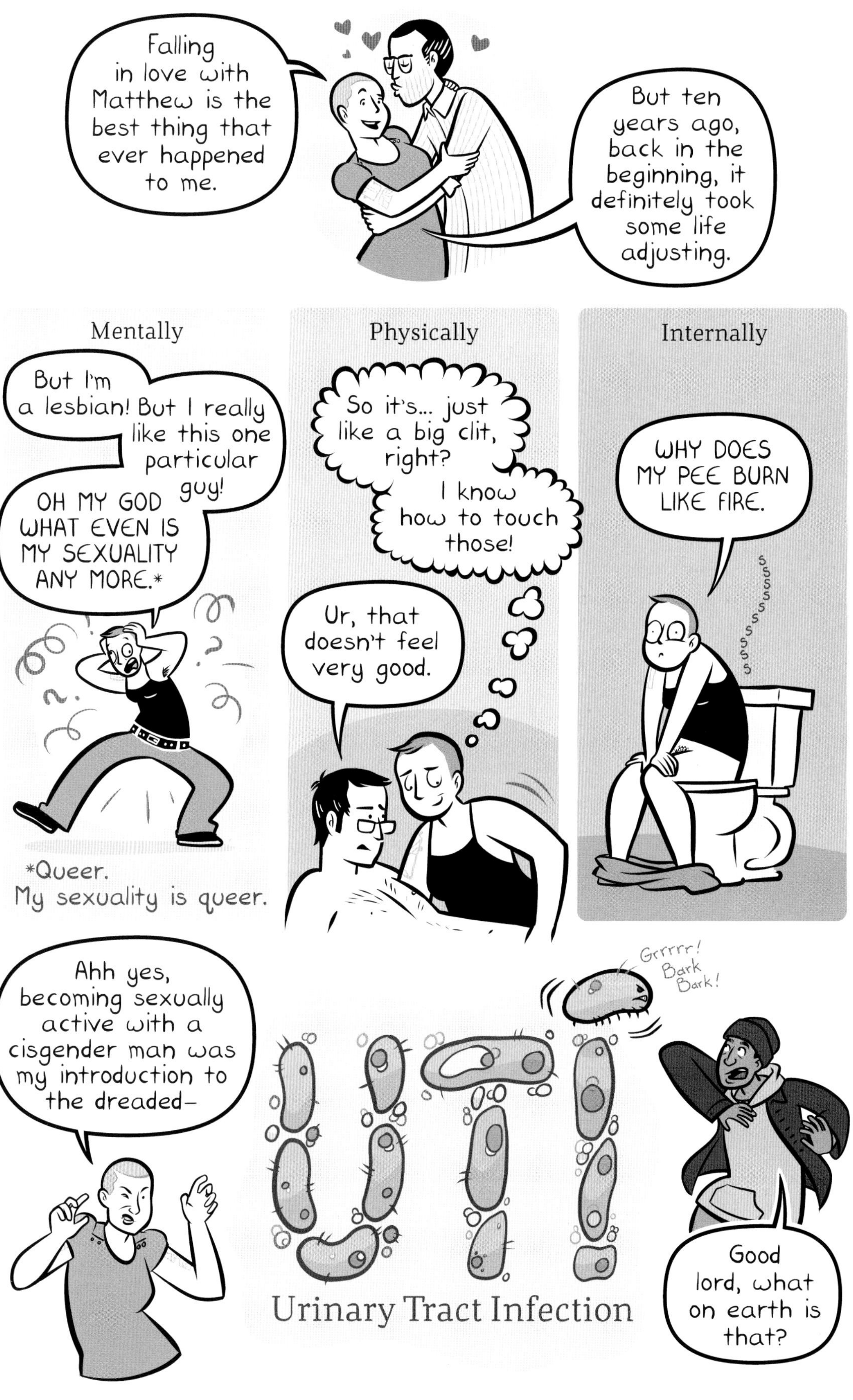

Falling in love with Matthew is the best thing that ever happened to me.
But ten years ago, back in the beginning, it definitely took some life adjusting.
Mentally
But I'm a lesbian! But I really like this one particular guy!
OH MY GOD WHAT EVEN IS MY SEXUALITY ANY MORE.*
*Queer. My sexuality is queer.
Physically
So it's... just like a big clit, right?
I know how to touch those!
Ur, that doesn't feel very good.
Internally
WHY DOES MY PEE BURN LIKE FIRE.
SSSSSSSSSS
Ahh yes, becoming sexually active with a cisgender man was my introduction to the dreaded–
Grrrrr! Bark Bark!
UTI!
Urinary Tract Infection
Good lord, what on earth is that?

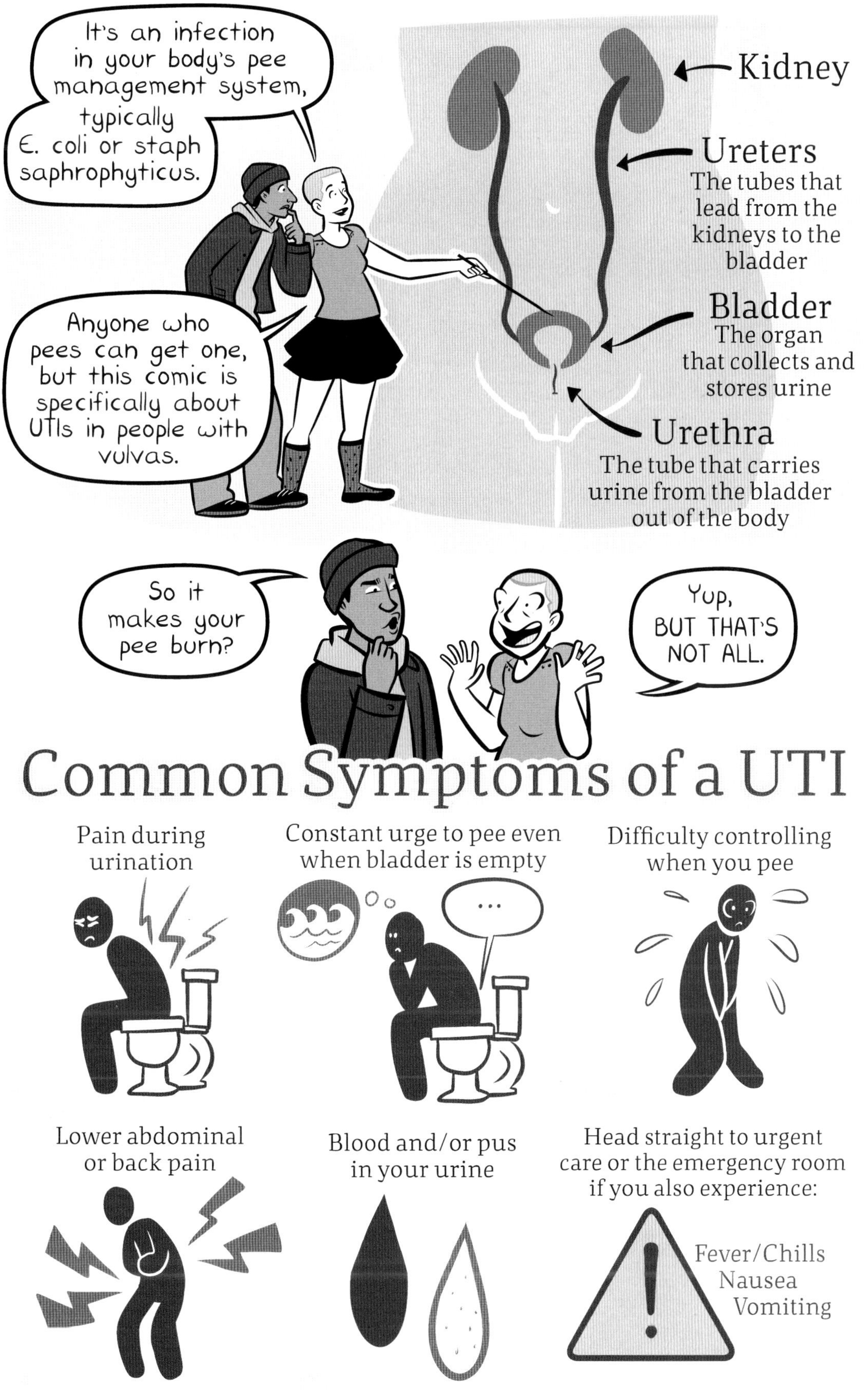
It's an infection in your body's pee management system, typically E. coli or staph saphrophyticus.
Kidney
Ureters
The tubes that lead from the kidneys to the bladder
Bladder
The organ that collects and stores urine
Urethra
The tube that carries urine from the bladder out of the body
Anyone who pees can get one, but this comic is specifically about UTIs in people with vulvas.
So it makes your pee burn?
Yup, BUT THAT'S NOT ALL.
Common Symptoms of a UTI
Pain during urination
Constant urge to pee even when bladder is empty
...
Difficulty controlling when you pee
Lower abdominal or back pain
Blood and/or pus in your urine
Head straight to urgent care or the emergency room if you also experience:
Fever/Chills
Nausea
Vomiting

I remember one particular flare up when I was on my way to interview for an apartment....

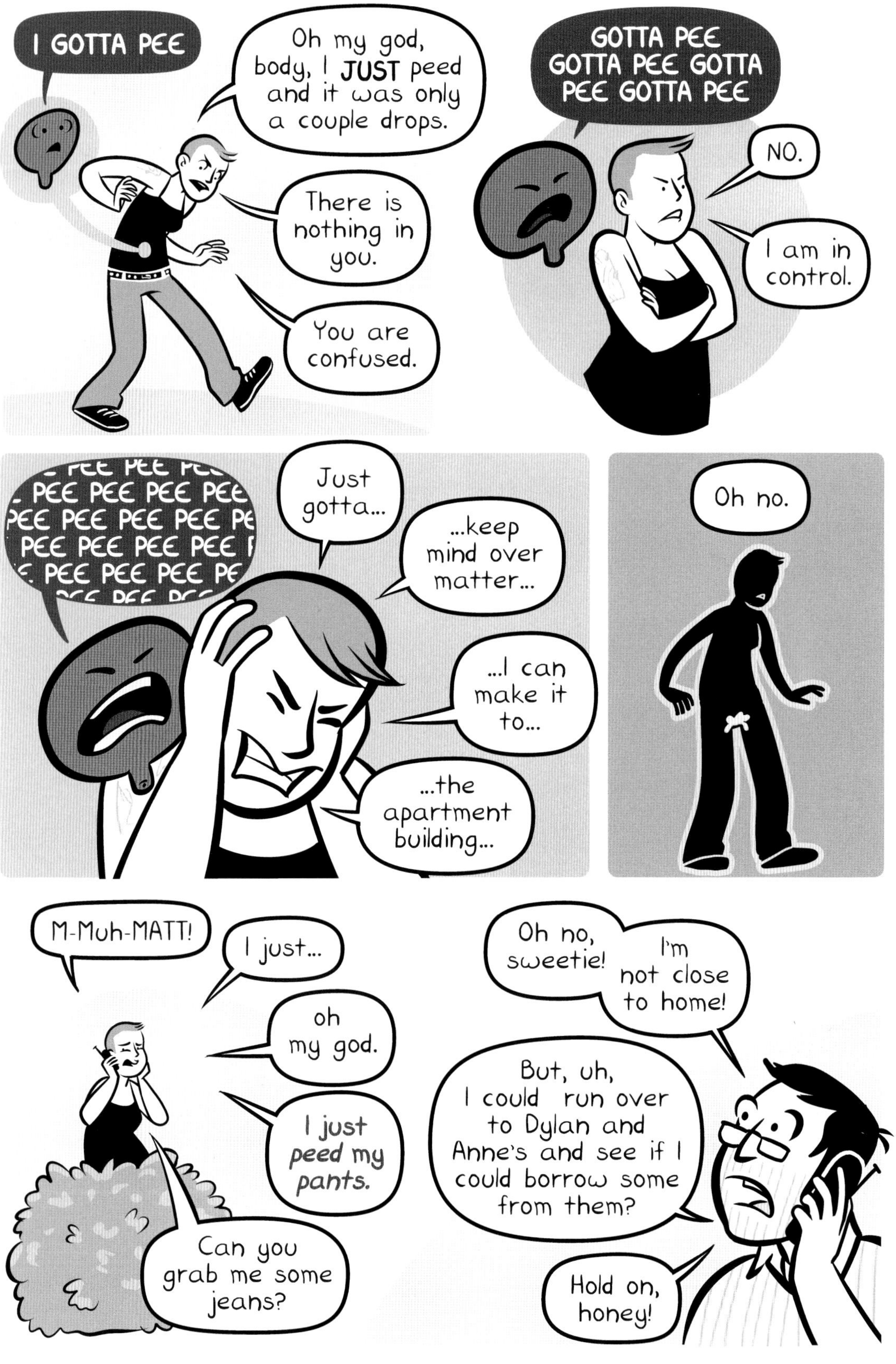
I GOTTA PEE
Oh my god, body, I **JUST** peed and it was only a couple drops.
There is nothing in you.
You are confused.
GOTTA PEE GOTTA PEE GOTTA PEE GOTTA PEE
NO.
I am in control.
PEE PEE PEE PEE PEE PEE PEE PEE PEE PEE PEE PEE PEE PEE PEE PEE
Just gotta...
...keep mind over matter...
...I can make it to...
...the apartment building...
Oh no.
M-Muh-MATT!
I just...
oh my god.
I just *peed* my *pants.*
Can you grab me some jeans?
Oh no, sweetie!
I'm not close to home!
But, uh, I could run over to Dylan and Anne's and see if I could borrow some from them?
Hold on, honey!

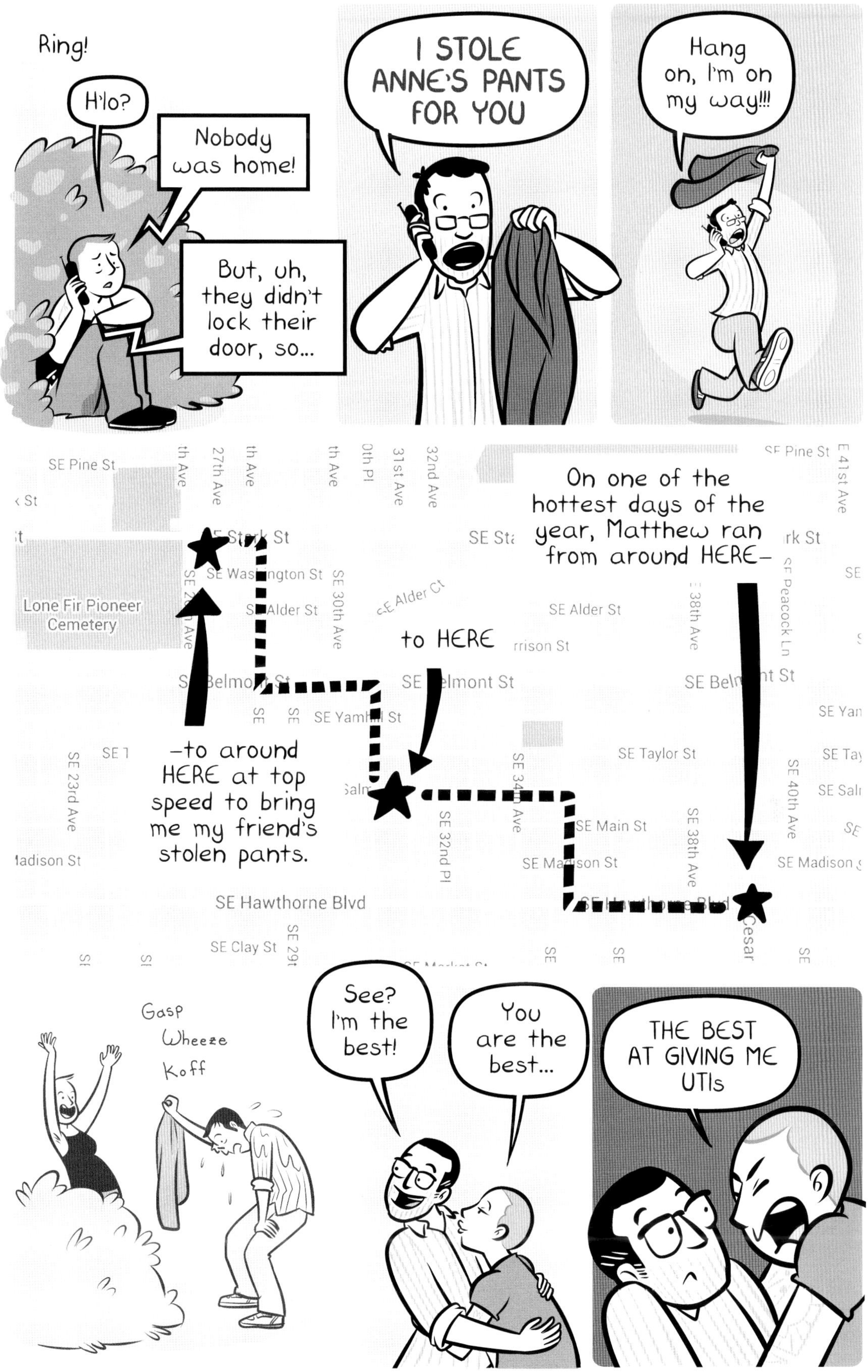
Ring!
H'lo?
Nobody was home!
But, uh, they didn't lock their door, so...
I STOLE ANNE'S PANTS FOR YOU
Hang on, I'm on my way!!!
On one of the hottest days of the year, Matthew ran from around HERE–
to HERE
–to around HERE at top speed to bring me my friend's stolen pants.
Gasp
Wheeze
Koff
See? I'm the best!
You are the best...
THE BEST AT GIVING ME UTIs

UTIs are AWFUL, but SO common.

All it takes is having your urethra coming into contact with bacteria.

It doesn't even have to be from sexual interactions!

And for us folks with a vulva, the urethra entrance is just RIGHT THERE where lots of action happens.

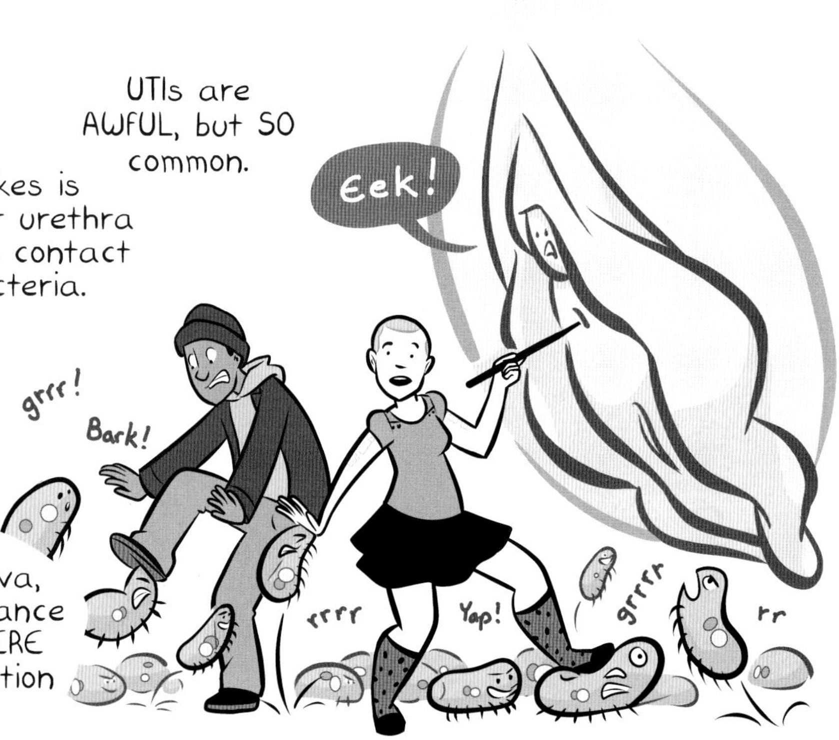
Eek!
grrr!
Bark!
rrrr
Yap!
grrrr
rr

Especially when a partner is rubbing their bits up against yours, it's the perfect scenario for bacteria to transfer off of them, or for your own bacteria to be pushed directly into your urethral opening, during all that grinding motion.

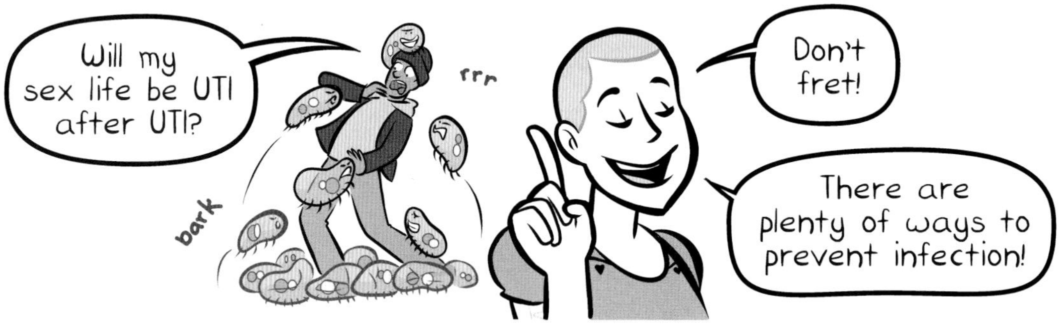
Will my sex life be UTI after UTI?
rrr
bark
Don't fret!
There are plenty of ways to prevent infection!

Stay well hydrated

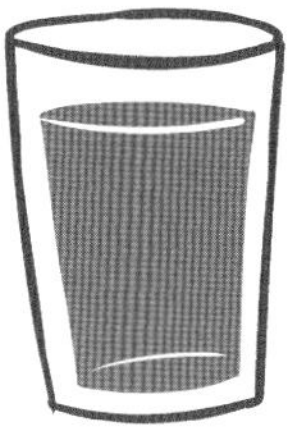

Pee as soon as you feel the urge (don't hold it!)

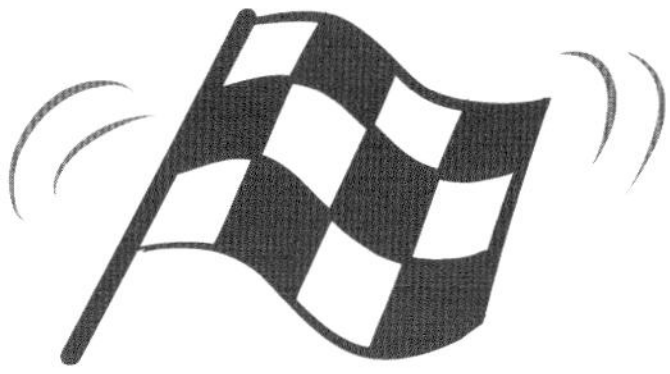

Wipe front (vulva) to back (anus) on the toilet

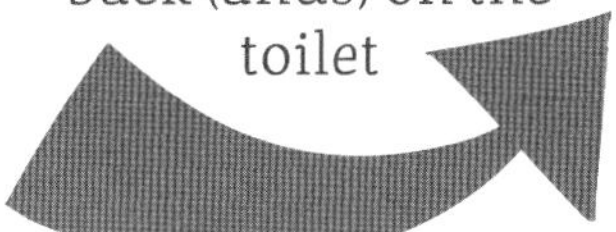

Avoid vulva-suffocating garments and g-strings

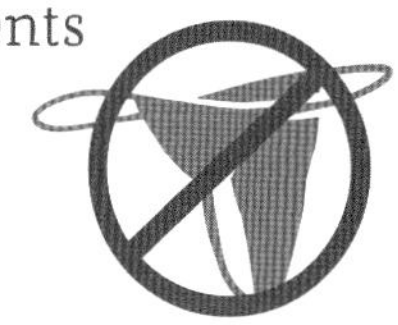

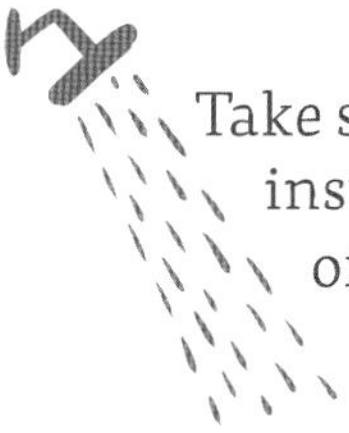

Take showers instead of baths

Use barriers during penetrative sex

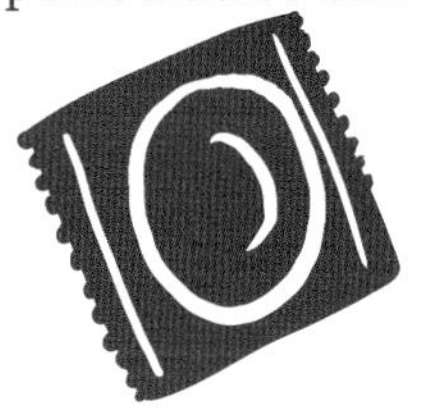

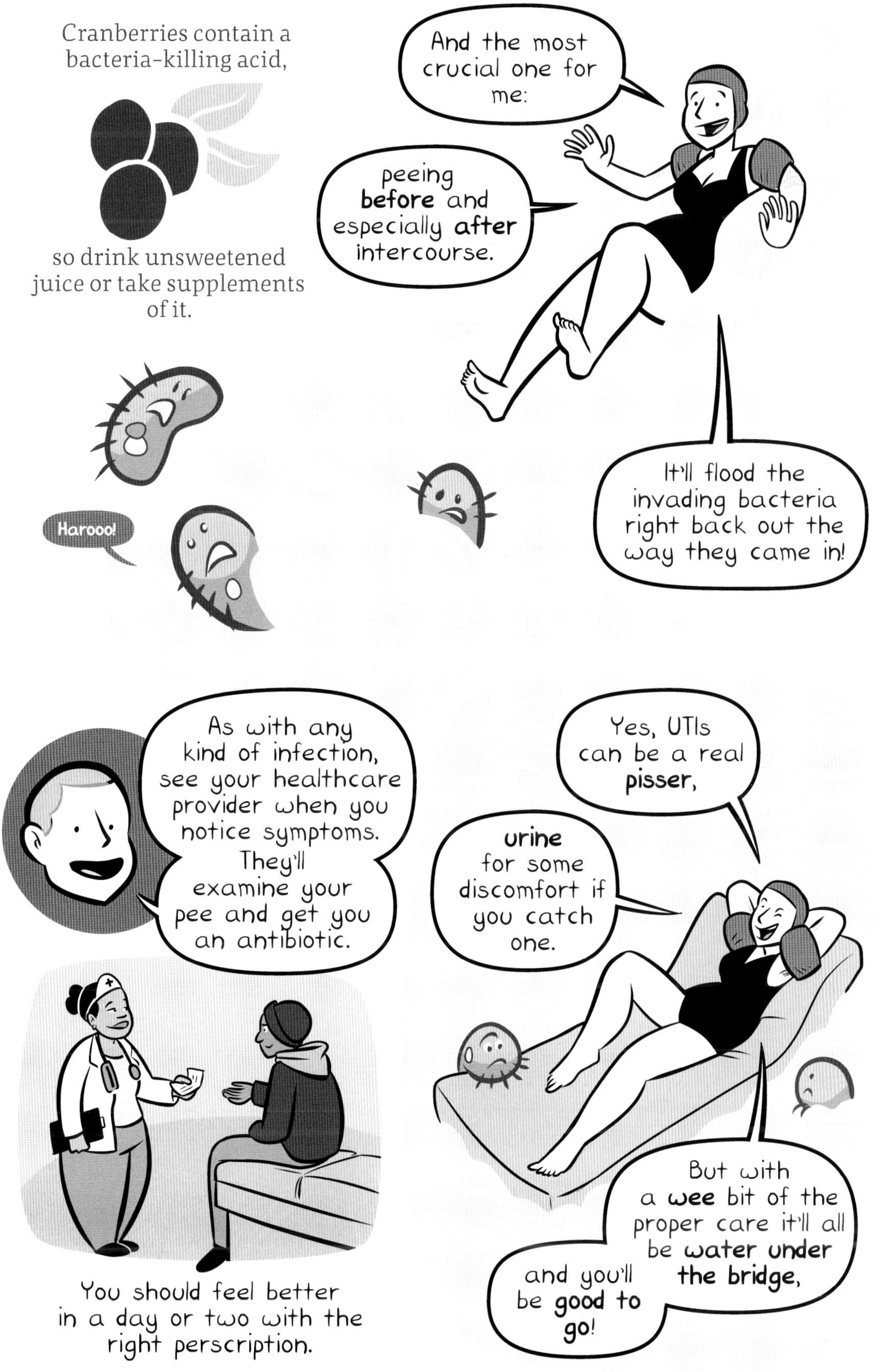
Cranberries contain a bacteria-killing acid,
so drink unsweetened juice or take supplements of it.
And the most crucial one for me:
peeing **before** and especially **after** intercourse.
Harooo!
It'll flood the invading bacteria right back out the way they came in!
As with any kind of infection, see your healthcare provider when you notice symptoms.
They'll examine your pee and get you an antibiotic.
You should feel better in a day or two with the right perscription.
Yes, UTIs can be a real **pisser**,
urine for some discomfort if you catch one.
But with a **wee** bit of the proper care it'll all be **water under the bridge**,
and you'll be **good to go**!

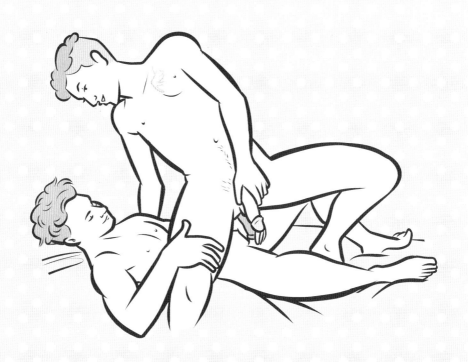

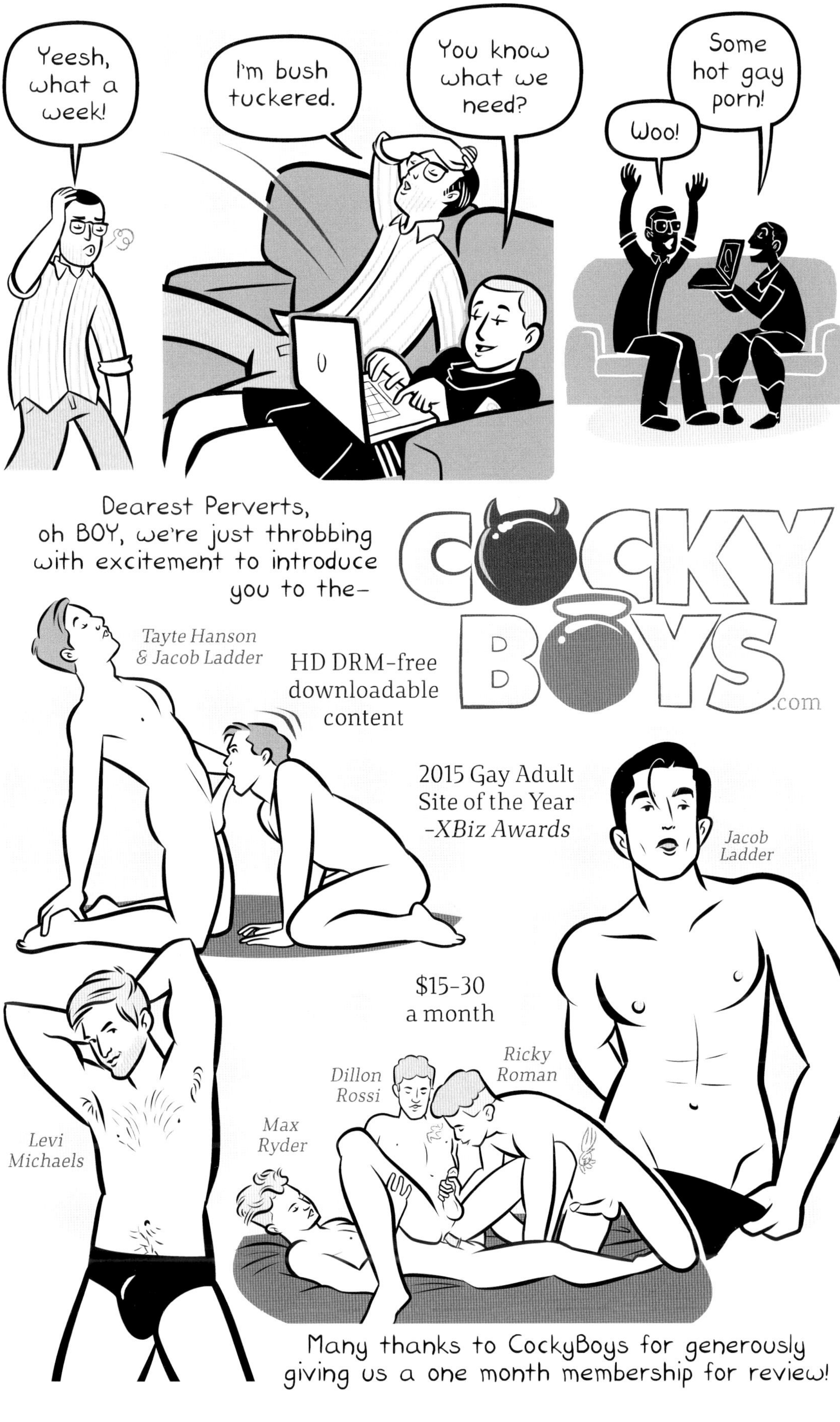
Yeesh, what a week!
I'm bush tuckered.
You know what we need?
Woo!
Some hot gay porn!
Dearest Perverts, oh BOY, we're just throbbing with excitement to introduce you to the–
COCKY BOYS.com
Tayte Hanson & Jacob Ladder
HD DRM-free downloadable content
2015 Gay Adult Site of the Year -XBiz Awards
Jacob Ladder
$15-30 a month
Levi Michaels
Max Ryder
Dillon Rossi
Ricky Roman
Many thanks to CockyBoys for generously giving us a one month membership for review!

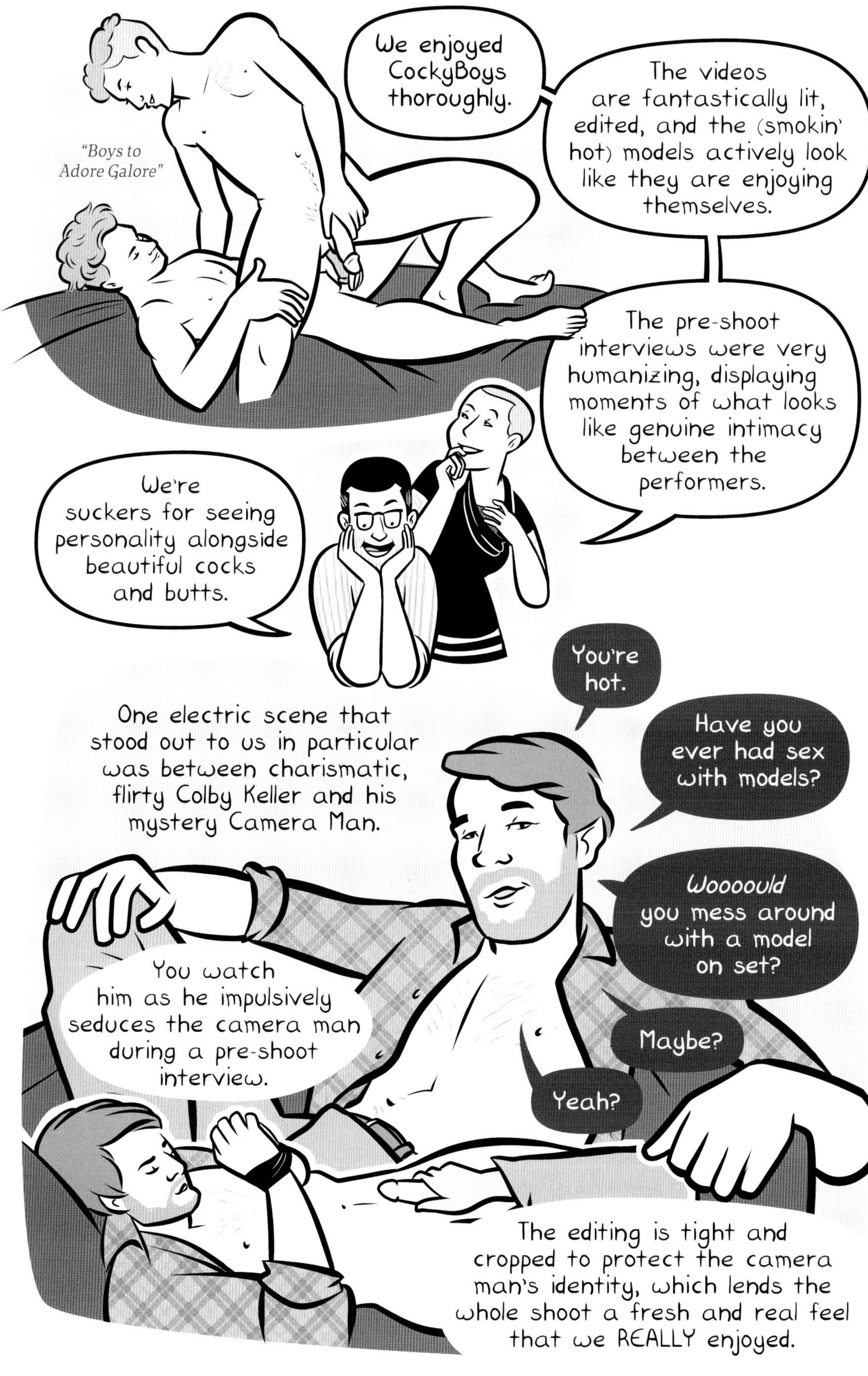
"Boys to Adore Galore"
We enjoyed CockyBoys thoroughly.
The videos are fantastically lit, edited, and the (smokin' hot) models actively look like they are enjoying themselves.
The pre-shoot interviews were very humanizing, displaying moments of what looks like genuine intimacy between the performers.
We're suckers for seeing personality alongside beautiful cocks and butts.
One electric scene that stood out to us in particular was between charismatic, flirty Colby Keller and his mystery Camera Man.
You're hot.
Have you ever had sex with models?
Wooooould you mess around with a model on set?
You watch him as he impulsively seduces the camera man during a pre-shoot interview.
Maybe?
Yeah?
The editing is tight and cropped to protect the camera man's identity, which lends the whole shoot a fresh and real feel that we REALLY enjoyed.

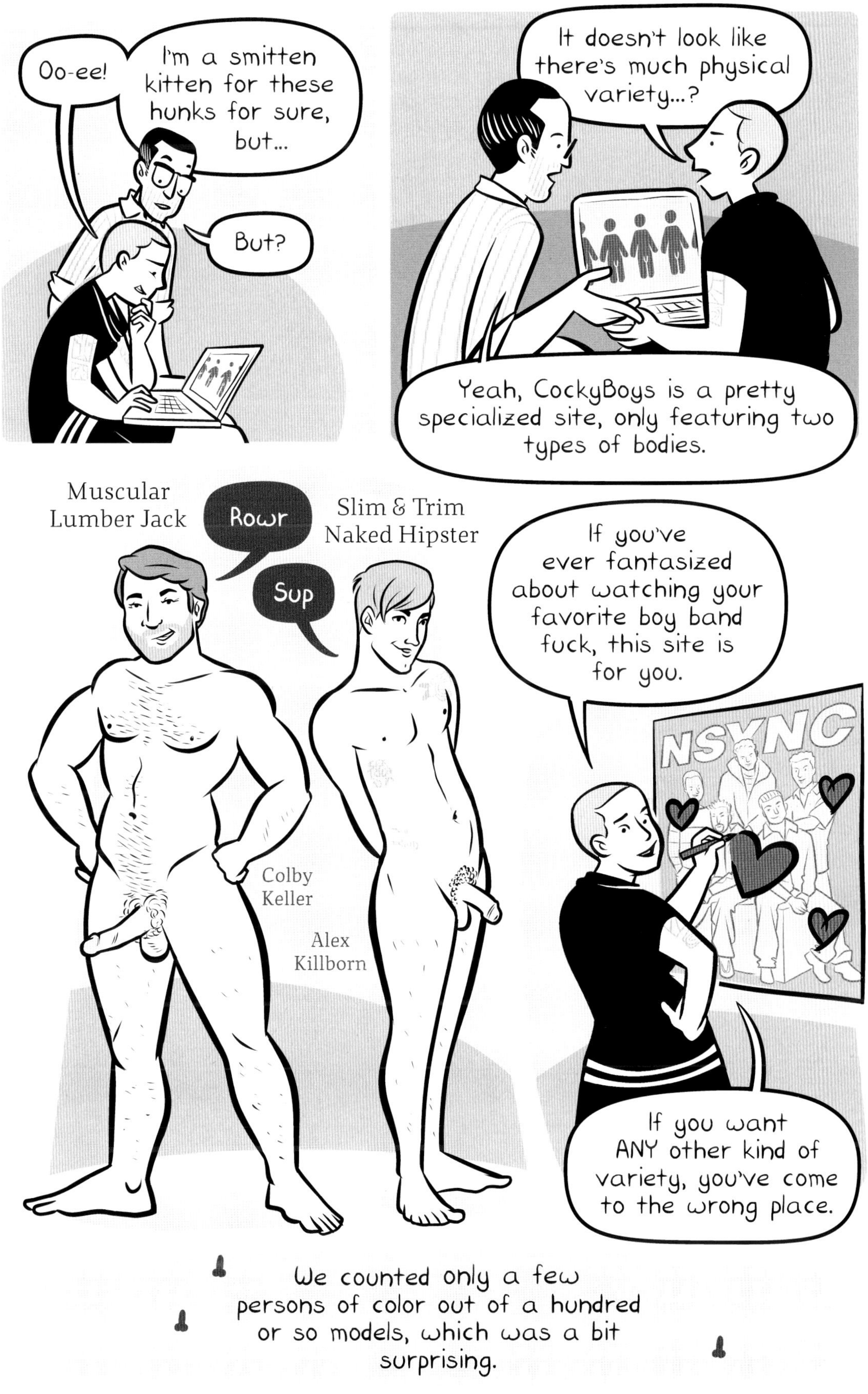

Oo-ee!
I'm a smitten kitten for these hunks for sure, but...
But?
It doesn't look like there's much physical variety...?
Yeah, CockyBoys is a pretty specialized site, only featuring two types of bodies.
Muscular Lumber Jack
Rowr
Slim & Trim Naked Hipster
Sup
Colby Keller
Alex Killborn
If you've ever fantasized about watching your favorite boy band fuck, this site is for you.
NSYNC
If you want ANY other kind of variety, you've come to the wrong place.
We counted only a few persons of color out of a hundred or so models, which was a bit surprising.

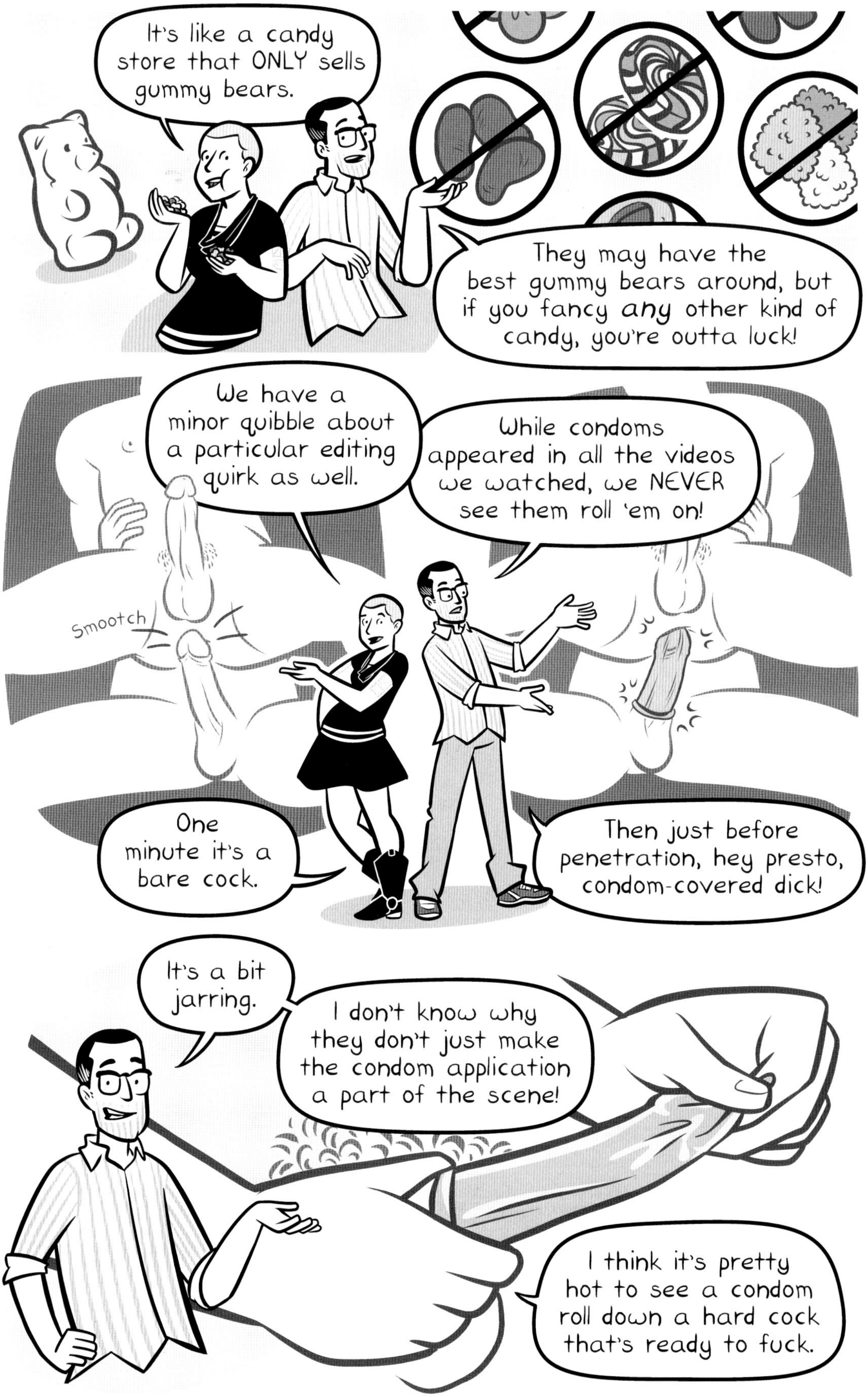
It's like a candy store that ONLY sells gummy bears.
They may have the best gummy bears around, but if you fancy *any* other kind of candy, you're outta luck!
We have a minor quibble about a particular editing quirk as well.
While condoms appeared in all the videos we watched, we NEVER see them roll 'em on!
Smootch
One minute it's a bare cock.
Then just before penetration, hey presto, condom-covered dick!
It's a bit jarring.
I don't know why they don't just make the condom application a part of the scene!
I think it's pretty hot to see a condom roll down a hard cock that's ready to fuck.

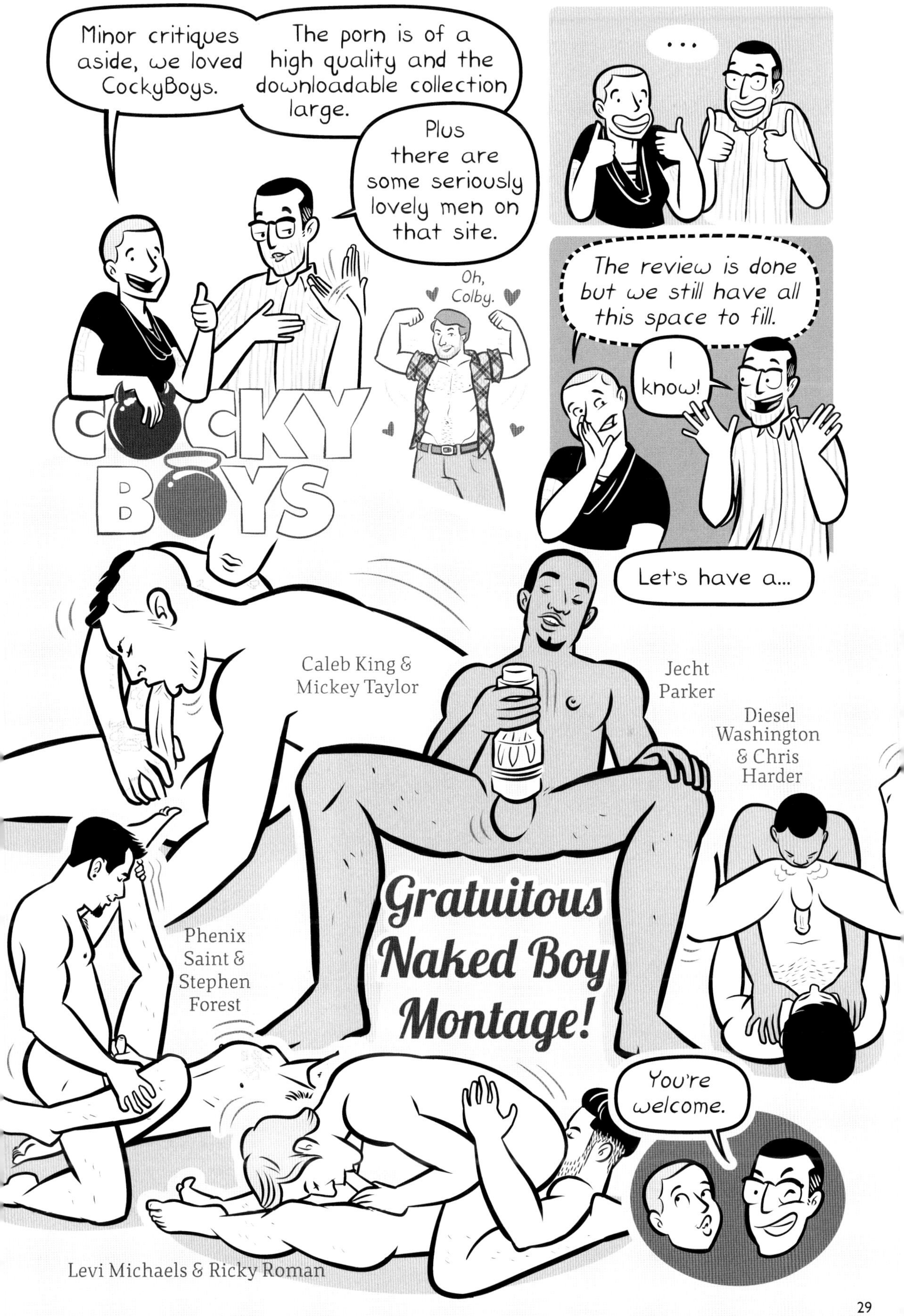

Minor critiques aside, we loved CockyBoys.
The porn is of a high quality and the downloadable collection large.
Plus there are some seriously lovely men on that site.
Oh, Colby.
COCKY BOYS
...
The review is done but we still have all this space to fill.
I know!
Let's have a...
Caleb King & Mickey Taylor
Jecht Parker
Diesel Washington & Chris Harder
Phenix Saint & Stephen Forest
Gratuitous Naked Boy Montage!
You're welcome.
Levi Michaels & Ricky Roman

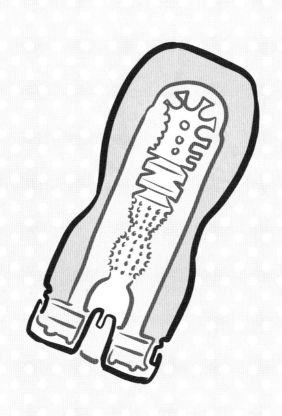

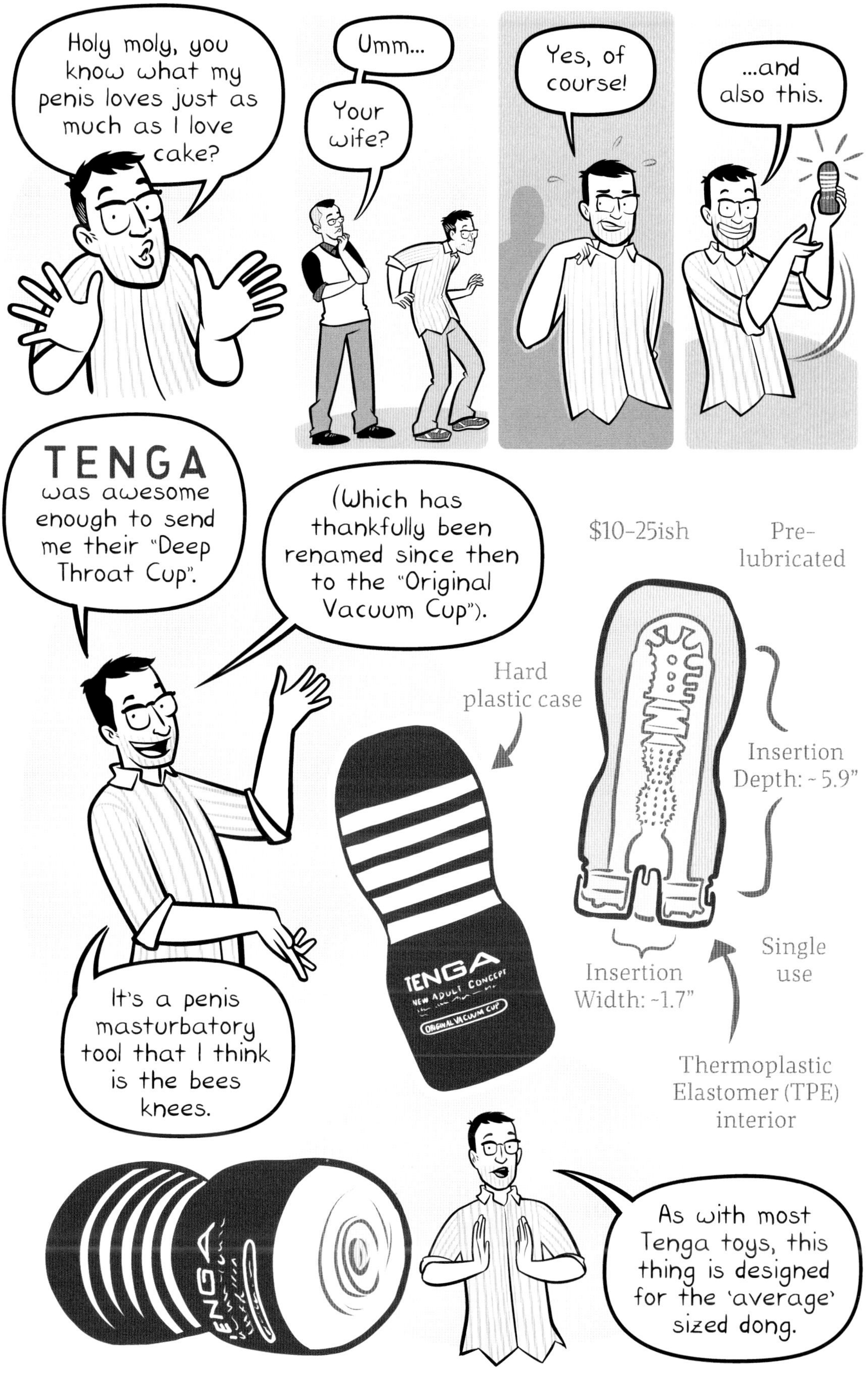
Holy moly, you know what my penis loves just as much as I love cake?
Umm...
Your wife?
Yes, of course!
...and also this.
TENGA was awesome enough to send me their "Deep Throat Cup".
(Which has thankfully been renamed since then to the "Original Vacuum Cup").
$10–25ish
Pre-lubricated
Hard plastic case
Insertion Depth: ~ 5.9"
TENGA NEW ADULT CONCEPT ORIGINAL VACUUM CUP
Insertion Width: ~1.7"
Single use
Thermoplastic Elastomer (TPE) interior
It's a penis masturbatory tool that I think is the bees knees.
As with most Tenga toys, this thing is designed for the 'average' sized dong.

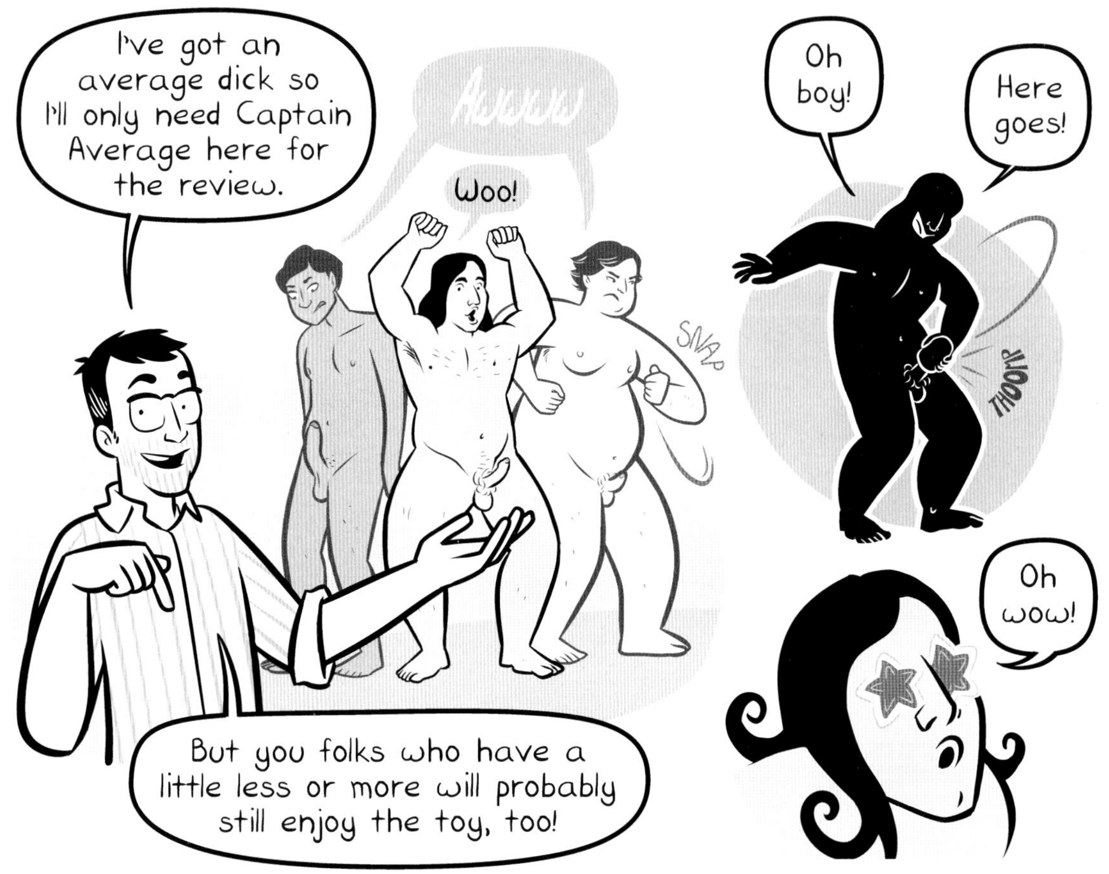
I've got an average dick so I'll only need Captain Average here for the review.
Woo!
SNAP
But you folks who have a little less or more will probably still enjoy the toy, too!
Oh boy!
Here goes!
THOOMP
Oh wow!

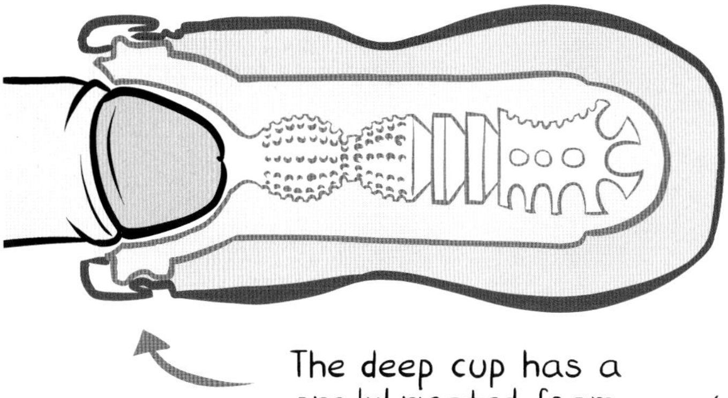

This Toy is SMALL and TIGHT, you're going to fill it up and that will put some wonderful pressure on your dick.

The deep cup has a pre-lubricated foam entrance...

...it's a smooth gritty wet-foam texture, that lubes you up and provides a contrasting sensation to the rest.

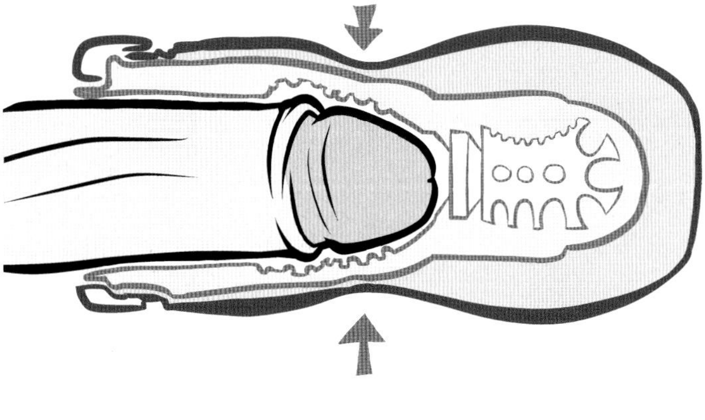

Past the entrance you meet the Deep Cup's smooth soft interior with its bumps, lumps, zigs and zags.

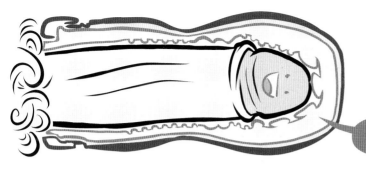

They add variation so it doesn't just end up feeling like a formless lump.

This is lovely!

But the real gem is the vacuum suction effect you get on your exit stroke.

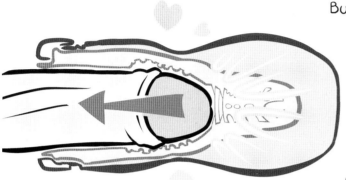

Due to its simple and clever design, the toy forces air out as you penetrate and grips as you pull back.

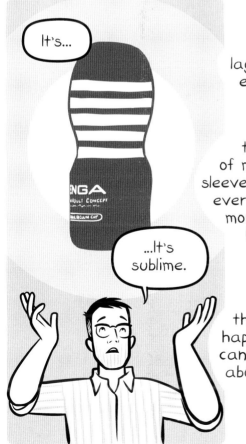

It's...

It has layers to the experience.

I've tried a lot of masturbation sleeves but nothing's ever surprised me more than the Deep Cup.

...It's sublime.

It's a toy that made me happy, how often can you say that about ANYTHING?

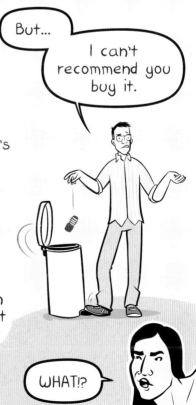

But...

I can't recommend you buy it.

WHAT!?

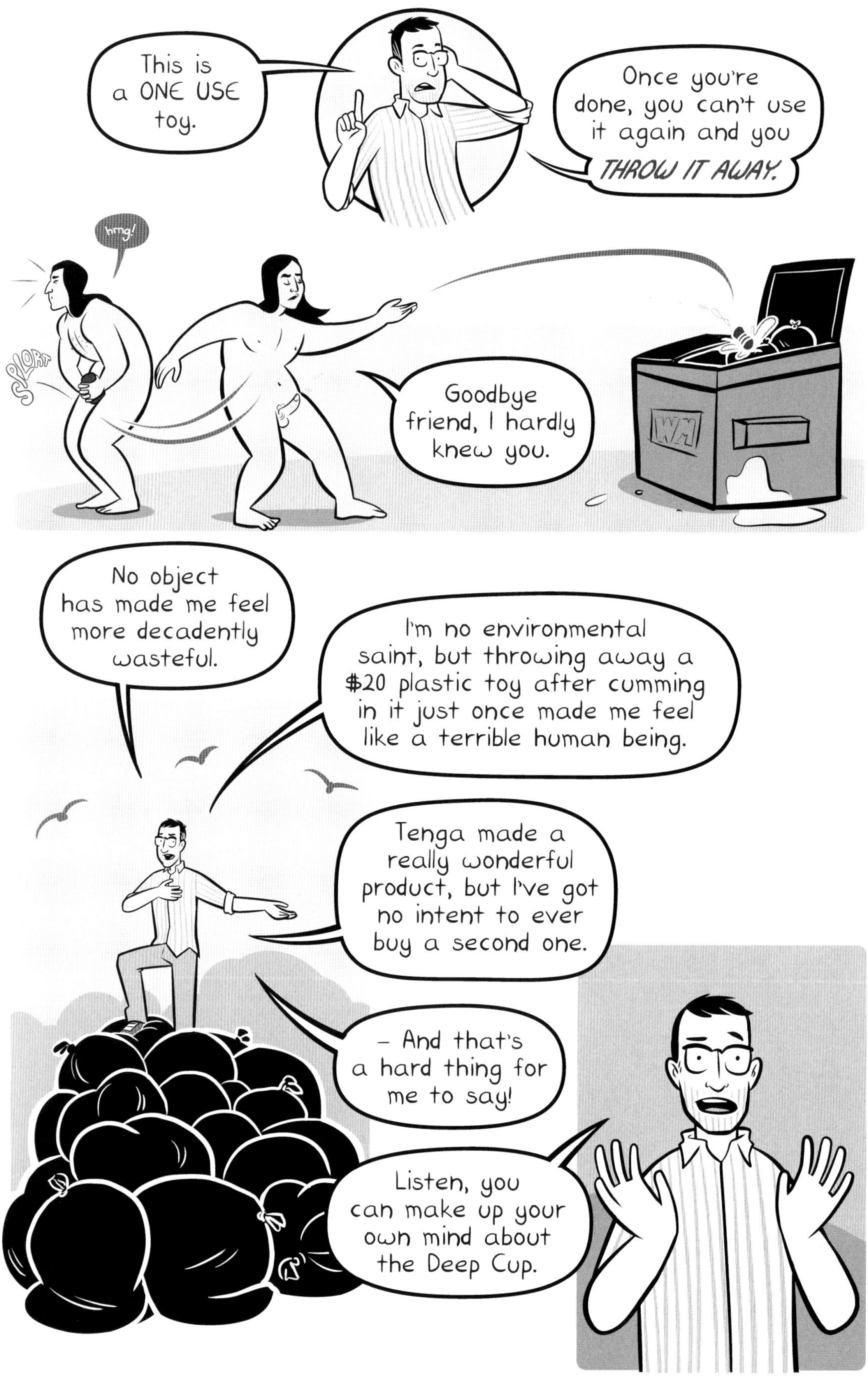
This is a ONE USE toy.
Once you're done, you can't use it again and you THROW IT AWAY.
hmg!
SPLORT
Goodbye friend, I hardly knew you.
WM
No object has made me feel more decadently wasteful.
I'm no environmental saint, but throwing away a $20 plastic toy after cumming in it just once made me feel like a terrible human being.
Tenga made a really wonderful product, but I've got no intent to ever buy a second one.
– And that's a hard thing for me to say!
Listen, you can make up your own mind about the Deep Cup.

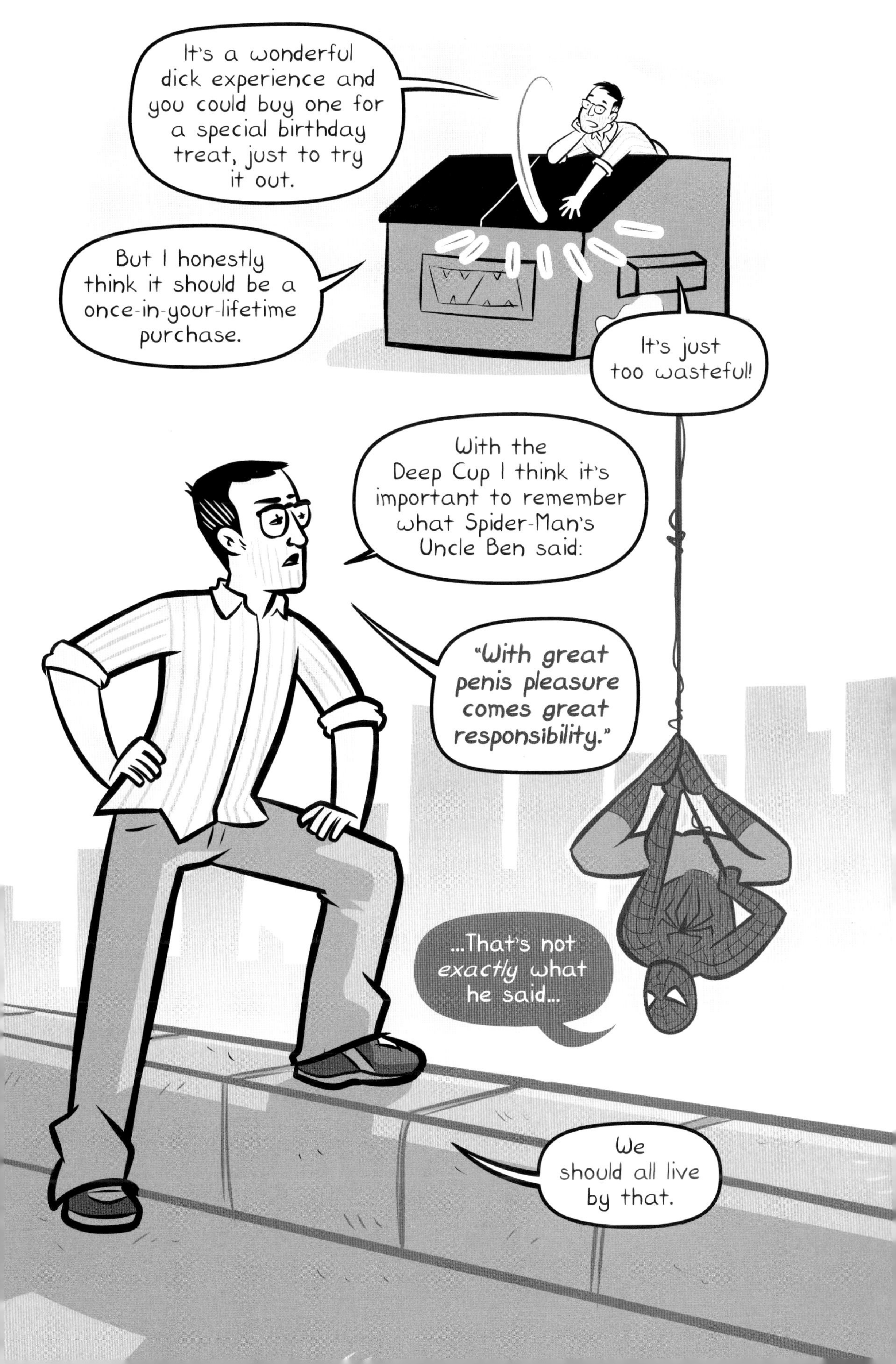
It's a wonderful dick experience and you could buy one for a special birthday treat, just to try it out.
But I honestly think it should be a once-in-your-lifetime purchase.
It's just too wasteful!
With the Deep Cup I think it's important to remember what Spider-Man's Uncle Ben said:
"With great penis pleasure comes great responsibility."
...That's not *exactly* what he said...
We should all live by that.

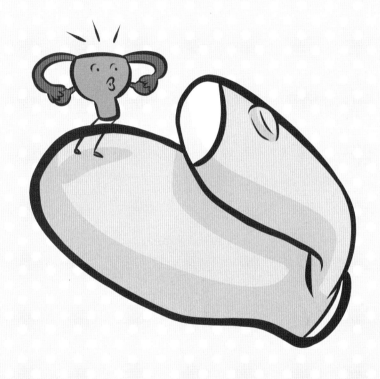

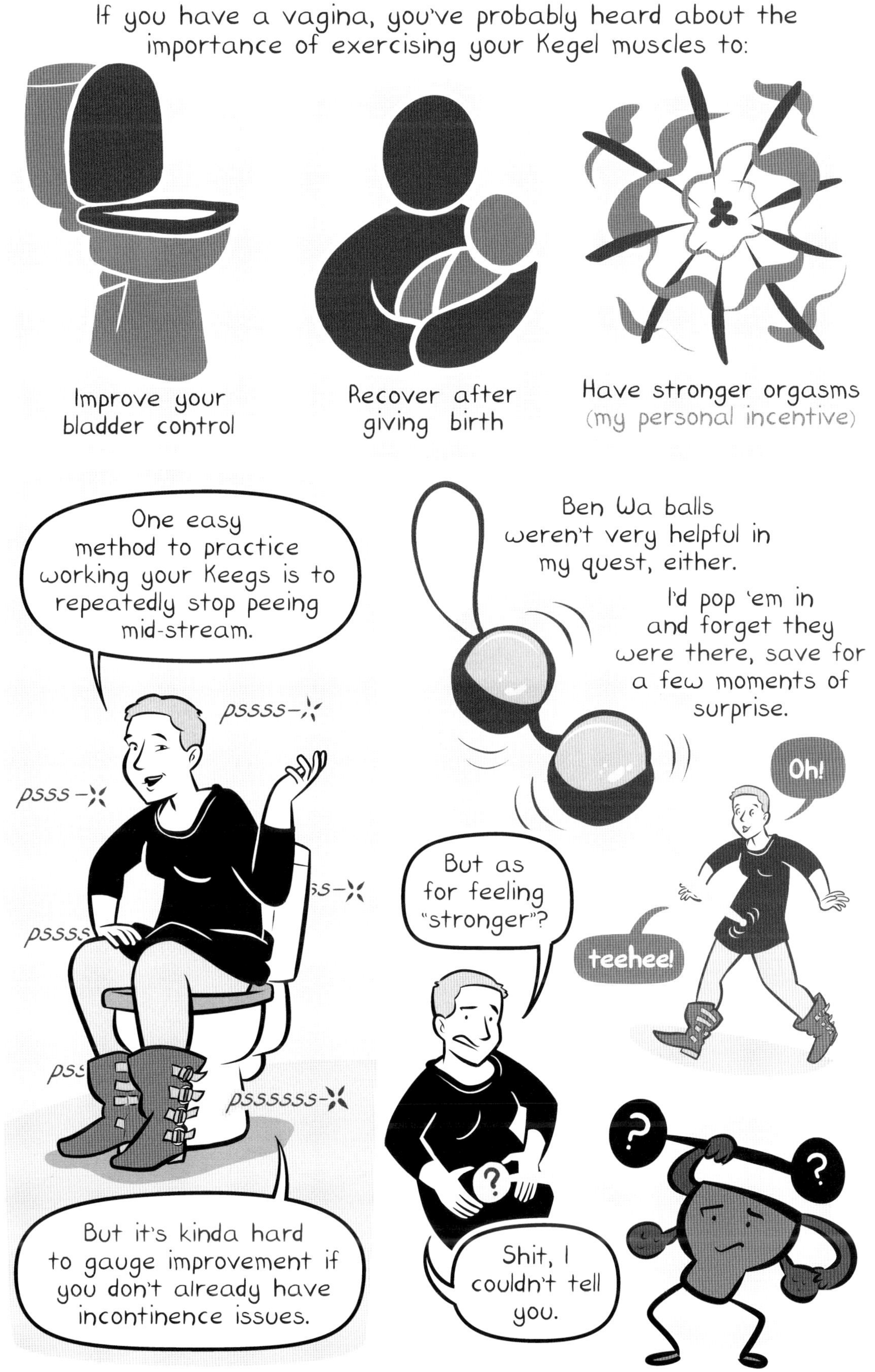
If you have a vagina, you've probably heard about the importance of exercising your Kegel muscles to:
Improve your bladder control
Recover after giving birth
Have stronger orgasms
(my personal incentive)
One easy method to practice working your Keegs is to repeatedly stop peeing mid-stream.
pssss-
psss -
ss-
pssss
pss
pssssss-
But it's kinda hard to gauge improvement if you don't already have incontinence issues.
Ben Wa balls weren't very helpful in my quest, either.
I'd pop 'em in and forget they were there, save for a few moments of surprise.
Oh!
teehee!
But as for feeling "stronger"?
Shit, I couldn't tell you.

Thing is, when you have no obvious feedback from flexing a muscle you can't see, you can't tell if you're making improvements.

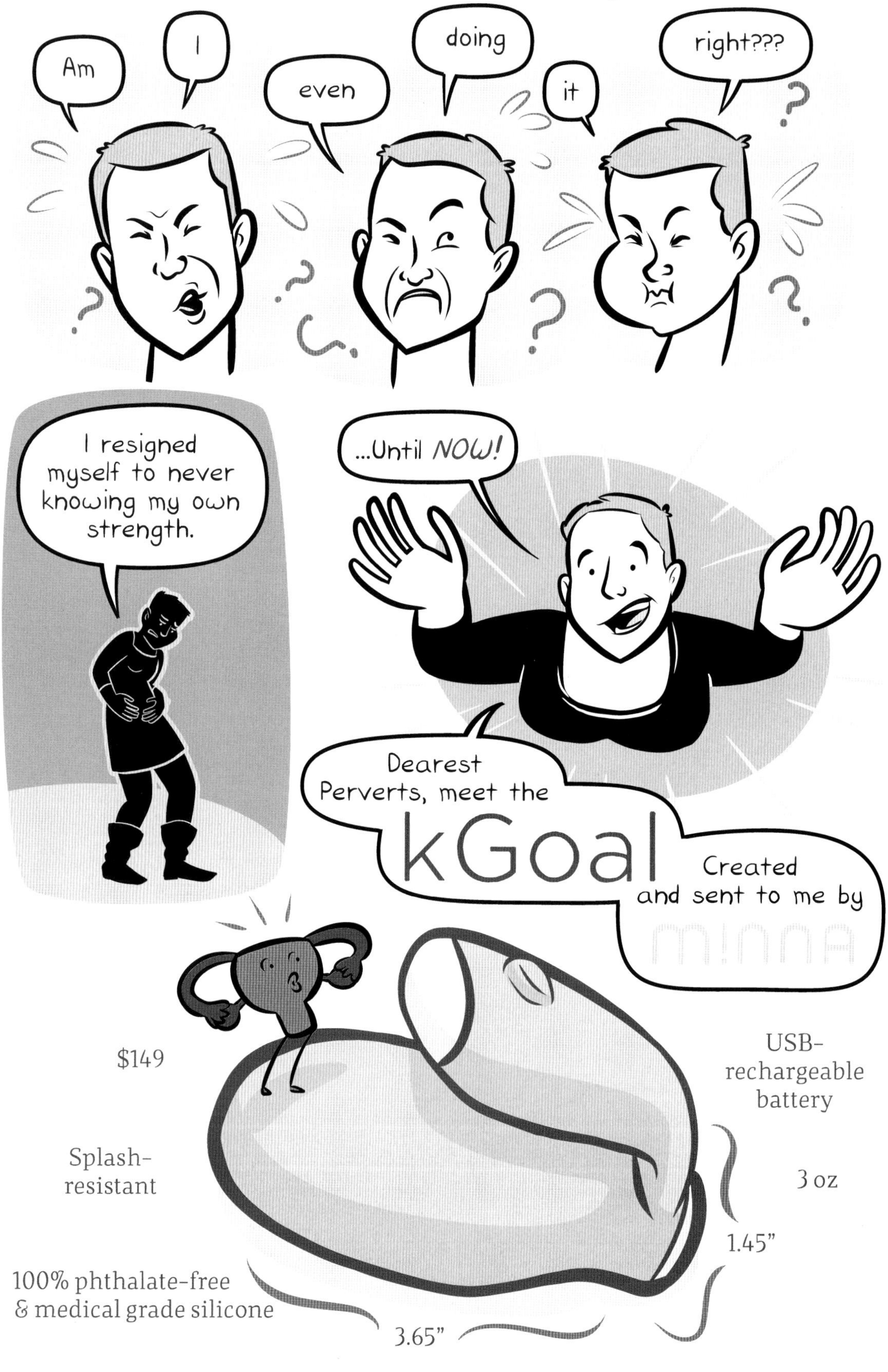

Am
I
even
doing
it
right???
I resigned myself to never knowing my own strength.
...Until *NOW!*
Dearest Perverts, meet the
kGoal
Created and sent to me by
m!nna
$149
Splash-resistant
100% phthalate-free & medical grade silicone
USB-rechargeable battery
3 oz
1.45"
3.65"

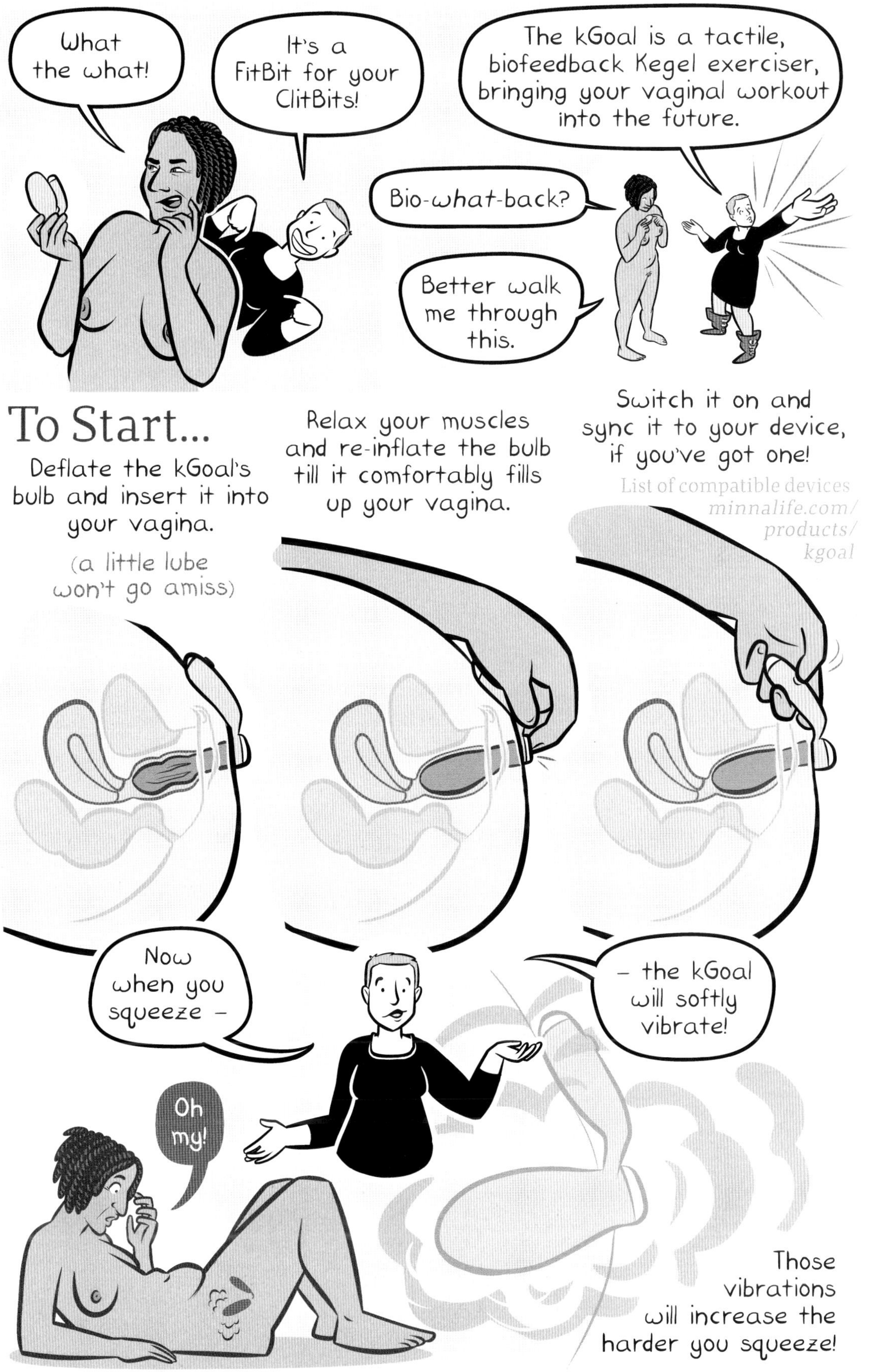
What the what!
It's a FitBit for your ClitBits!
The kGoal is a tactile, biofeedback Kegel exerciser, bringing your vaginal workout into the future.
Bio-what-back?
Better walk me through this.
To Start...
Deflate the kGoal's bulb and insert it into your vagina.
(a little lube won't go amiss)
Relax your muscles and re-inflate the bulb till it comfortably fills up your vagina.
Switch it on and sync it to your device, if you've got one!
List of compatible devices minnalife.com/products/kgoal
Now when you squeeze –
– the kGoal will softly vibrate!
Oh my!
Those vibrations will increase the harder you squeeze!

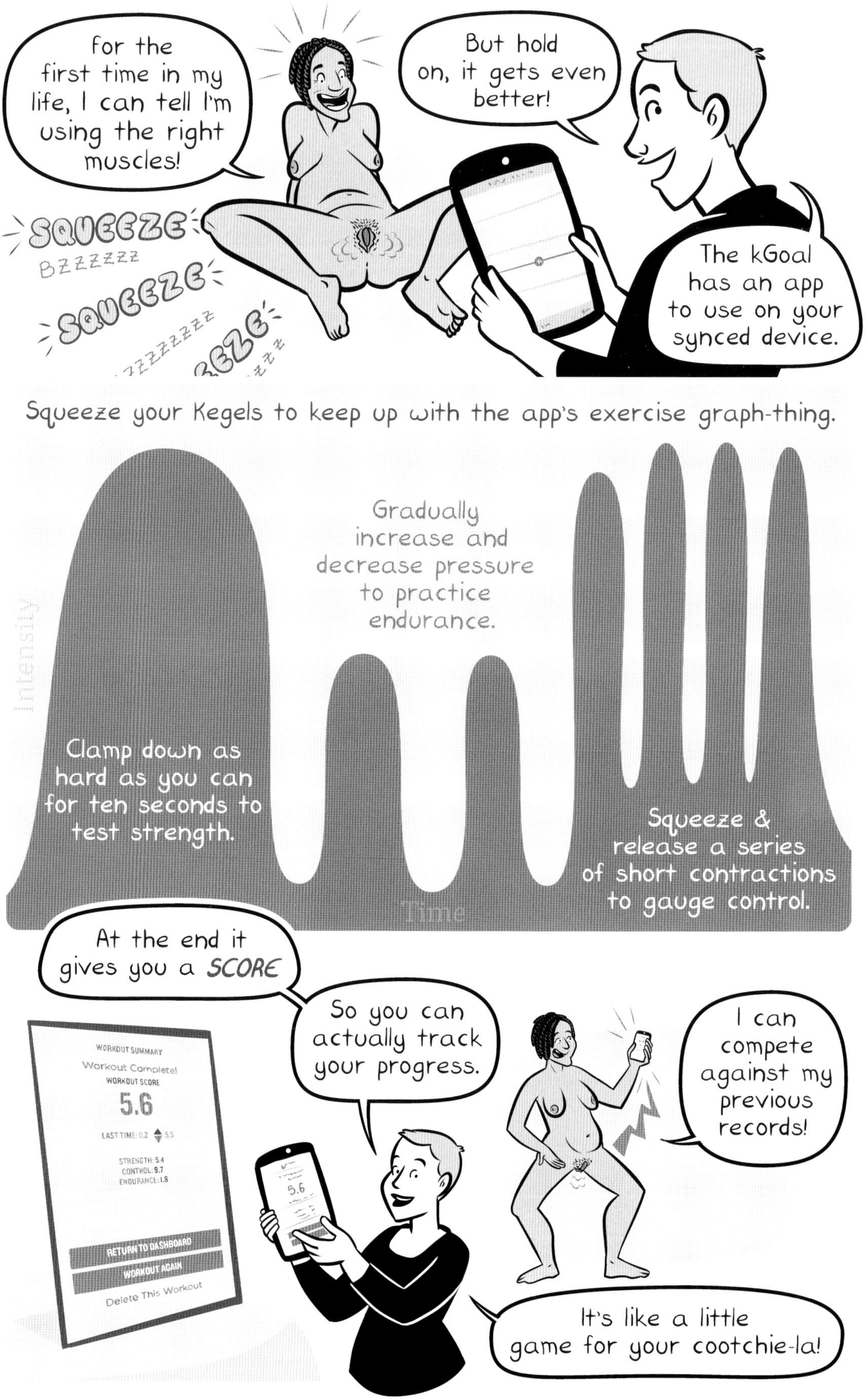
For the first time in my life, I can tell I'm using the right muscles!
SQUEEZE
BZZZZZZ
SQUEEZE
ZZZZZZZZZ
But hold on, it gets even better!
The kGoal has an app to use on your synced device.
Squeeze your Kegels to keep up with the app's exercise graph-thing.
Intensity
Clamp down as hard as you can for ten seconds to test strength.
Gradually increase and decrease pressure to practice endurance.
Squeeze & release a series of short contractions to gauge control.
Time
At the end it gives you a SCORE
So you can actually track your progress.
WORKOUT SUMMARY
Workout Complete!
WORKOUT SCORE
5.6
LAST TIME: 0.2
5.5
STRENGTH: 5.4
CONTROL: 9.7
ENDURANCE: 1.8
RETURN TO DASHBOARD
WORKOUT AGAIN
Delete This Workout
5.6
I can compete against my previous records!
It's like a little game for your cootchie-la!

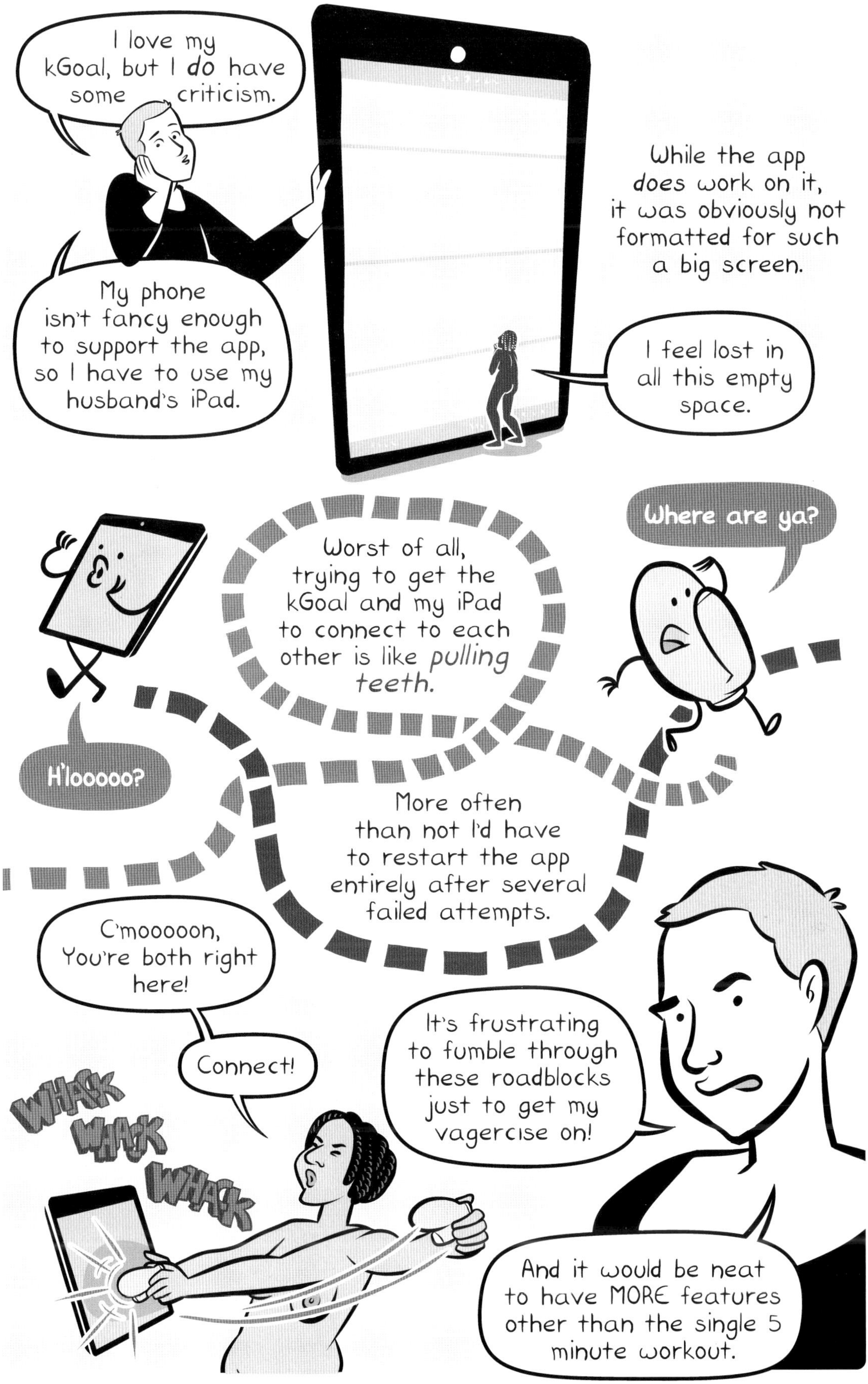
I love my kGoal, but I *do* have some criticism.
My phone isn't fancy enough to support the app, so I have to use my husband's iPad.
While the app *does* work on it, it was obviously not formatted for such a big screen.
I feel lost in all this empty space.
Worst of all, trying to get the kGoal and my iPad to connect to each other is like *pulling teeth.*
Where are ya?
H'looooo?
More often than not I'd have to restart the app entirely after several failed attempts.
C'moooooon, You're both right here!
Connect!
WHAK
WHAK
WHAK
It's frustrating to fumble through these roadblocks just to get my vagercise on!
And it would be neat to have MORE features other than the single 5 minute workout.

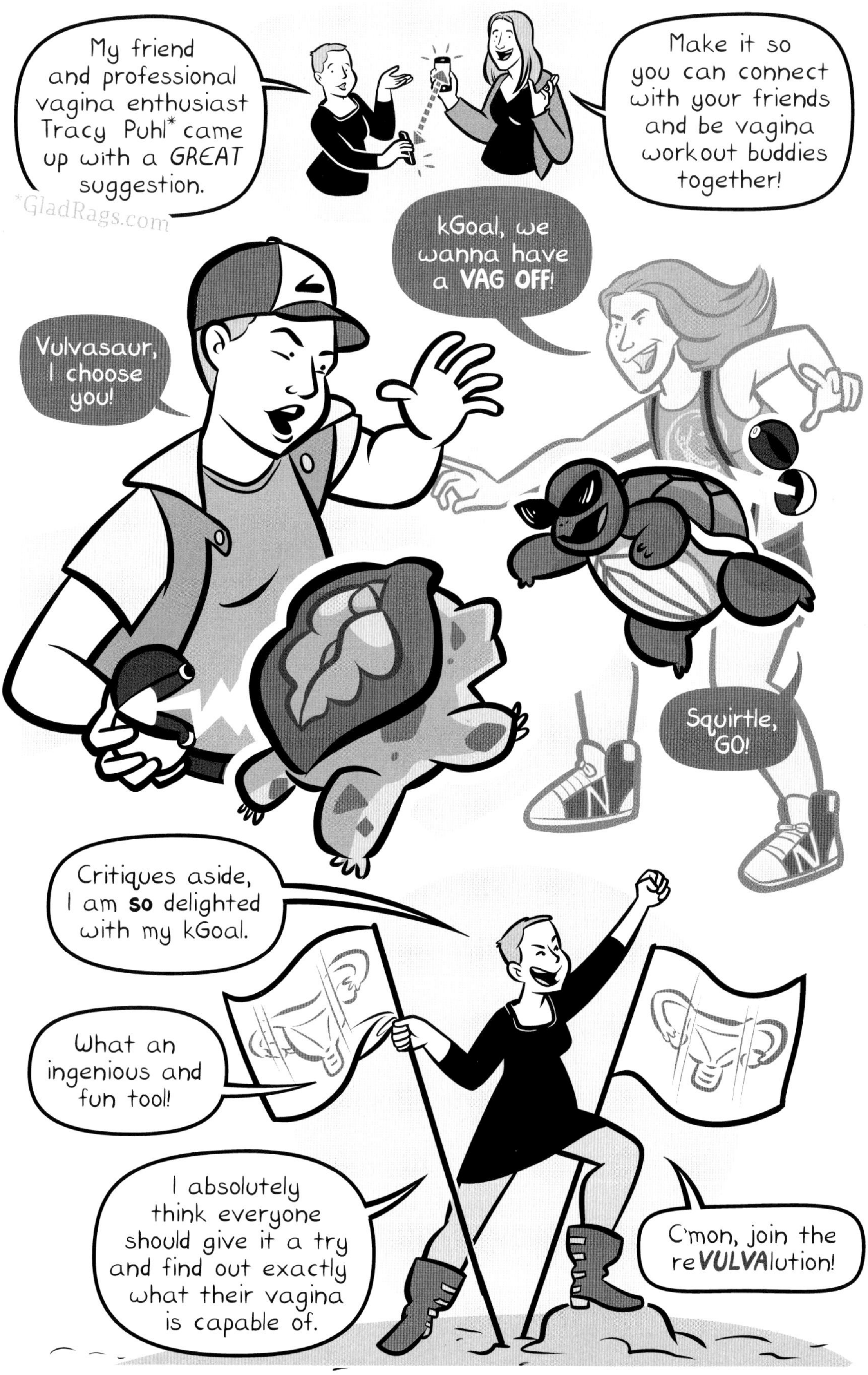
My friend and professional vagina enthusiast Tracy Puhl* came up with a GREAT suggestion.
*GladRags.com
Make it so you can connect with your friends and be vagina workout buddies together!
kGoal, we wanna have a VAG OFF!
Vulvasaur, I choose you!
Squirtle, GO!
Critiques aside, I am so delighted with my kGoal.
What an ingenious and fun tool!
I absolutely think everyone should give it a try and find out exactly what their vagina is capable of.
C'mon, join the reVULVAlution!

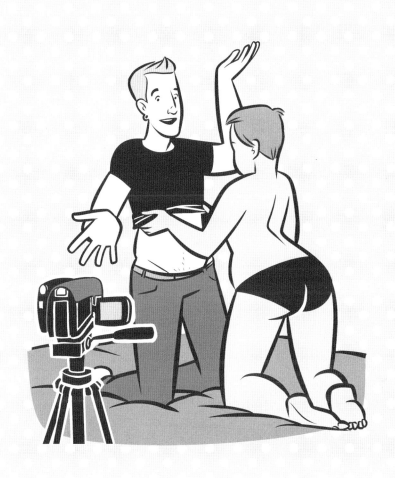

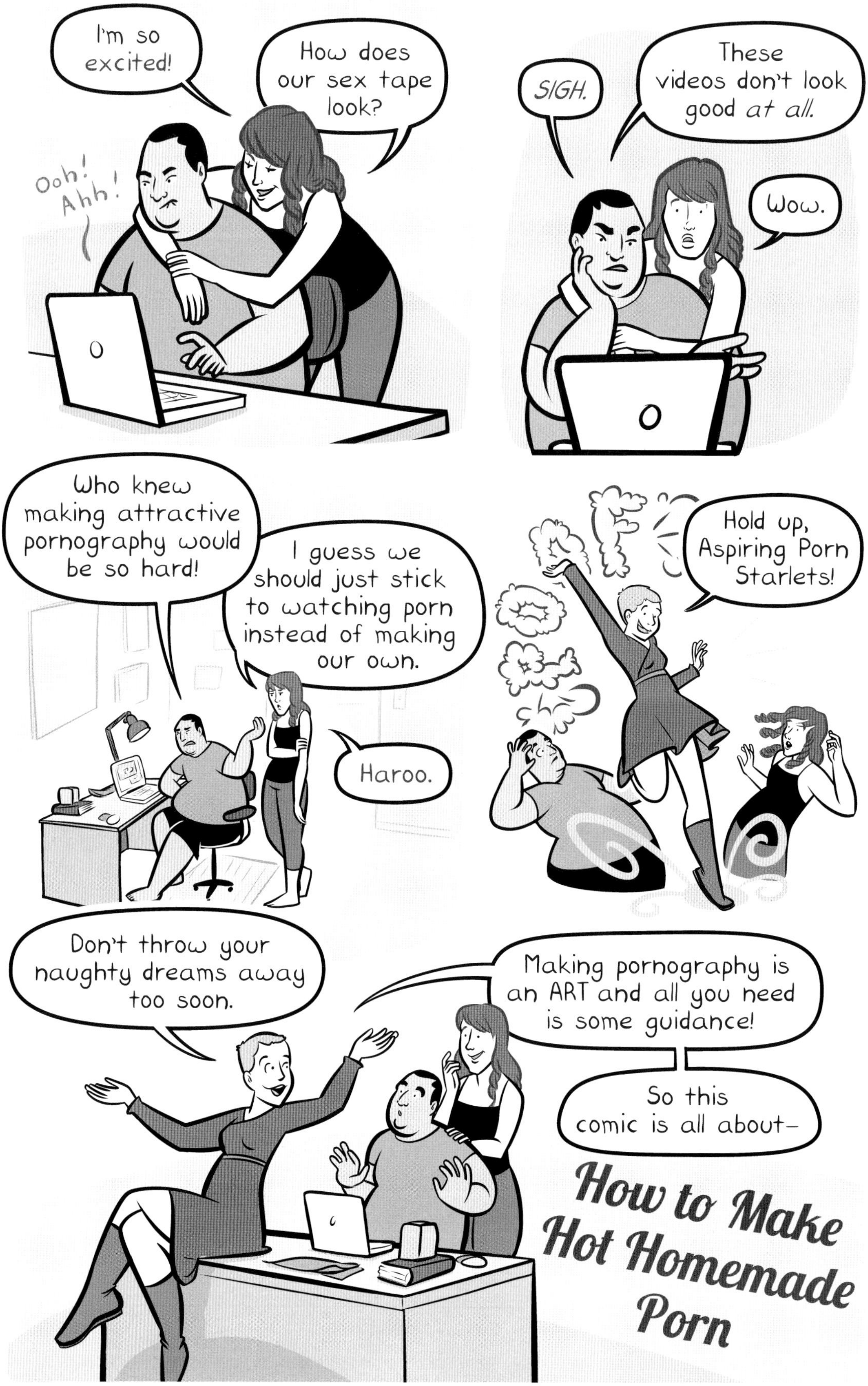
I'm so excited!
How does our sex tape look?
Ooh! Ahh!
SIGH.
These videos don't look good *at all.*
Wow.
Who knew making attractive pornography would be so hard!
I guess we should just stick to watching porn instead of making our own.
Haroo.
Hold up, Aspiring Porn Starlets!
Don't throw your naughty dreams away too soon.
Making pornography is an ART and all you need is some guidance!
So this comic is all about–
How to Make Hot Homemade Porn

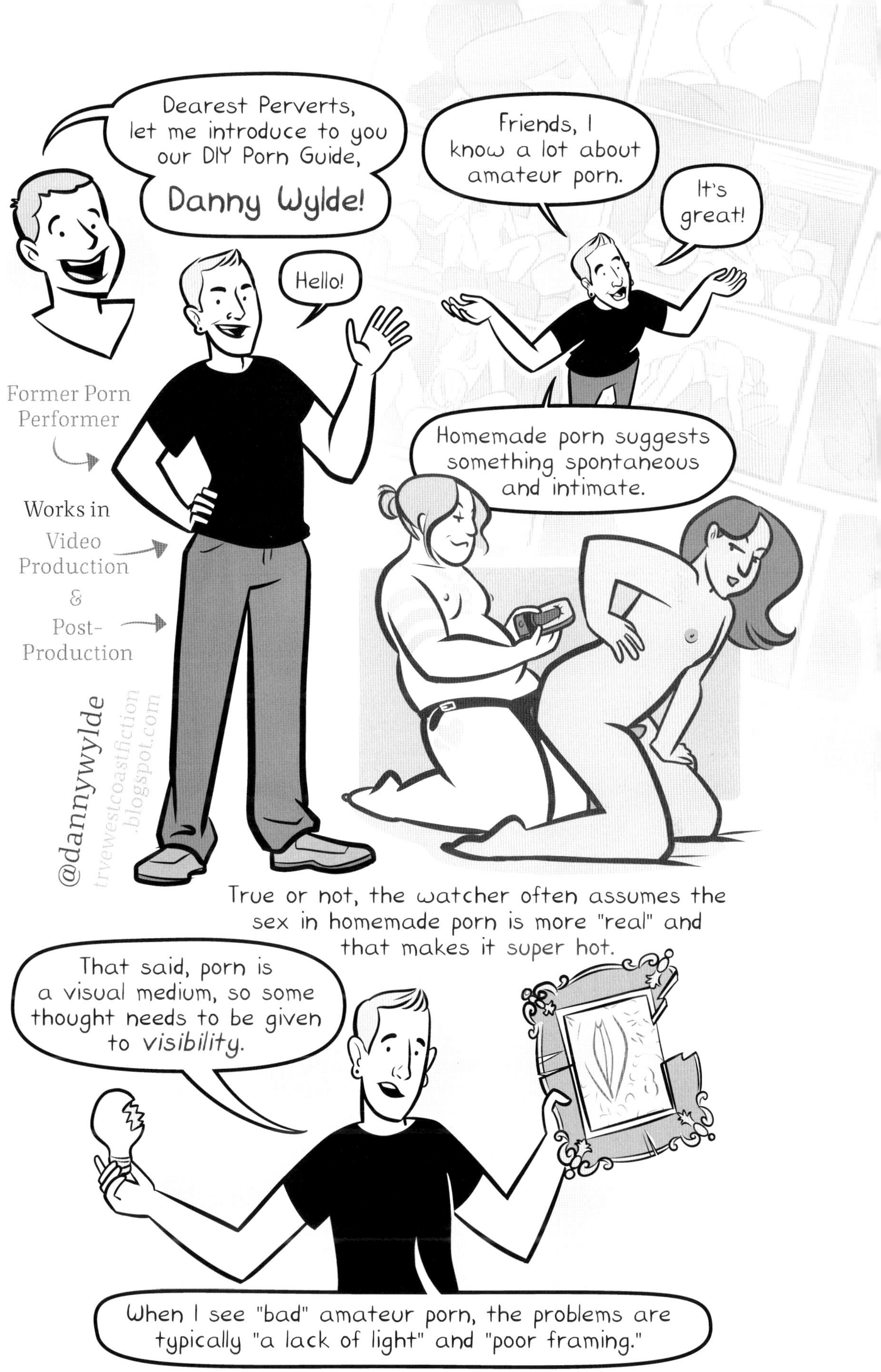
Dearest Perverts, let me introduce to you our DIY Porn Guide,
Danny Wylde!
Hello!
Former Porn Performer
Works in Video Production & Post-Production
@dannywylde
trvewestcoastfiction.blogspot.com
Friends, I know a lot about amateur porn.
It's great!
Homemade porn suggests something spontaneous and intimate.
True or not, the watcher often assumes the sex in homemade porn is more "real" and that makes it super hot.
That said, porn is a visual medium, so some thought needs to be given to visibility.
When I see "bad" amateur porn, the problems are typically "a lack of light" and "poor framing."

Upping Your Lighting Game

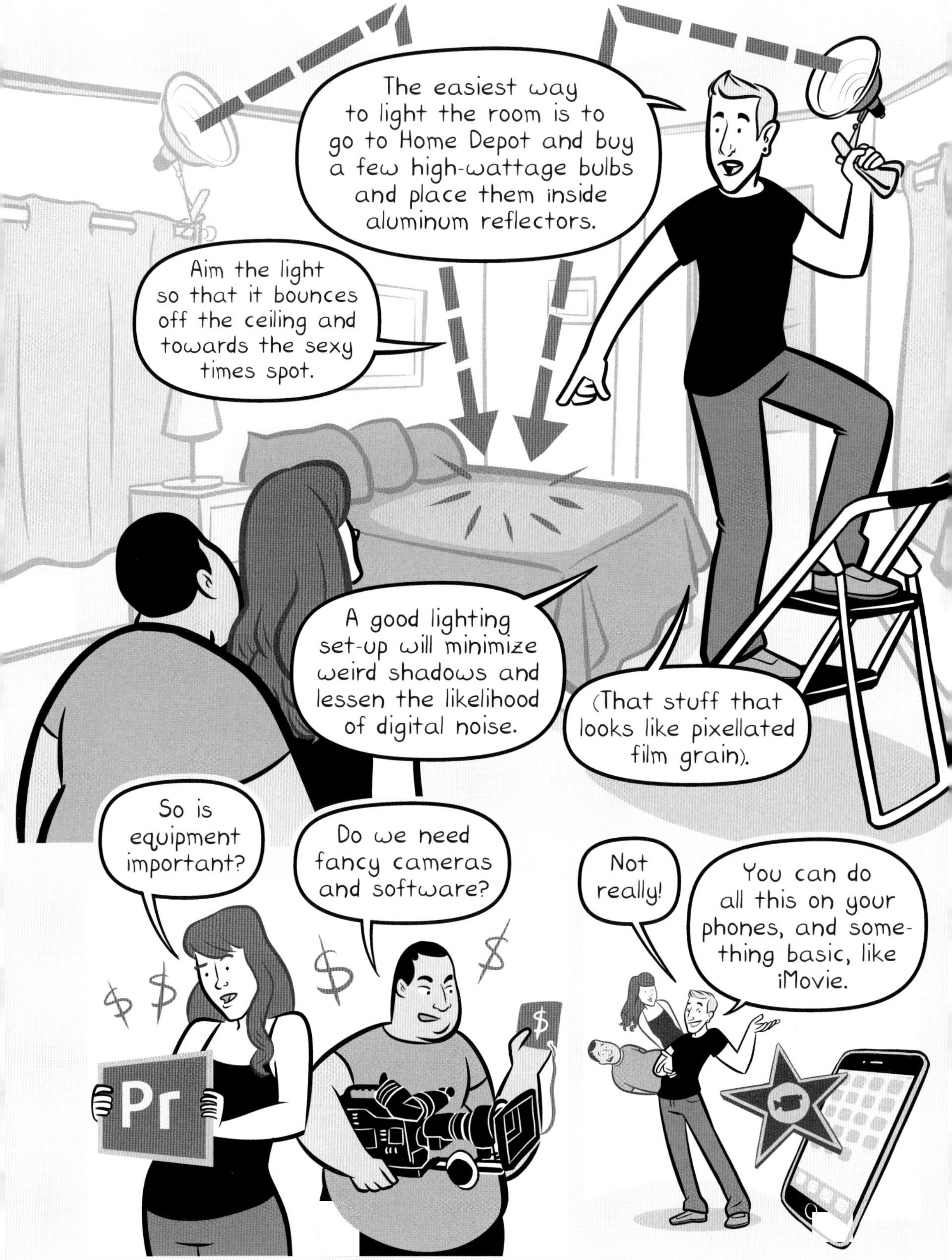

The easiest way to light the room is to go to Home Depot and buy a few high-wattage bulbs and place them inside aluminum reflectors.
Aim the light so that it bounces off the ceiling and towards the sexy times spot.
A good lighting set-up will minimize weird shadows and lessen the likelihood of digital noise.
(That stuff that looks like pixellated film grain).
So is equipment important?
Do we need fancy cameras and software?
Not really!
You can do all this on your phones, and something basic, like iMovie.
Pr

Time to Freshen Up Your Framing

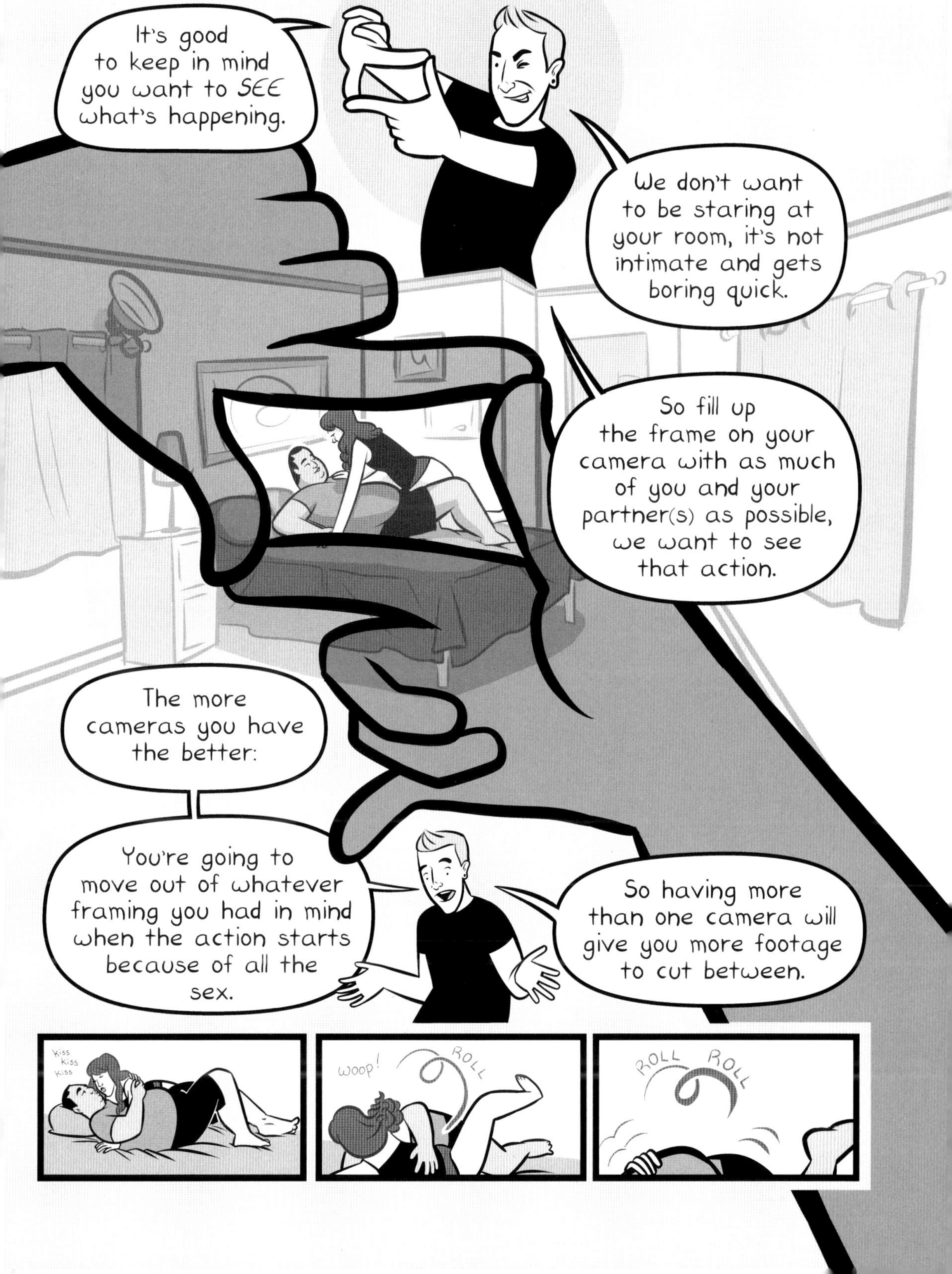

It's good to keep in mind you want to SEE what's happening.
We don't want to be staring at your room, it's not intimate and gets boring quick.
So fill up the frame on your camera with as much of you and your partner(s) as possible, we want to see that action.
The more cameras you have the better:
You're going to move out of whatever framing you had in mind when the action starts because of all the sex.
So having more than one camera will give you more footage to cut between.
Kiss Kiss Kiss
Woop!
ROLL
ROLL ROLL

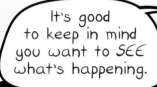

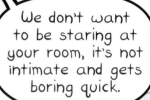

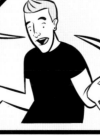

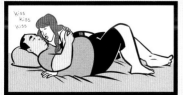

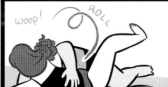

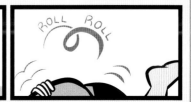

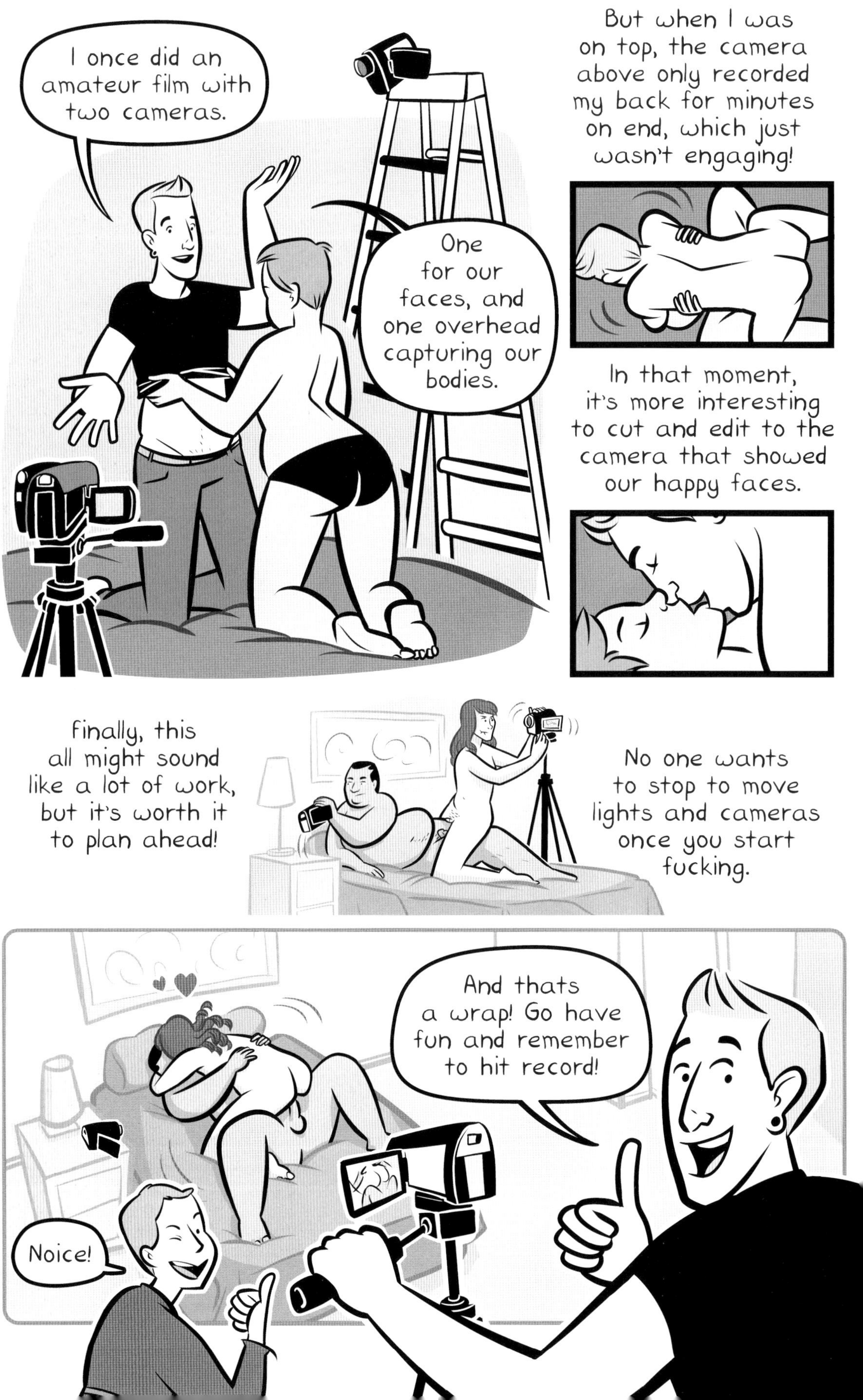
I once did an amateur film with two cameras.
One for our faces, and one overhead capturing our bodies.
But when I was on top, the camera above only recorded my back for minutes on end, which just wasn't engaging!
In that moment, it's more interesting to cut and edit to the camera that showed our happy faces.
Finally, this all might sound like a lot of work, but it's worth it to plan ahead!
No one wants to stop to move lights and cameras once you start fucking.
And thats a wrap! Go have fun and remember to hit record!
Noice!

Magic Wand®
Rechargeable

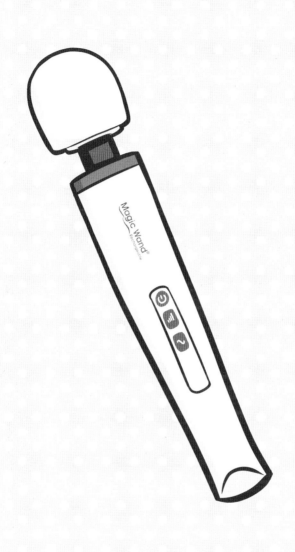

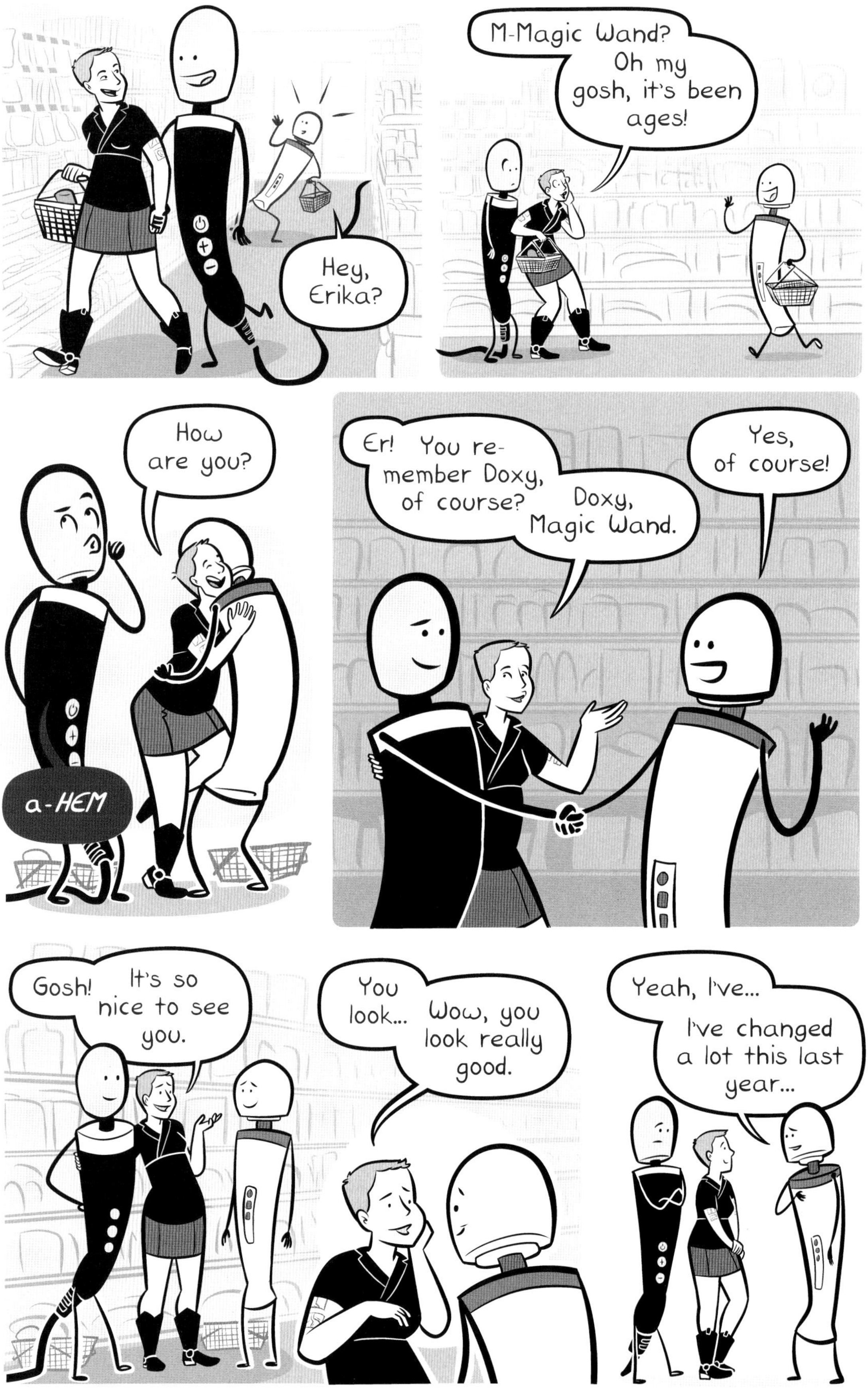
Hey, Erika?
M-Magic Wand? Oh my gosh, it's been ages!
How are you?
a-HEM
Er! You re-member Doxy, of course?
Doxy, Magic Wand.
Yes, of course!
Gosh!
It's so nice to see you.
You look...
Wow, you look really good.
Yeah, I've...
I've changed a lot this last year...

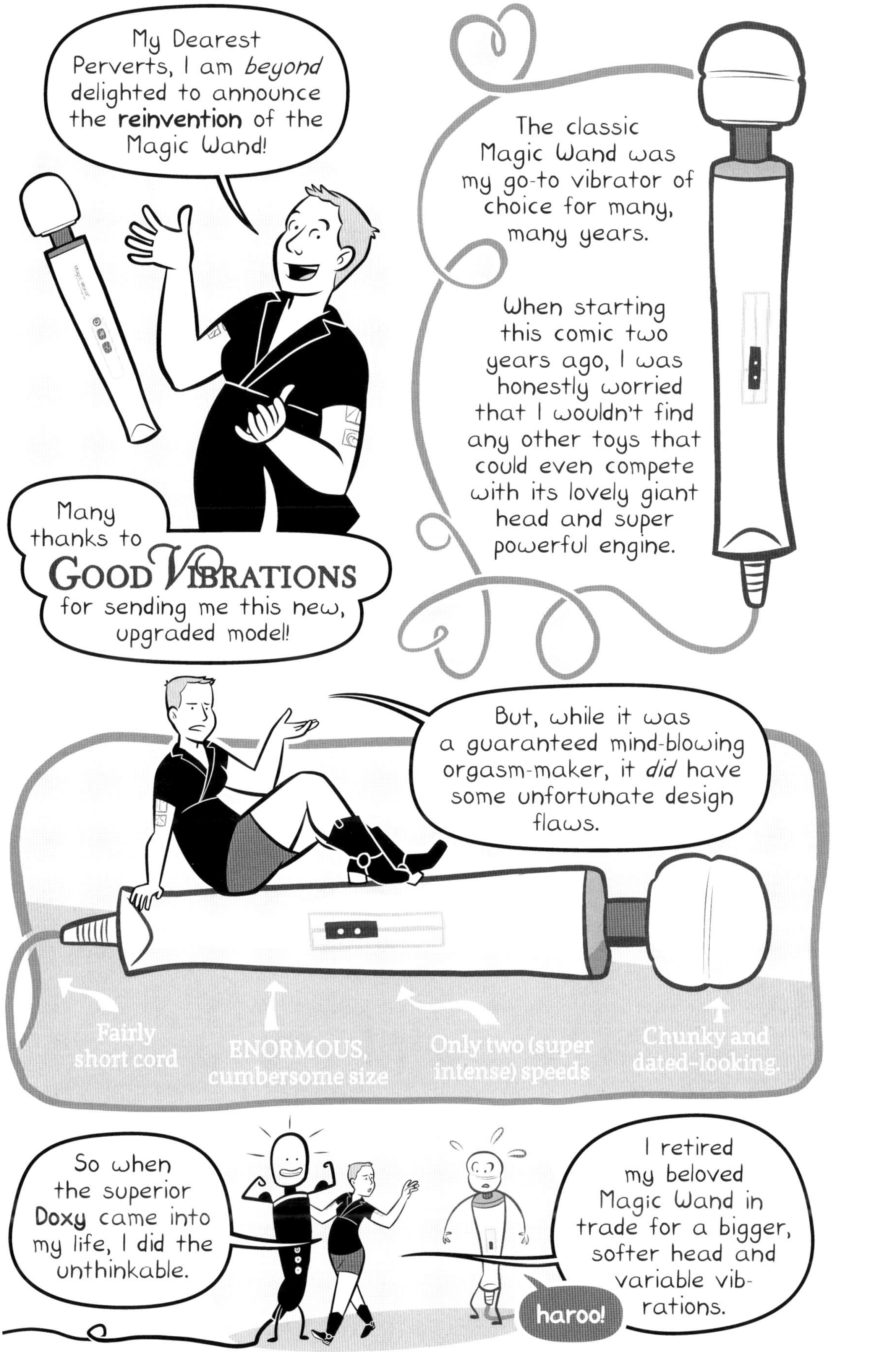

My Dearest Perverts, I am *beyond* delighted to announce the **reinvention** of the Magic Wand!
The classic Magic Wand was my go-to vibrator of choice for many, many years.
When starting this comic two years ago, I was honestly worried that I wouldn't find any other toys that could even compete with its lovely giant head and super powerful engine.
Many thanks to GOOD VIBRATIONS for sending me this new, upgraded model!
But, while it was a guaranteed mind-blowing orgasm-maker, it *did* have some unfortunate design flaws.
Fairly short cord
ENORMOUS, cumbersome size
Only two (super intense) speeds
Chunky and dated-looking.
So when the superior **Doxy** came into my life, I **did** the unthinkable.
I retired my beloved Magic Wand in trade for a bigger, softer head and variable vibrations.
haroo!

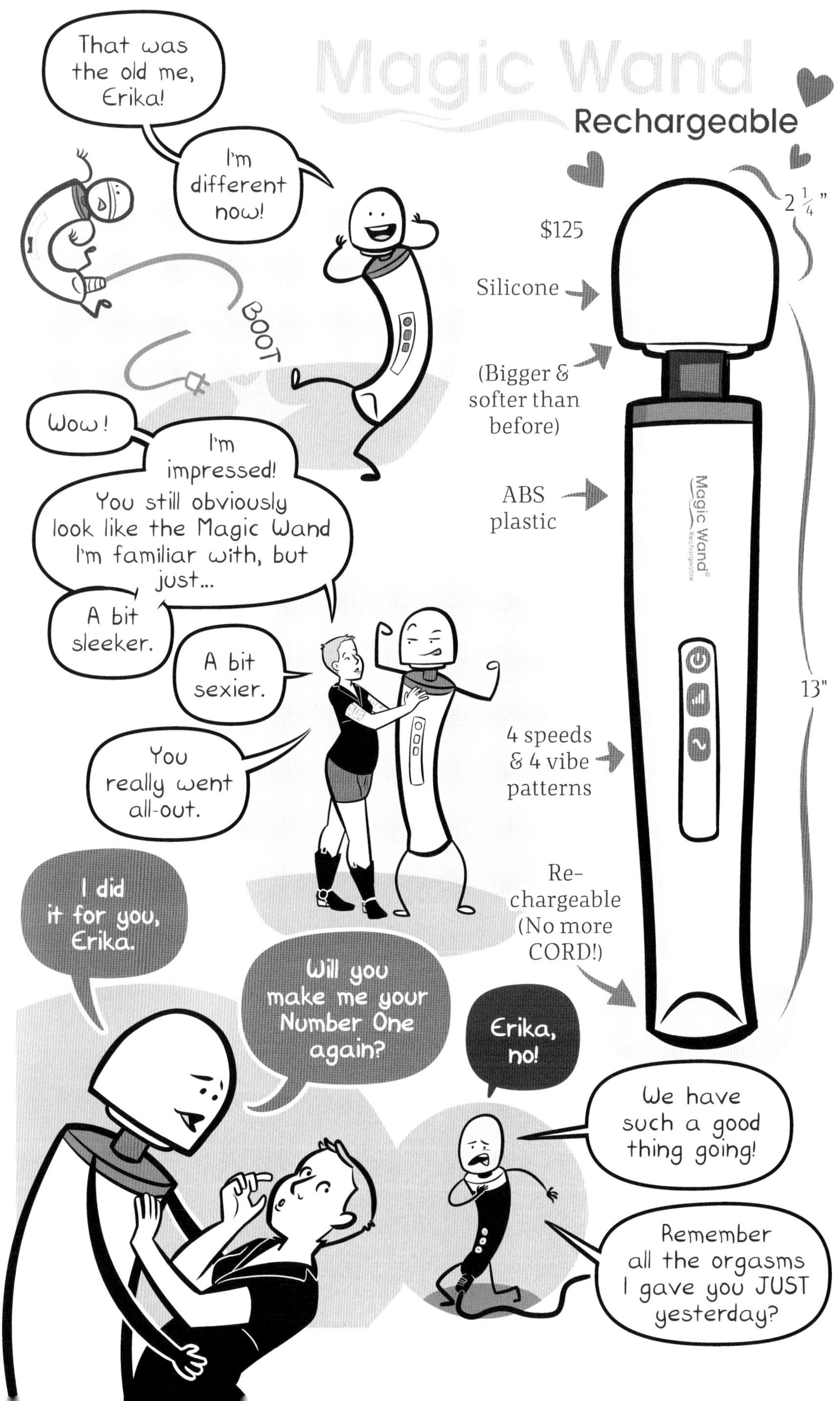

Magic Wand
Rechargeable
That was the old me, Erika!
I'm different now!
BOOT
$125
Silicone
(Bigger & softer than before)
2 1/4"
ABS plastic
Magic Wand Rechargeable
Wow!
I'm impressed! You still obviously look like the Magic Wand I'm familiar with, but just...
A bit sleeker.
A bit sexier.
You really went all-out.
13"
4 speeds & 4 vibe patterns
Re-chargeable (No more CORD!)
I did it for you, Erika.
Will you make me your Number One again?
Erika, no!
We have such a good thing going!
Remember all the orgasms I gave you JUST yesterday?

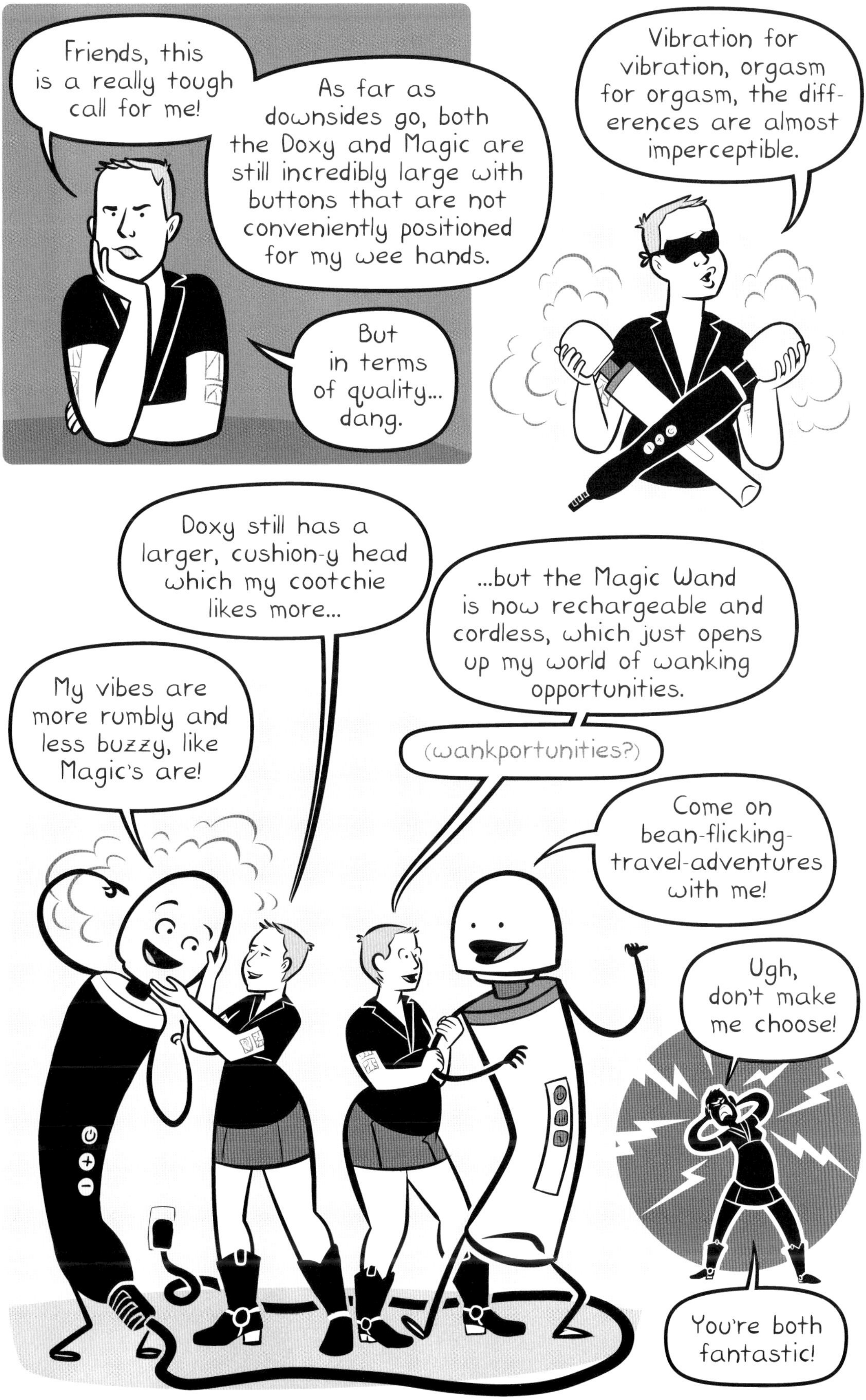
Friends, this is a really tough call for me!
As far as downsides go, both the Doxy and Magic are still incredibly large with buttons that are not conveniently positioned for my wee hands.
But in terms of quality... dang.
Vibration for vibration, orgasm for orgasm, the diff-erences are almost imperceptible.
Doxy still has a larger, cushion-y head which my cootchie likes more...
...but the Magic Wand is now rechargeable and cordless, which just opens up my world of wanking opportunities.
(wankportunities?)
My vibes are more rumbly and less buzzy, like Magic's are!
Come on bean-flicking-travel-adventures with me!
Ugh, don't make me choose!
You're both fantastic!

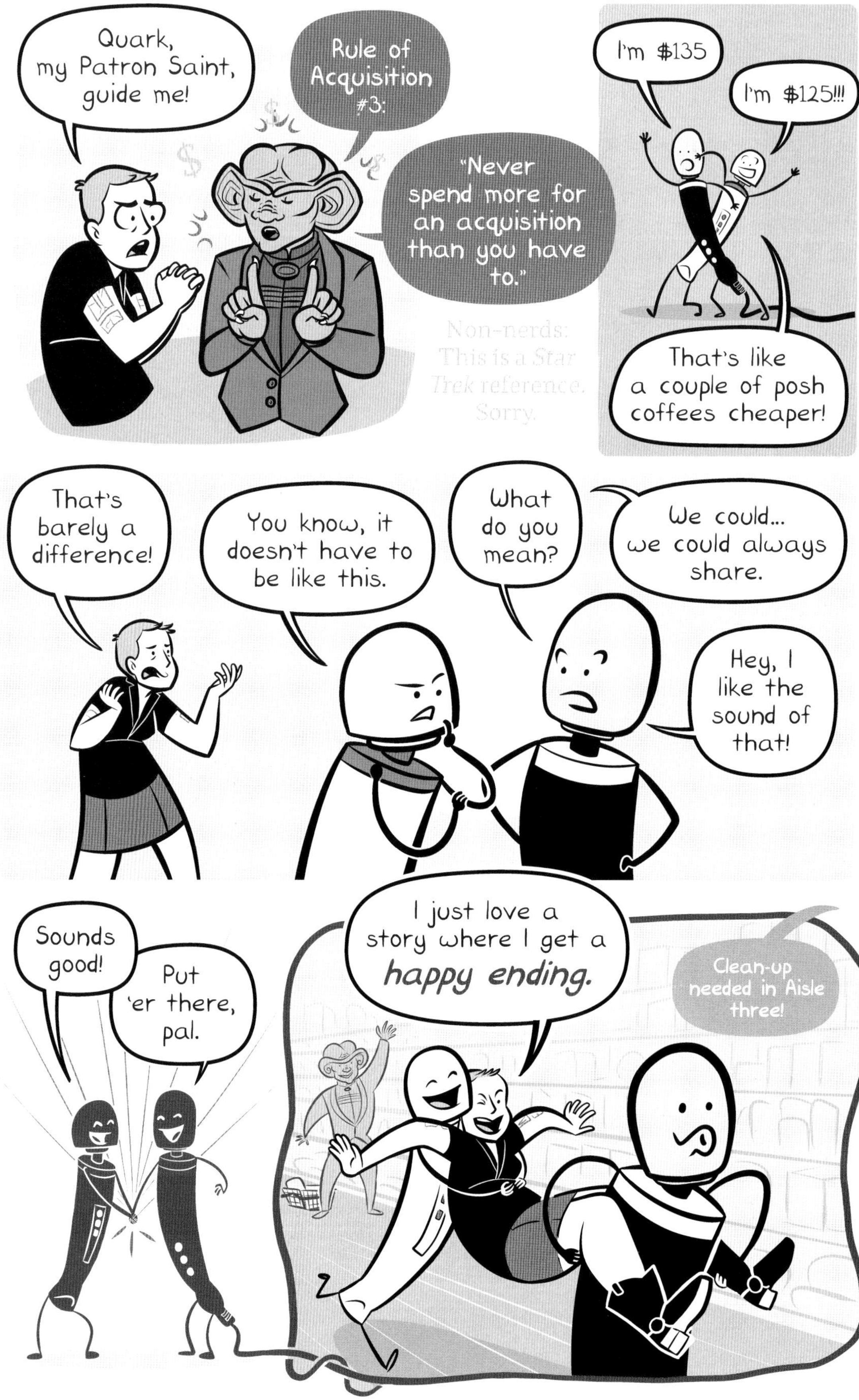

Quark, my Patron Saint, guide me!
Rule of Acquisition #3:
"Never spend more for an acquisition than you have to."
Non-nerds: This is a *Star Trek* reference. Sorry.
I'm $135
I'm $125!!!
That's like a couple of posh coffees cheaper!
That's barely a difference!
You know, it doesn't have to be like this.
What do you mean?
We could... we could always share.
Hey, I like the sound of that!
Sounds good!
Put 'er there, pal.
I just love a story where I get a ***happy ending.***
Clean-up needed in Aisle three!

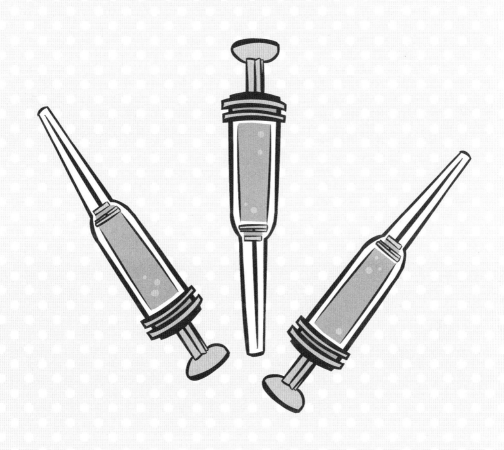

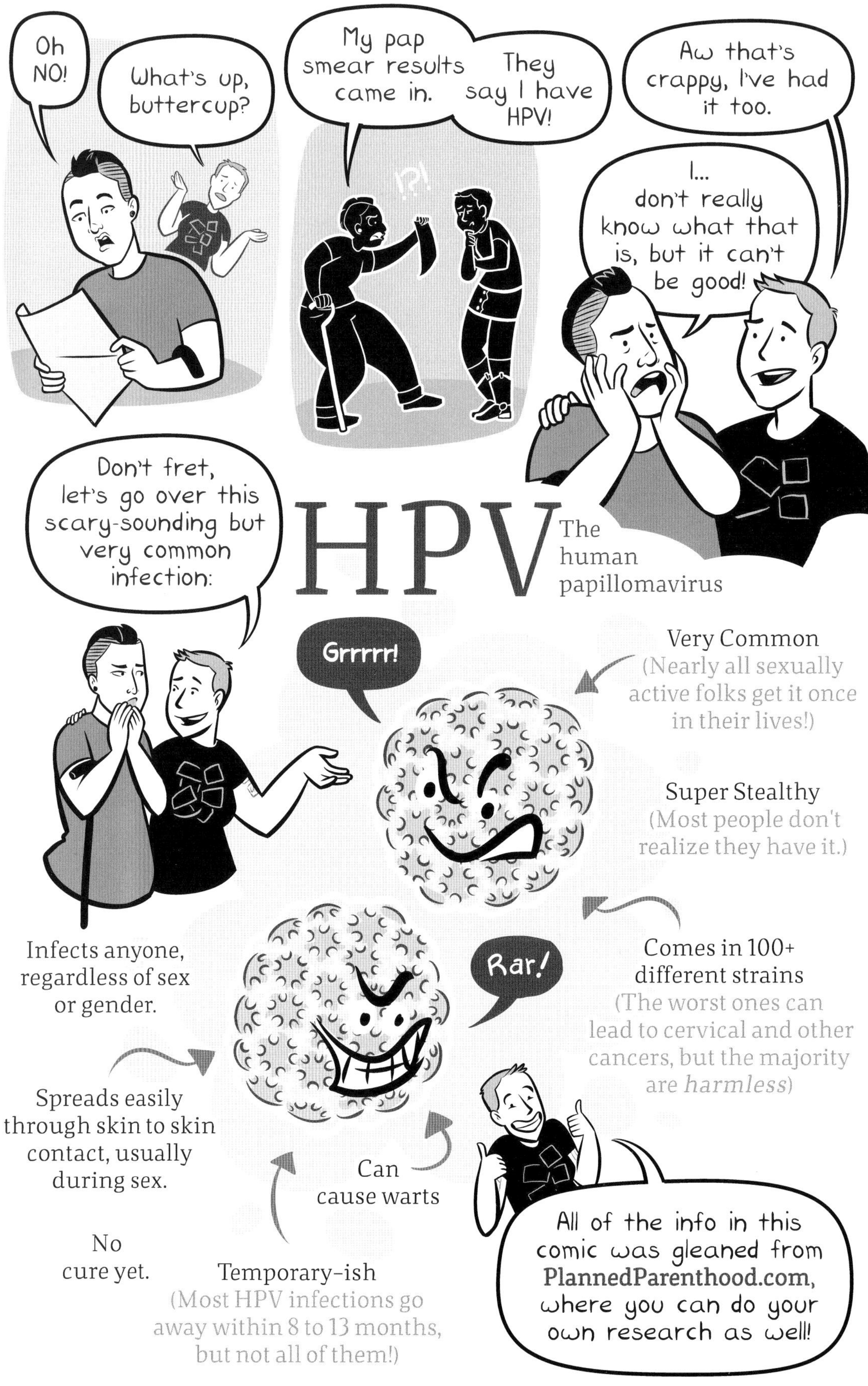

Oh NO!
What's up, buttercup?
My pap smear results came in.
They say I have HPV!
!?!
Aw that's crappy, I've had it too.
I... don't really know what that is, but it can't be good!
Don't fret, let's go over this scary-sounding but very common infection:
HPV
The human papillomavirus
Grrrrr!
Very Common
(Nearly all sexually active folks get it once in their lives!)
Super Stealthy
(Most people don't realize they have it.)
Rar!
Comes in 100+ different strains
(The worst ones can lead to cervical and other cancers, but the majority are *harmless*)
Infects anyone, regardless of sex or gender.
Spreads easily through skin to skin contact, usually during sex.
Can cause warts
No cure yet.
Temporary-ish
(Most HPV infections go away within 8 to 13 months, but not all of them!)
All of the info in this comic was gleaned from **PlannedParenthood.com**, where you can do your own research as well!

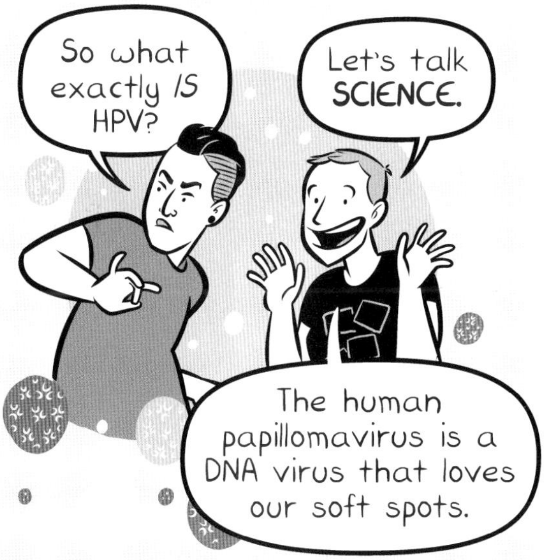
So what exactly IS HPV?
Let's talk SCIENCE.
The human papillomavirus is a DNA virus that loves our soft spots.

Your cervix, vagina, vulva, anus, penis, and throat are its favorite places to hang.

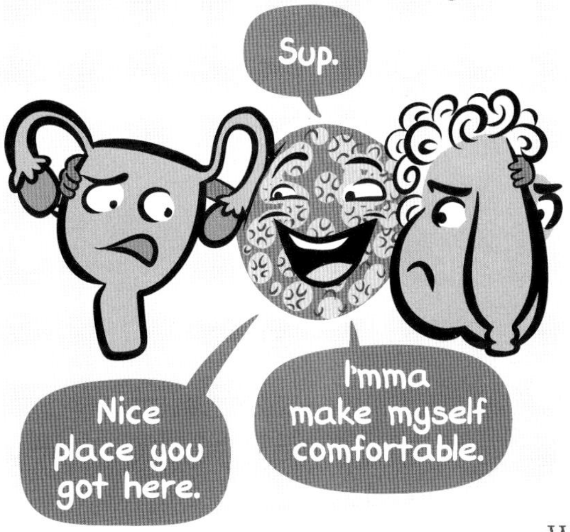
Sup.
Nice place you got here.
I'mma make myself comfortable.

Like any infection, it likes to hunker down and try to duke it out with our body's immune system.

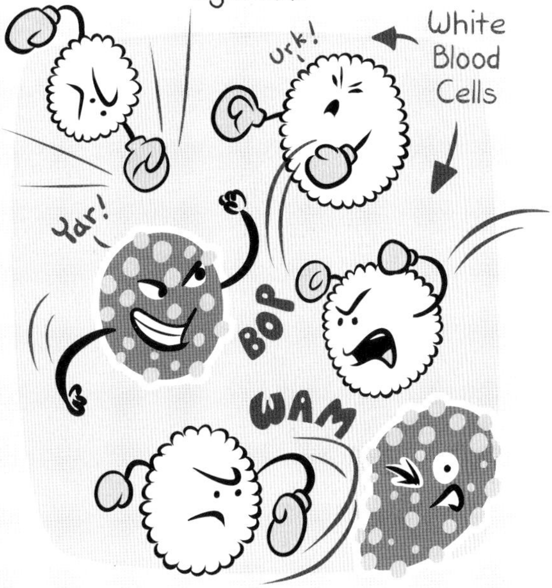
White Blood Cells
Urk!
Yar!
BOP
WAM

While we almost always clear the virus out naturally in **8-13 months** without any symptoms or issues, there are some unlucky few who will get the longer lasting strains or ones that cause genital warts or nasty cancers.

Those cancer-producing strains are no joke.

Fortunately, it's extra easy for your gynecologist to detect on your cervix.

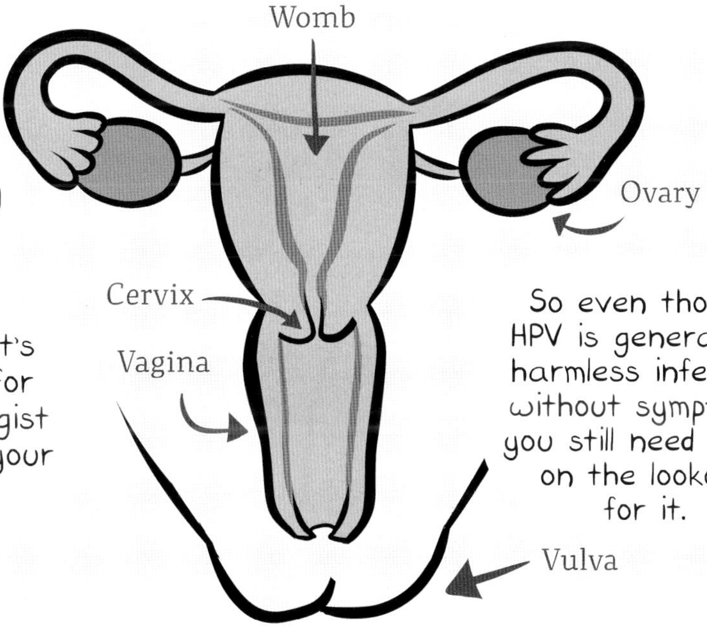
Womb
Ovary
Cervix
Vagina
Vulva

So even though HPV is generally a harmless infection without symptoms, you still need to be on the lookout for it.

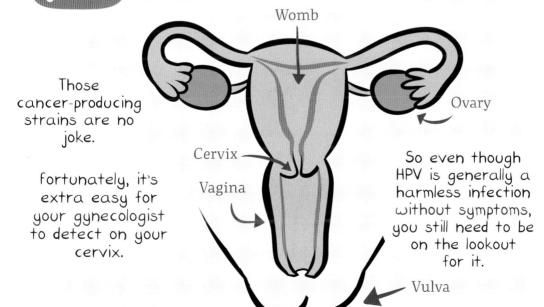

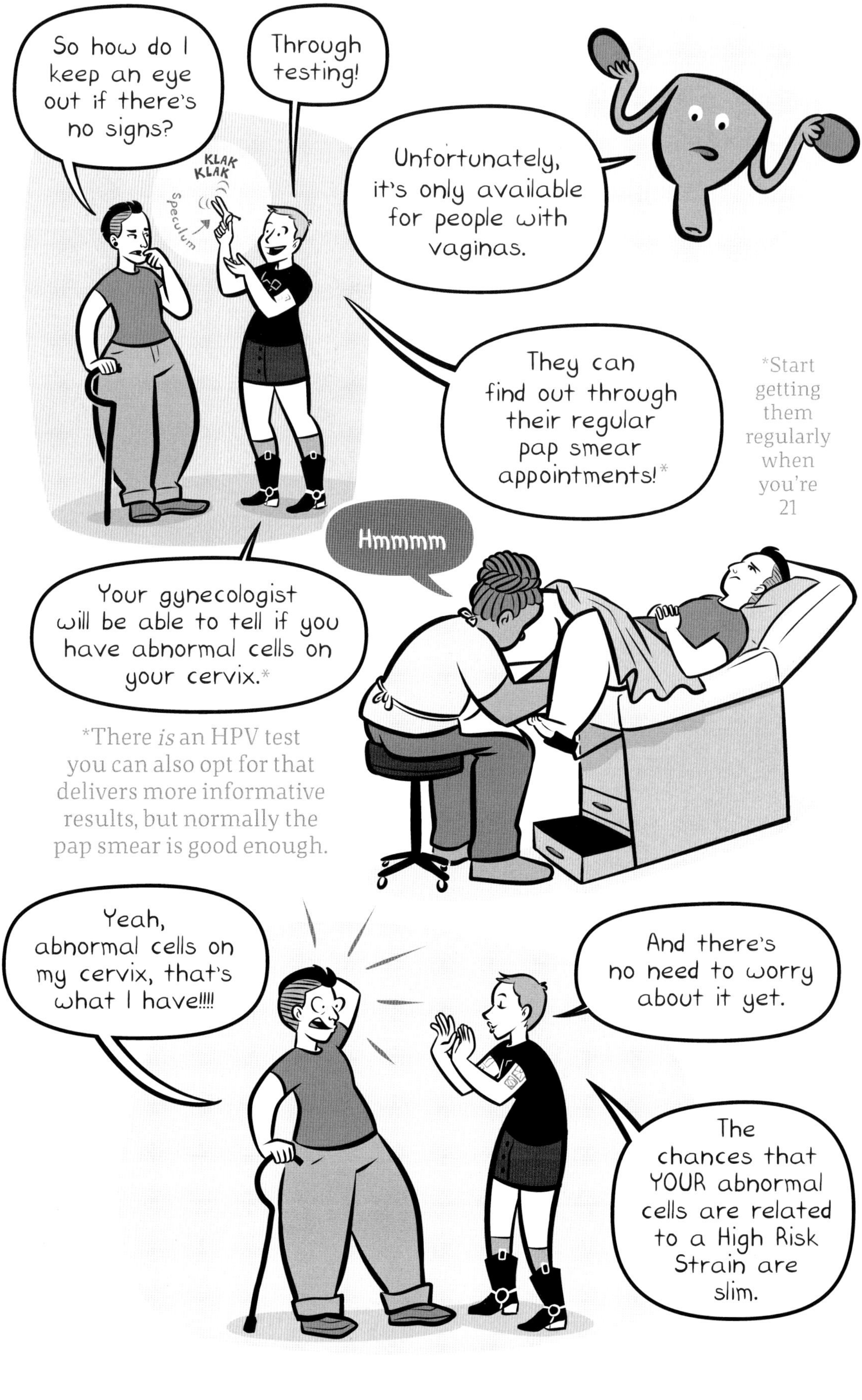
So how do I keep an eye out if there's no signs?
Through testing!
KLAK KLAK
Speculum
Unfortunately, it's only available for people with vaginas.
They can find out through their regular pap smear appointments!*
*Start getting them regularly when you're 21
Hmmmm
Your gynecologist will be able to tell if you have abnormal cells on your cervix.*
*There *is* an HPV test you can also opt for that delivers more informative results, but normally the pap smear is good enough.
Yeah, abnormal cells on my cervix, that's what I have!!!!
And there's no need to worry about it yet.
The chances that YOUR abnormal cells are related to a High Risk Strain are slim.

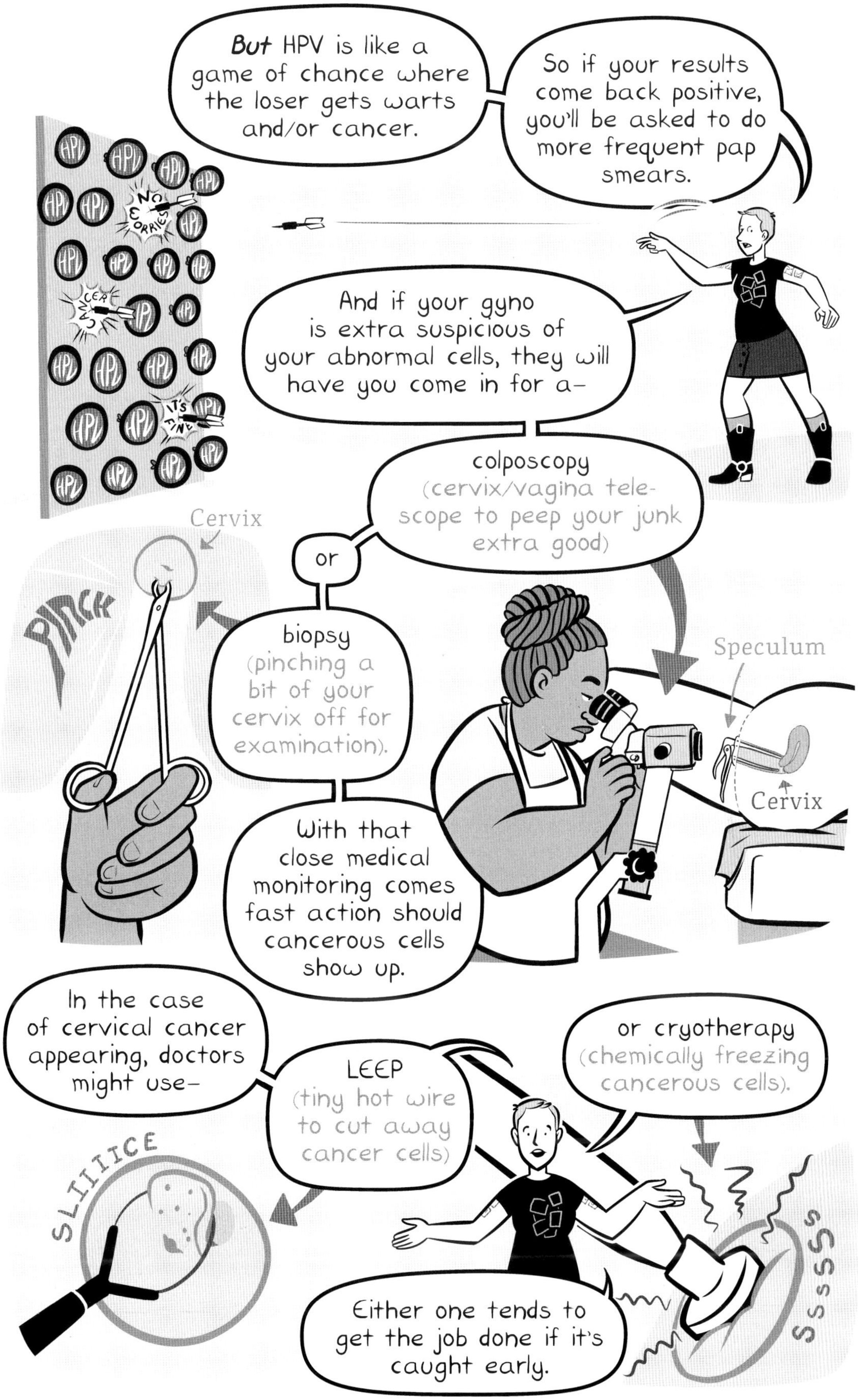

But HPV is like a game of chance where the loser gets warts and/or cancer.
So if your results come back positive, you'll be asked to do more frequent pap smears.
NO WORRIES
CANCER
IT'S FINE
And if your gyno is extra suspicious of your abnormal cells, they will have you come in for a–
colposcopy (cervix/vagina tele-scope to peep your junk extra good)
or
biopsy (pinching a bit of your cervix off for examination).
Cervix
PINCH
Speculum
Cervix
With that close medical monitoring comes fast action should cancerous cells show up.
In the case of cervical cancer appearing, doctors might use–
LEEP (tiny hot wire to cut away cancer cells)
or cryotherapy (chemically freezing cancerous cells).
SLIIIICE
Ssssss
Either one tends to get the job done if it's caught early.

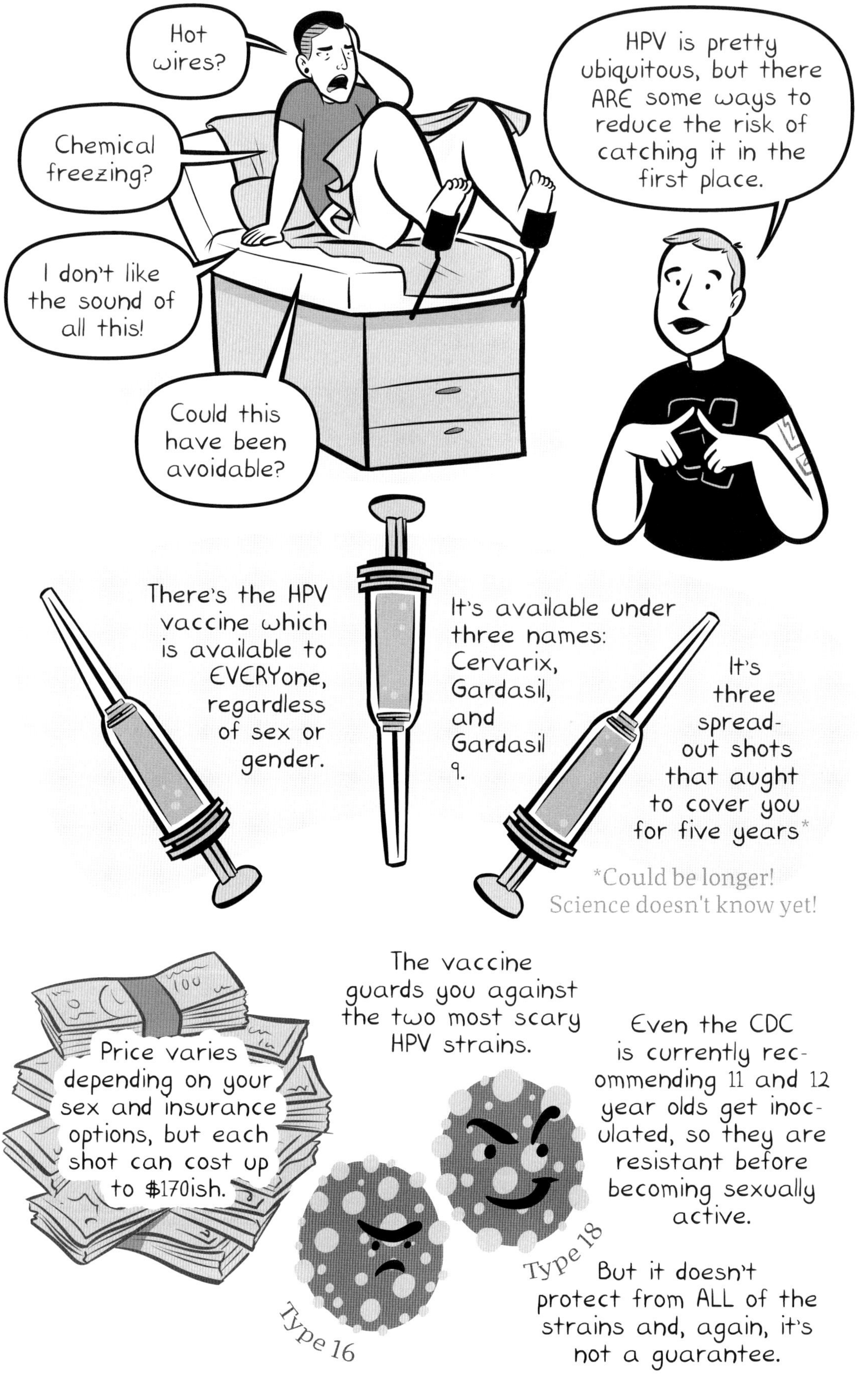
Hot wires?
Chemical freezing?
I don't like the sound of all this!
Could this have been avoidable?
HPV is pretty ubiquitous, but there ARE some ways to reduce the risk of catching it in the first place.
There's the HPV vaccine which is available to EVERYone, regardless of sex or gender.
It's available under three names: Cervarix, Gardasil, and Gardasil 9.
It's three spread-out shots that aught to cover you for five years*
*Could be longer! Science doesn't know yet!
100
Price varies depending on your sex and insurance options, but each shot can cost up to $170ish.
The vaccine guards you against the two most scary HPV strains.
Type 16
Type 18
Even the CDC is currently recommending 11 and 12 year olds get inoculated, so they are resistant before becoming sexually active.
But it doesn't protect from ALL of the strains and, again, it's not a guarantee.

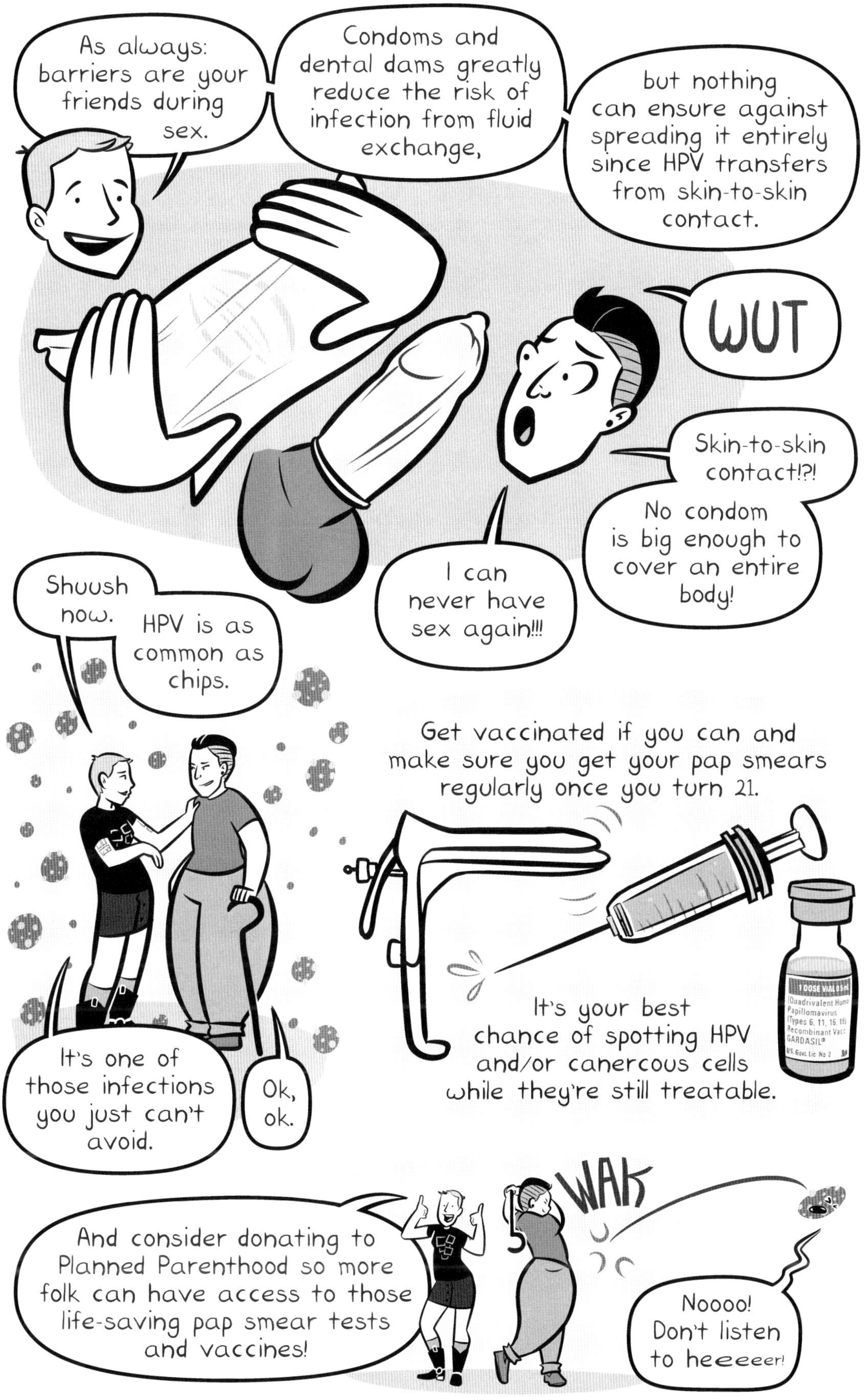
As always: barriers are your friends during sex.
Condoms and dental dams greatly reduce the risk of infection from fluid exchange,
but nothing can ensure against spreading it entirely since HPV transfers from skin-to-skin contact.
WUT
Skin-to-skin contact!?!
No condom is big enough to cover an entire body!
I can never have sex again!!!
Shuush now.
HPV is as common as chips.
It's one of those infections you just can't avoid.
Ok, ok.
Get vaccinated if you can and make sure you get your pap smears regularly once you turn 21.
Papillomavirus
GARDASIL®
It's your best chance of spotting HPV and/or canercous cells while they're still treatable.
And consider donating to Planned Parenthood so more folk can have access to those life-saving pap smear tests and vaccines!
WAK
Noooo! Don't listen to heeeeer!

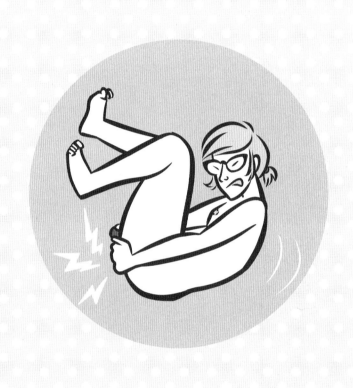

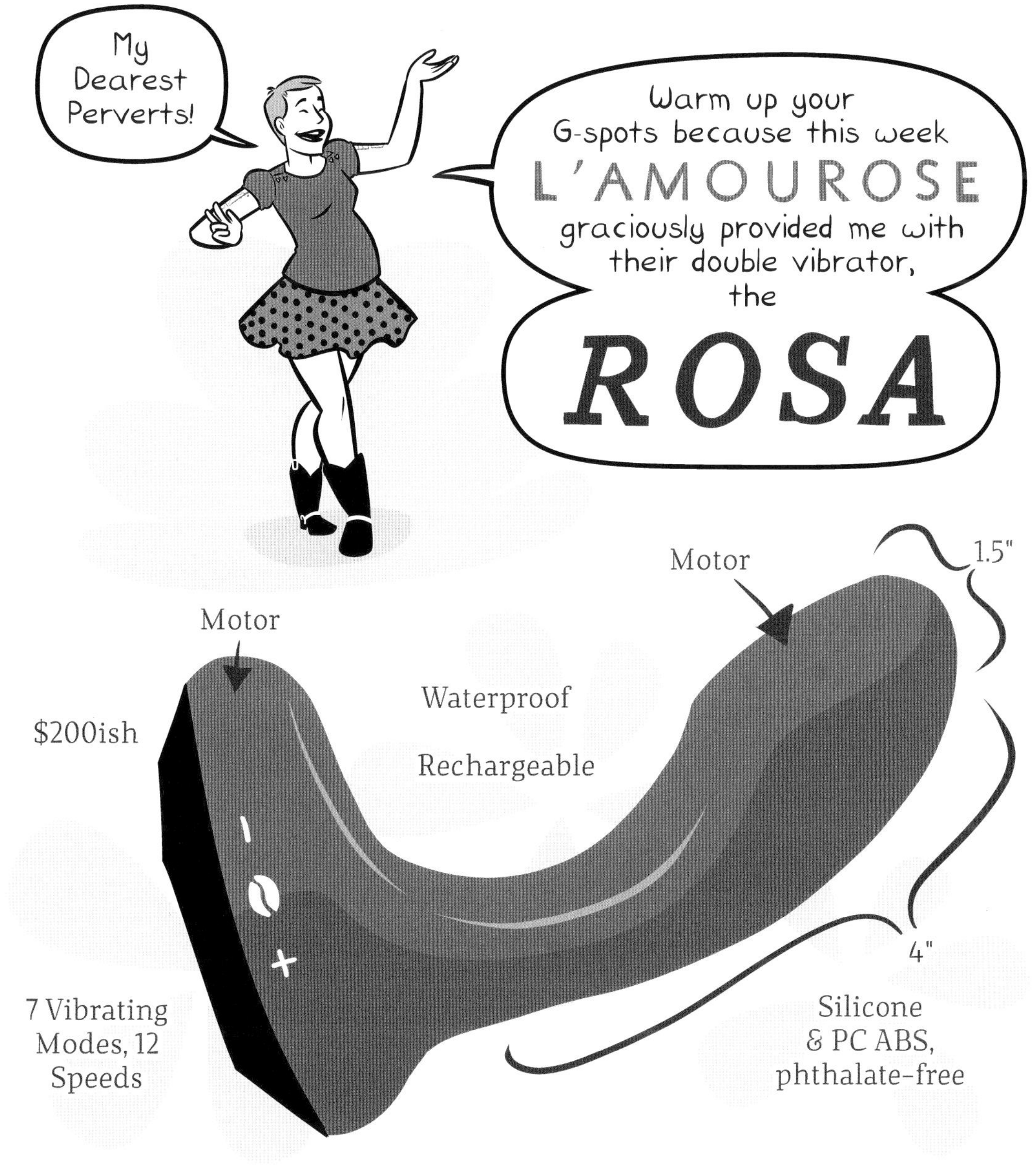
My Dearest Perverts!
Warm up your G-spots because this week L'AMOUROSE graciously provided me with their double vibrator, the ROSA
Motor
Motor
1.5"
$200ish
Waterproof
Rechargeable
4"
7 Vibrating Modes, 12 Speeds
Silicone & PC ABS, phthalate-free

This expensive toy gives you a variety of stimulation to choose from.

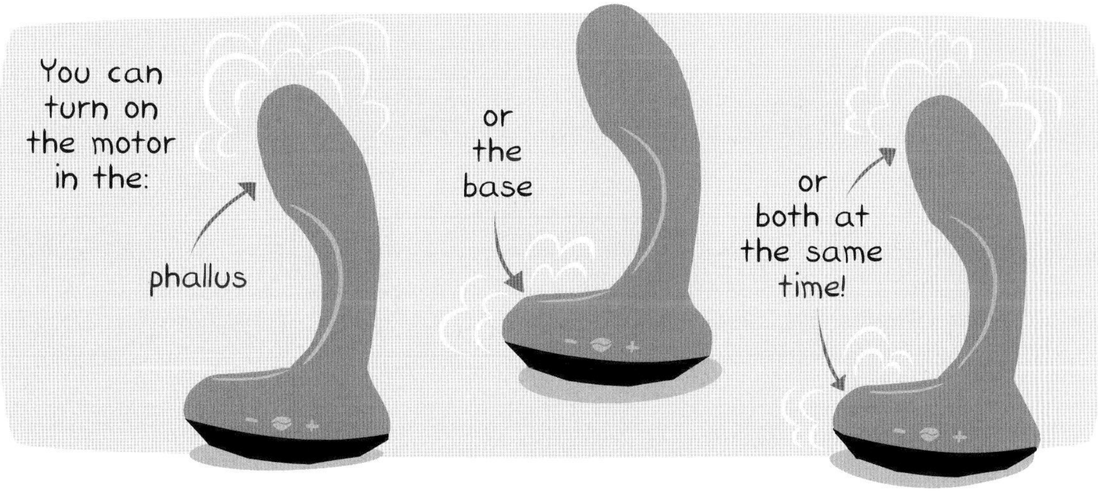
You can turn on the motor in the:
phallus
or the base
or both at the same time!

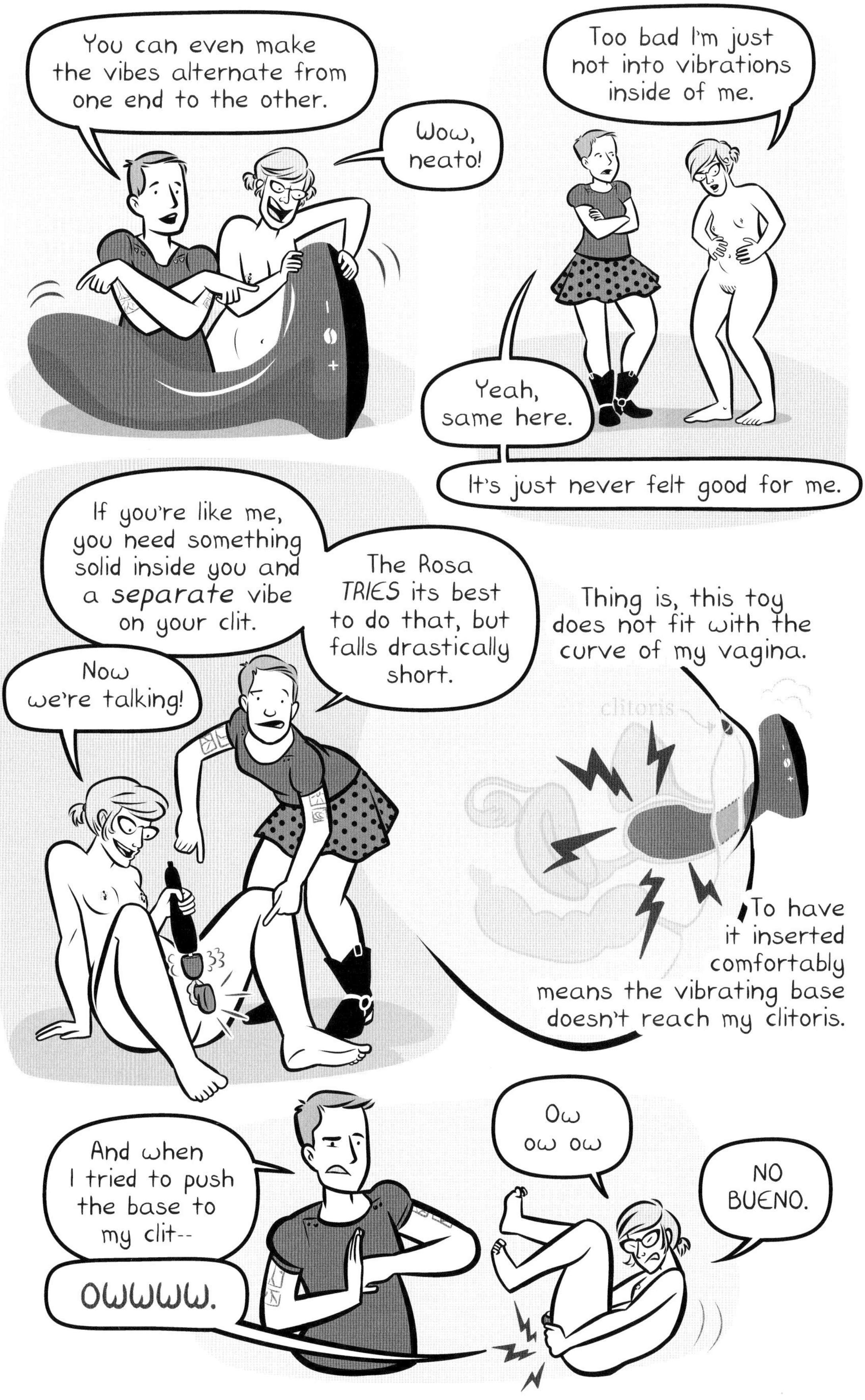

You can even make the vibes alternate from one end to the other.
Wow, neato!
Too bad I'm just not into vibrations inside of me.
Yeah, same here.
It's just never felt good for me.
If you're like me, you need something solid inside you and a *separate* vibe on your clit.
The Rosa *TRIES* its best to do that, but falls drastically short.
Now we're talking!
Thing is, this toy does not fit with the curve of my vagina.
clitoris
To have it inserted comfortably means the vibrating base doesn't reach my clitoris.
And when I tried to push the base to my clit--
OWWWW.
Ow ow ow
NO BUENO.

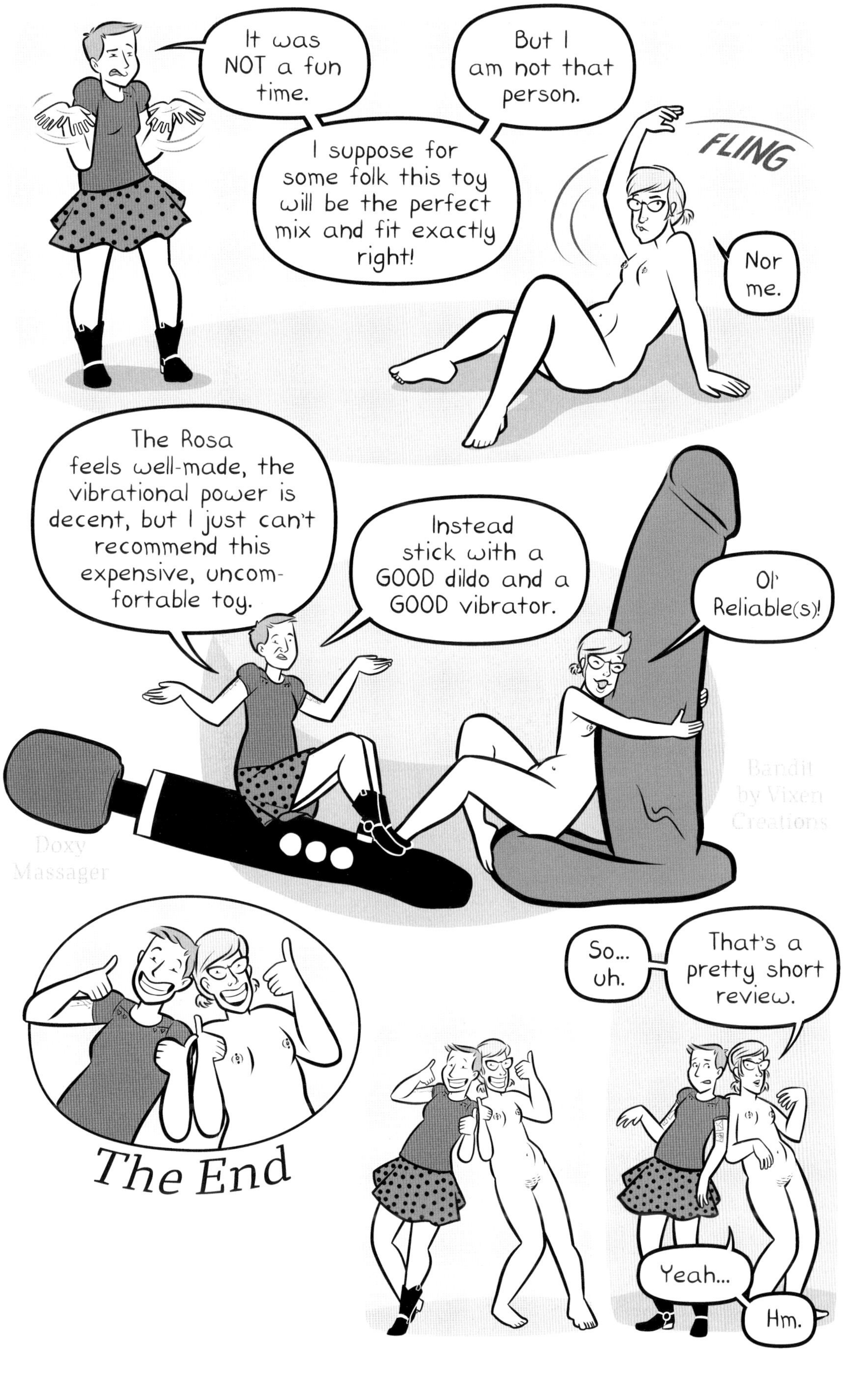
It was NOT a fun time.
But I am not that person.
I suppose for some folk this toy will be the perfect mix and fit exactly right!
FLING
Nor me.
The Rosa feels well-made, the vibrational power is decent, but I just can't recommend this expensive, uncom-fortable toy.
Instead stick with a GOOD dildo and a GOOD vibrator.
Ol' Reliable(s)!
Doxy Massager
Bandit by Vixen Creations
The End
So... uh.
That's a pretty short review.
Yeah...
Hm.

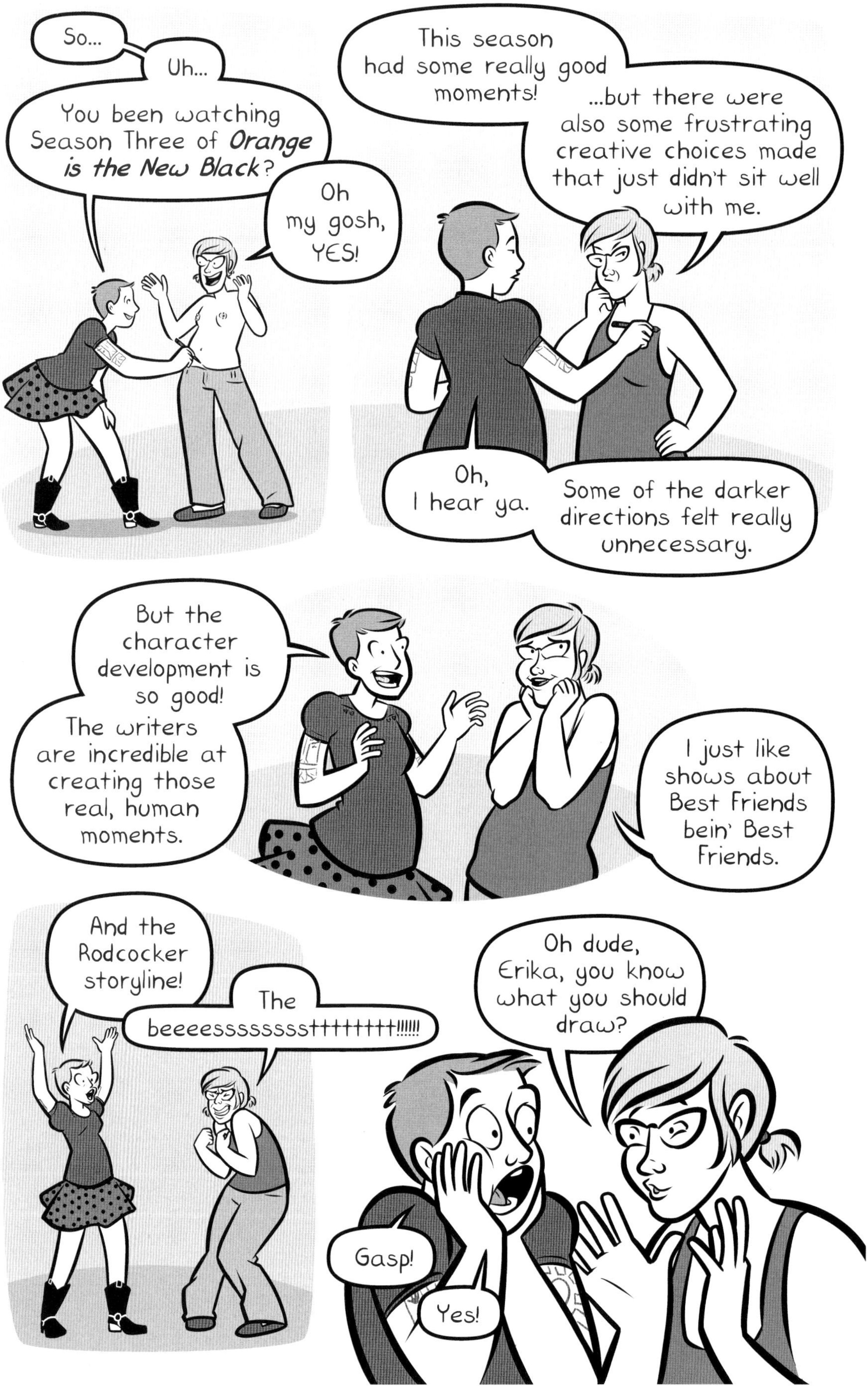
So...
Uh...
You been watching Season Three of *Orange is the New Black*?
Oh my gosh, YES!
This season had some really good moments!
...but there were also some frustrating creative choices made that just didn't sit well with me.
Oh, I hear ya.
Some of the darker directions felt really unnecessary.
But the character development is so good!
The writers are incredible at creating those real, human moments.
I just like shows about Best Friends bein' Best Friends.
And the Rodcocker storyline!
The beeeessssssssttttttttt!!!!!!
Oh dude, Erika, you know what you should draw?
Gasp!
Yes!

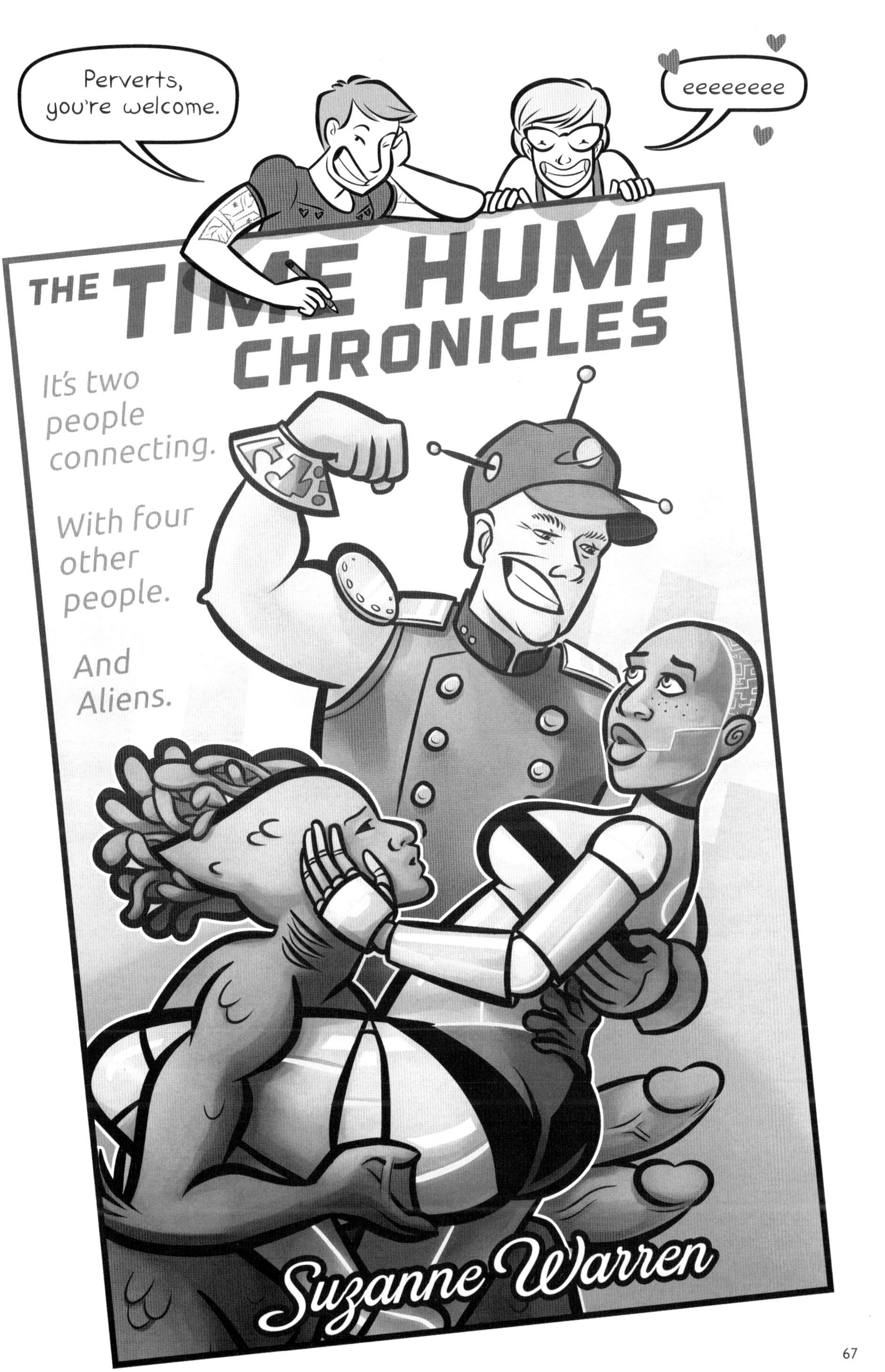
Perverts, you're welcome.
eeeeeeee
THE TIME HUMP CHRONICLES
It's two people connecting.
With four other people.
And Aliens.
Suzanne Warren

Oh my!

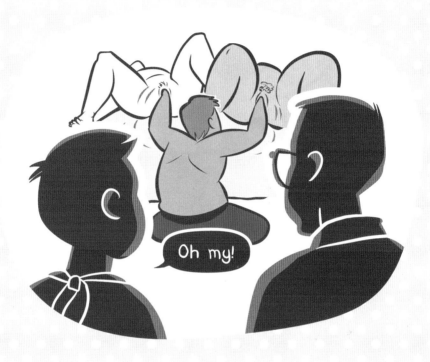

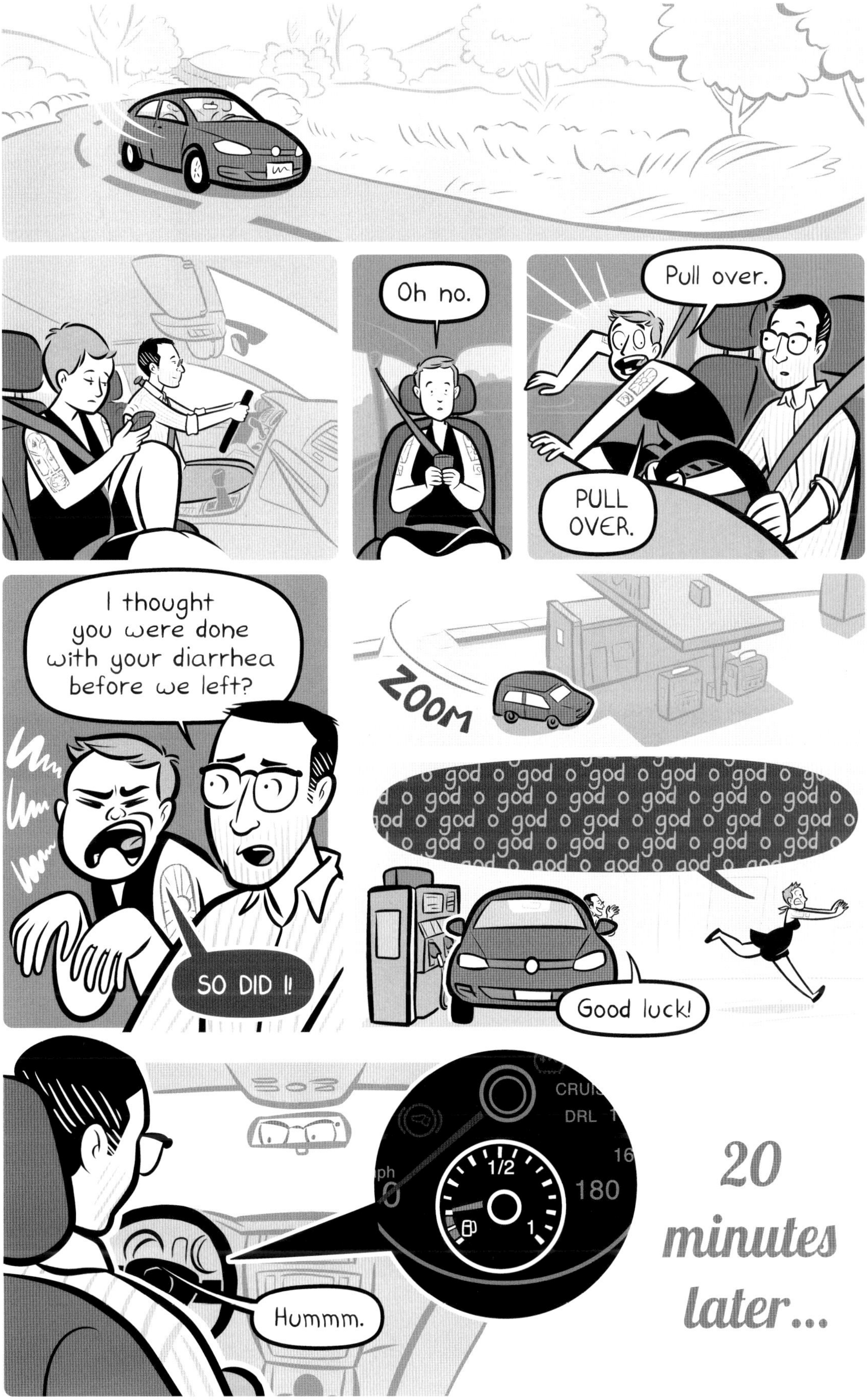
Oh no.
Pull over.
PULL OVER.
I thought you were done with your diarrhea before we left?
SO DID I!
ZOOM
o god o god
Good luck!
CRUIS
DRL
1/2
180
Hummm.
20 minutes later...

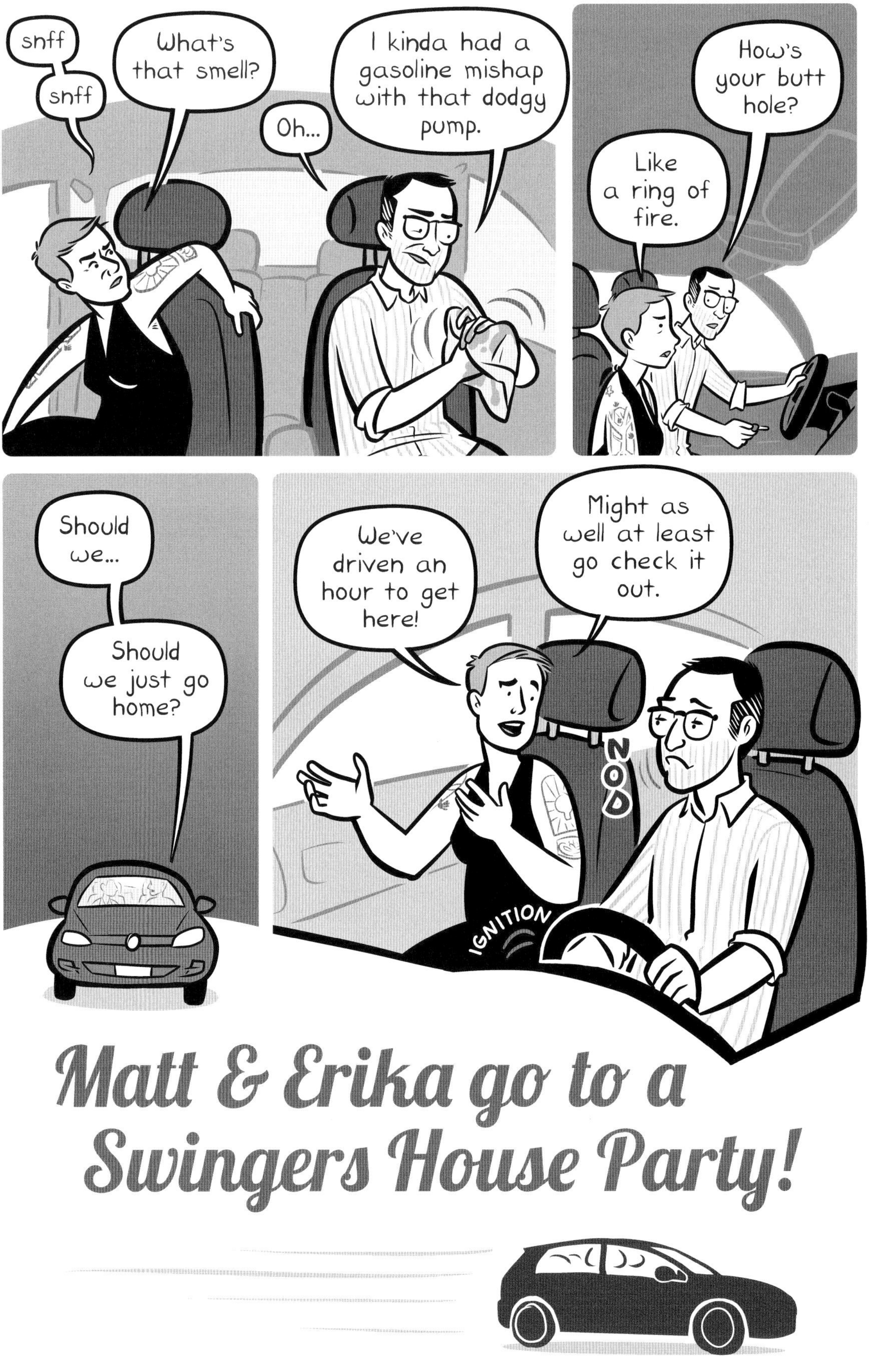
snff
snff
What's that smell?
Oh...
I kinda had a gasoline mishap with that dodgy pump.
How's your butt hole?
Like a ring of fire.
Should we...
Should we just go home?
We've driven an hour to get here!
Might as well at least go check it out.
NOD
IGNITION
Matt & Erika go to a Swingers House Party!

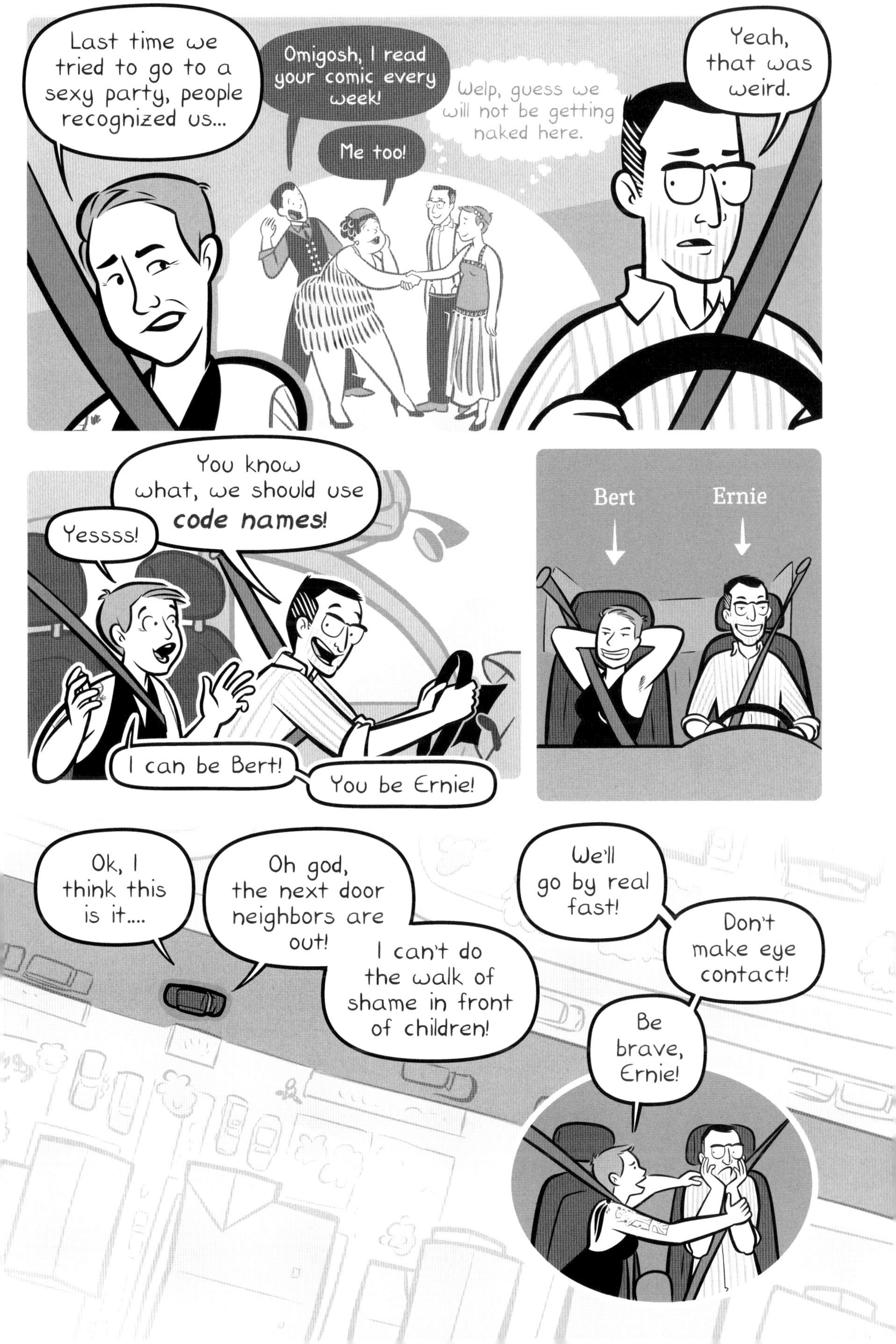
Last time we tried to go to a sexy party, people recognized us...
Omigosh, I read your comic every week!
Me too!
Welp, guess we will not be getting naked here.
Yeah, that was weird.
You know what, we should use **code names**!
Yessss!
I can be Bert!
You be Ernie!
Bert
Ernie
Ok, I think this is it....
Oh god, the next door neighbors are out!
I can't do the walk of shame in front of children!
We'll go by real fast!
Don't make eye contact!
Be brave, Ernie!

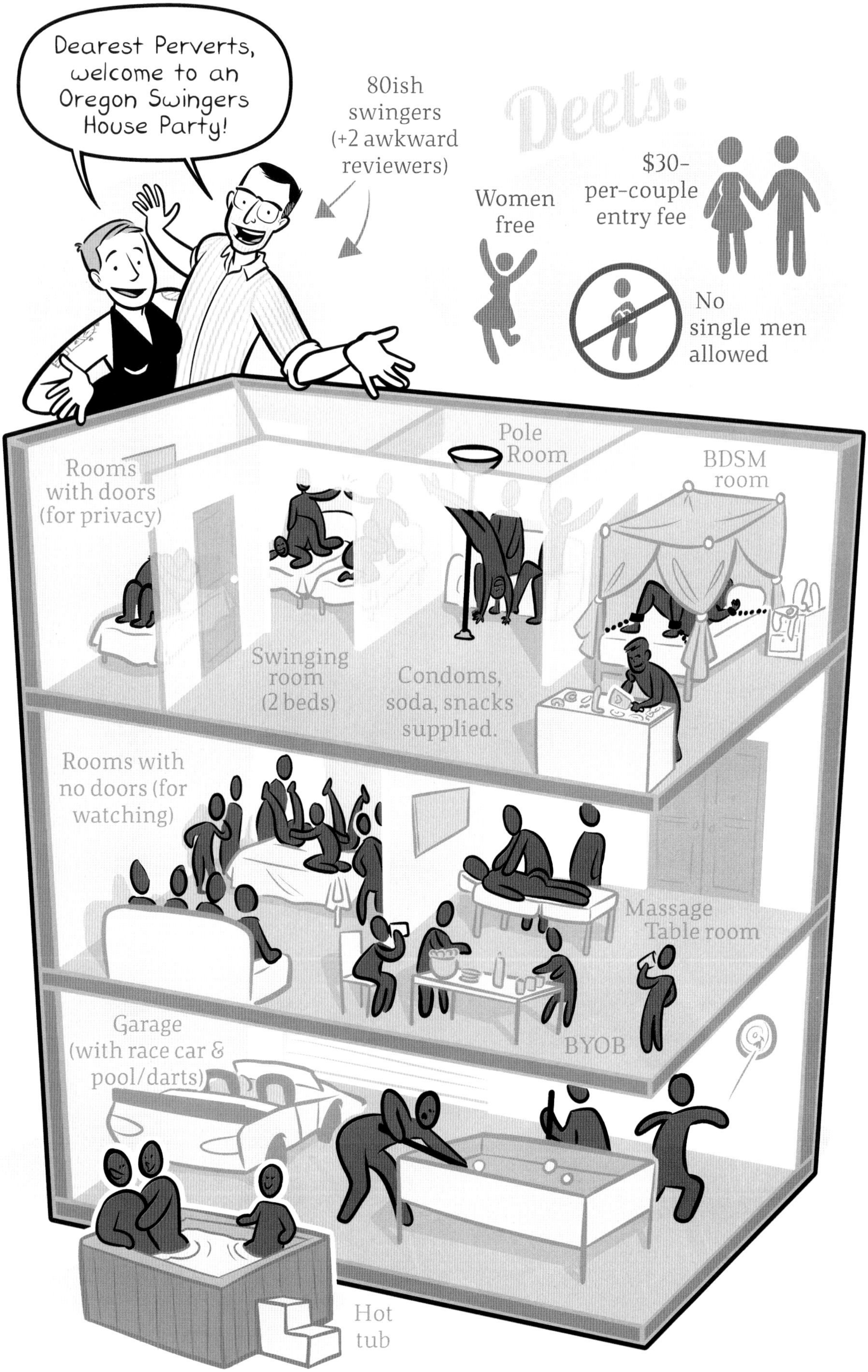
Dearest Perverts, welcome to an Oregon Swingers House Party!
80ish swingers (+2 awkward reviewers)
Deets:
Women free
$30-per-couple entry fee
No single men allowed
Rooms with doors (for privacy)
Pole Room
BDSM room
Swinging room (2 beds)
Condoms, soda, snacks supplied.
Rooms with no doors (for watching)
Massage Table room
BYOB
Garage (with race car & pool/darts)
Hot tub

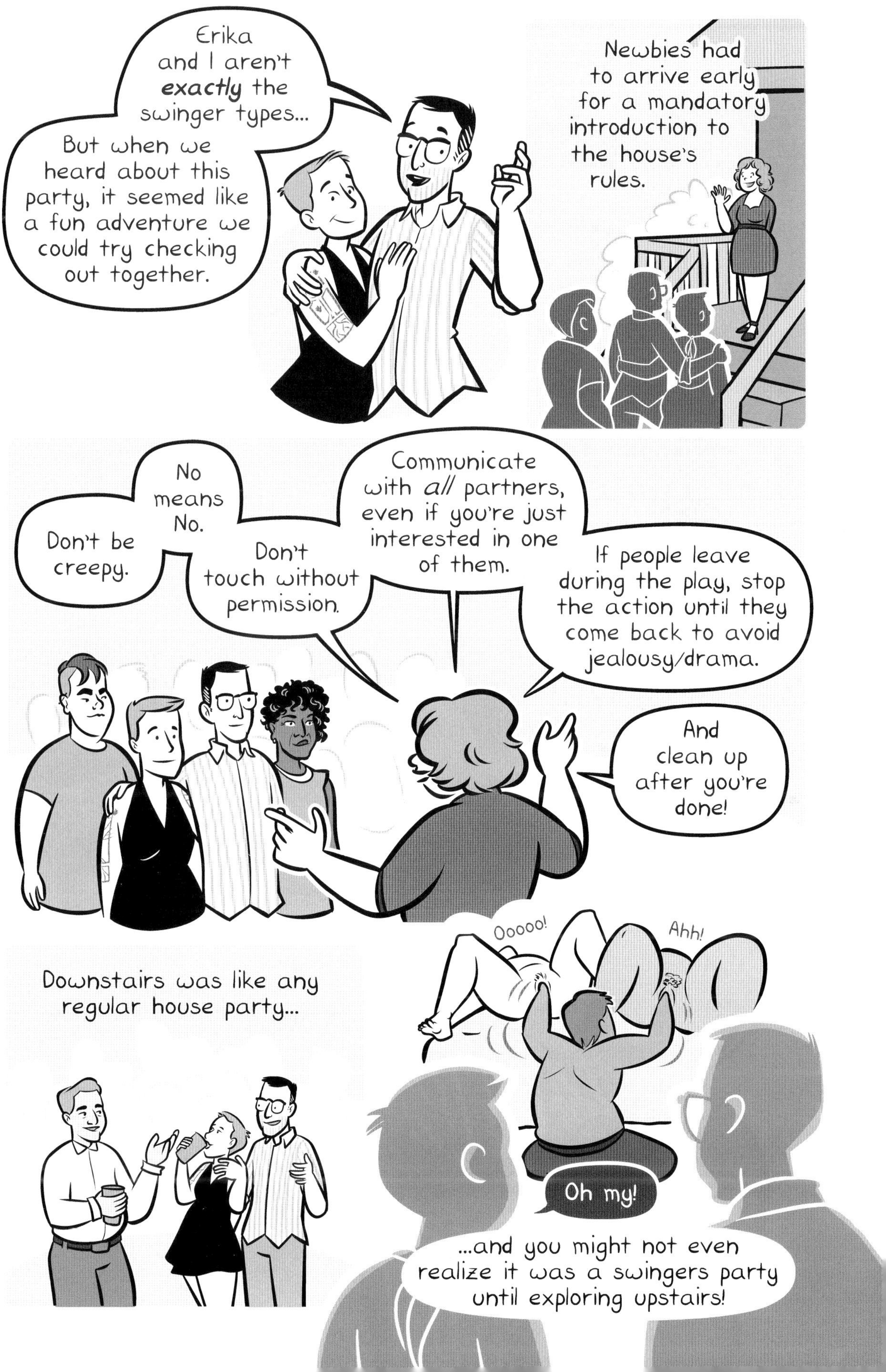
Erika and I aren't *exactly* the swinger types...
But when we heard about this party, it seemed like a fun adventure we could try checking out together.
Newbies had to arrive early for a mandatory introduction to the house's rules.
Don't be creepy.
No means No.
Don't touch without permission.
Communicate with *all* partners, even if you're just interested in one of them.
If people leave during the play, stop the action until they come back to avoid jealousy/drama.
And clean up after you're done!
Downstairs was like any regular house party...
Ooooo!
Ahh!
Oh my!
...and you might not even realize it was a swingers party until exploring upstairs!

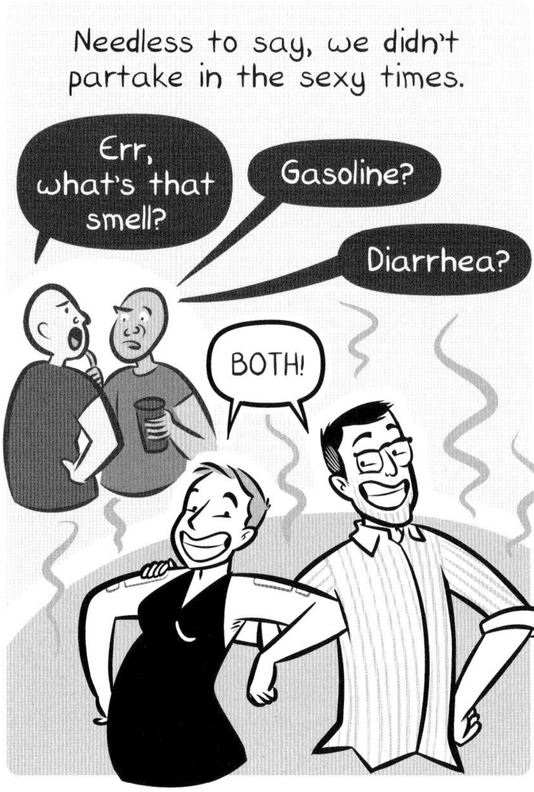
Needless to say, we didn't partake in the sexy times.
Err, what's that smell?
Gasoline?
Diarrhea?
BOTH!

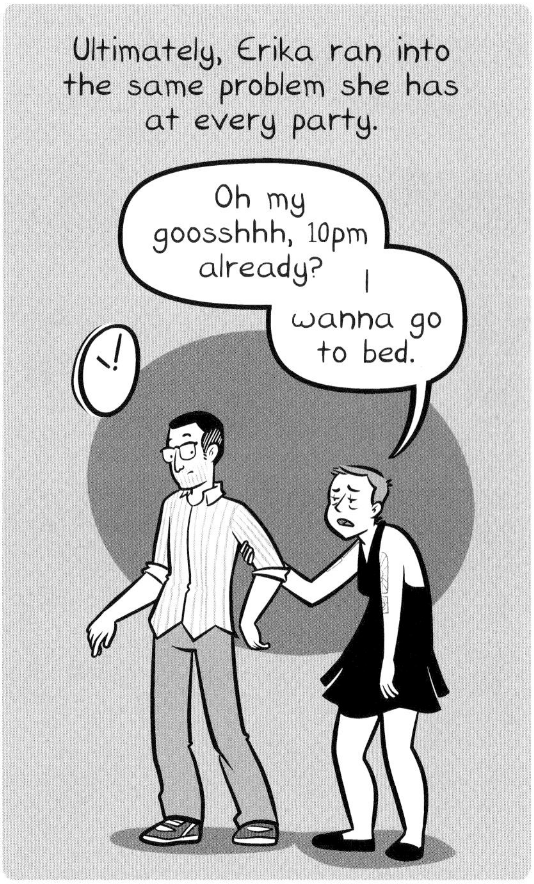
Ultimately, Erika ran into the same problem she has at every party.
Oh my goossshhh, 10pm already?
I wanna go to bed.

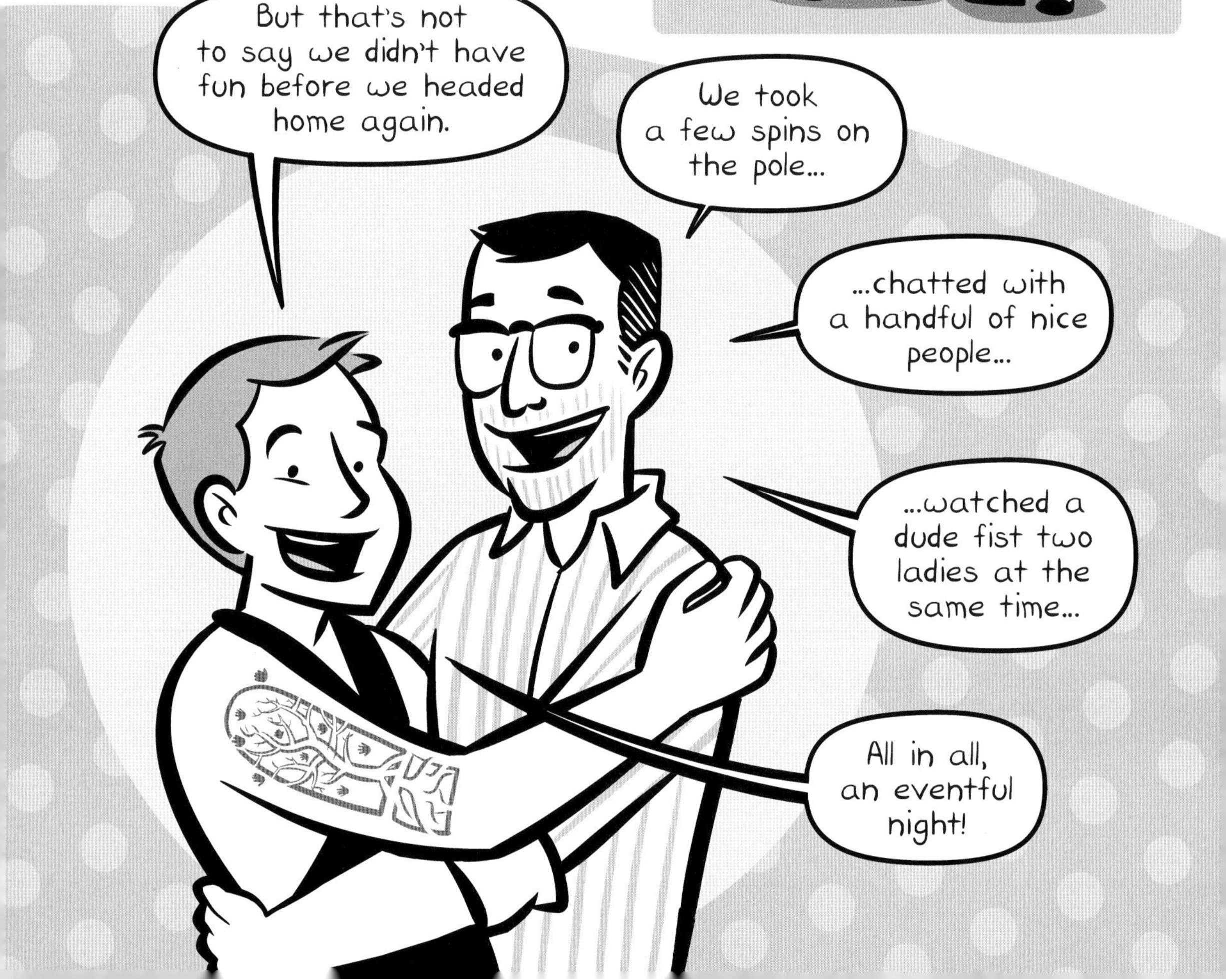
But that's not to say we didn't have fun before we headed home again.
We took a few spins on the pole...
...chatted with a handful of nice people...
...watched a dude fist two ladies at the same time...
All in all, an eventful night!

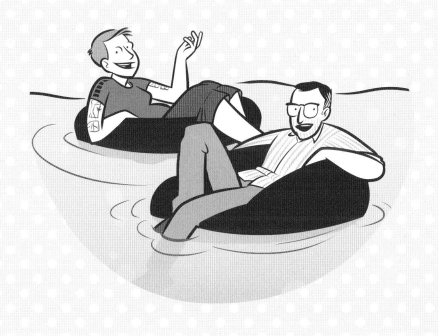

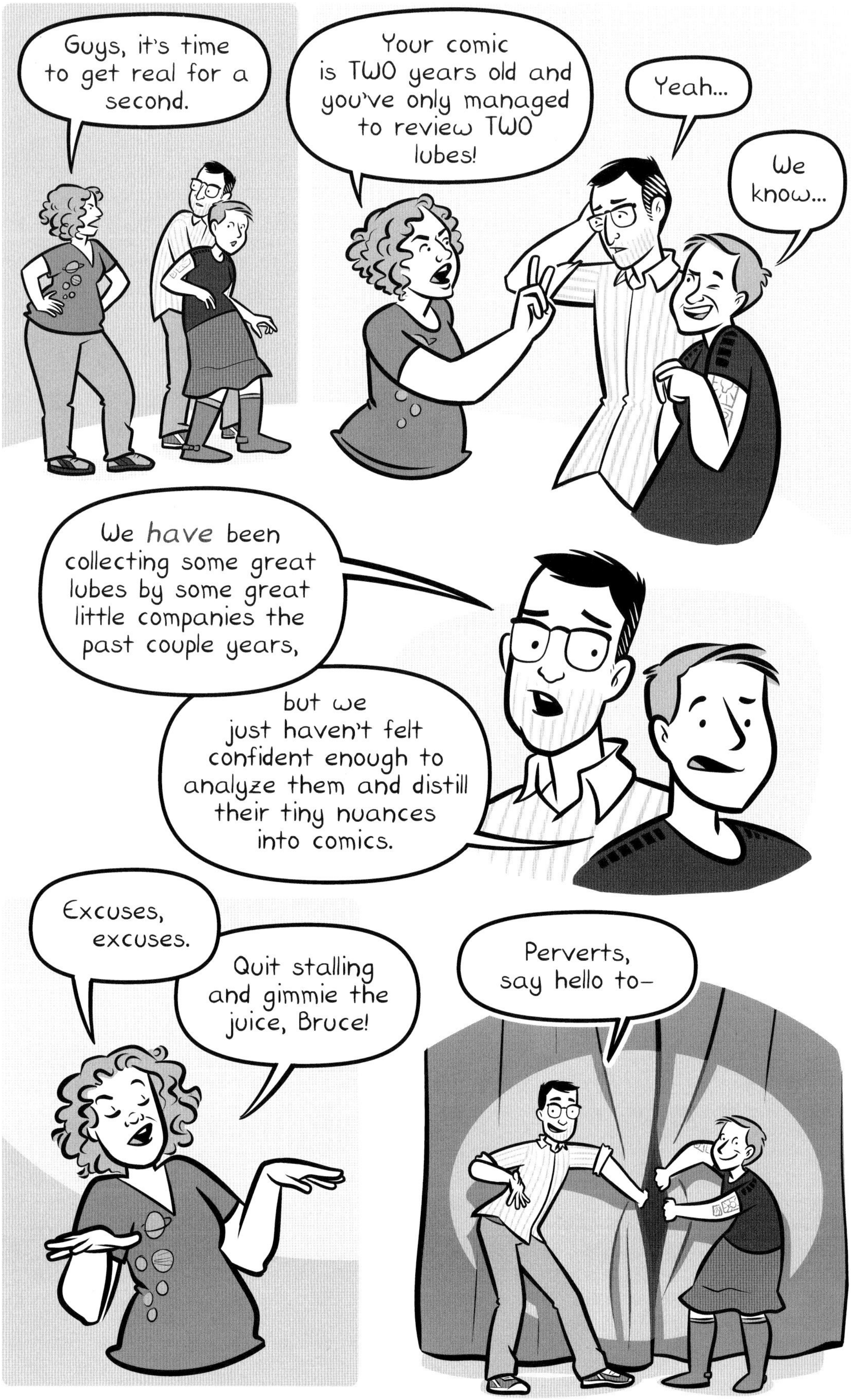
Guys, it's time to get real for a second.
Your comic is TWO years old and you've only managed to review TWO lubes!
Yeah...
We know...
We *have* been collecting some great lubes by some great little companies the past couple years,
but we just haven't felt confident enough to analyze them and distill their tiny nuances into comics.
Excuses, excuses.
Quit stalling and gimmie the juice, Bruce!
Perverts, say hello to—

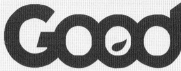

yes ®

water-based
intimate lubricant

And

Good
clean love
ALMOST NAKED
Personal Lubricant

Organic

Kinda
expensive,
$22ish for
75ml

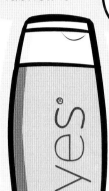

Thank you to the companies of the same names who sent them to us!

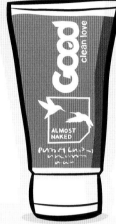

Vegan

Made
in Oregon
(nice!)

$16 for
118ml

Ingredients: water, Aloe vera, Guar Gum, Locust Bean Gum, Flax extract, Phenoxyethanol, Potassium Sorbate, Xanthan Gum, Citric acid.

Ingredients: water, Aloe Vera, Xanthan Gum, seaweed, Potassium Sorbate, Sodium Benzoate, Sodium Lactate, Benzyl Alcohol, Lactic Acid, Natural lemon and vanilla Flavors

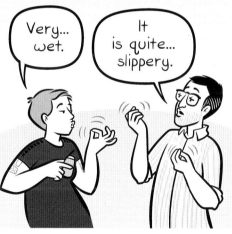

Very... wet.

It is quite... slippery.

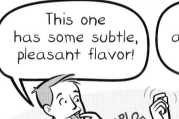
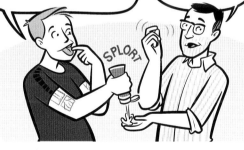

This one has some subtle, pleasant flavor!

It is also... quite slippery!

SPLORT

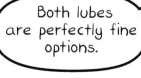
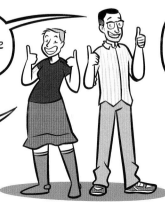

Both lubes are perfectly fine options.

We totally recommend them.

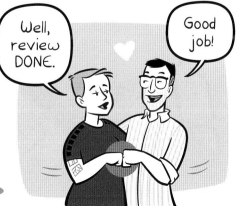

Well, review DONE.

Good job!

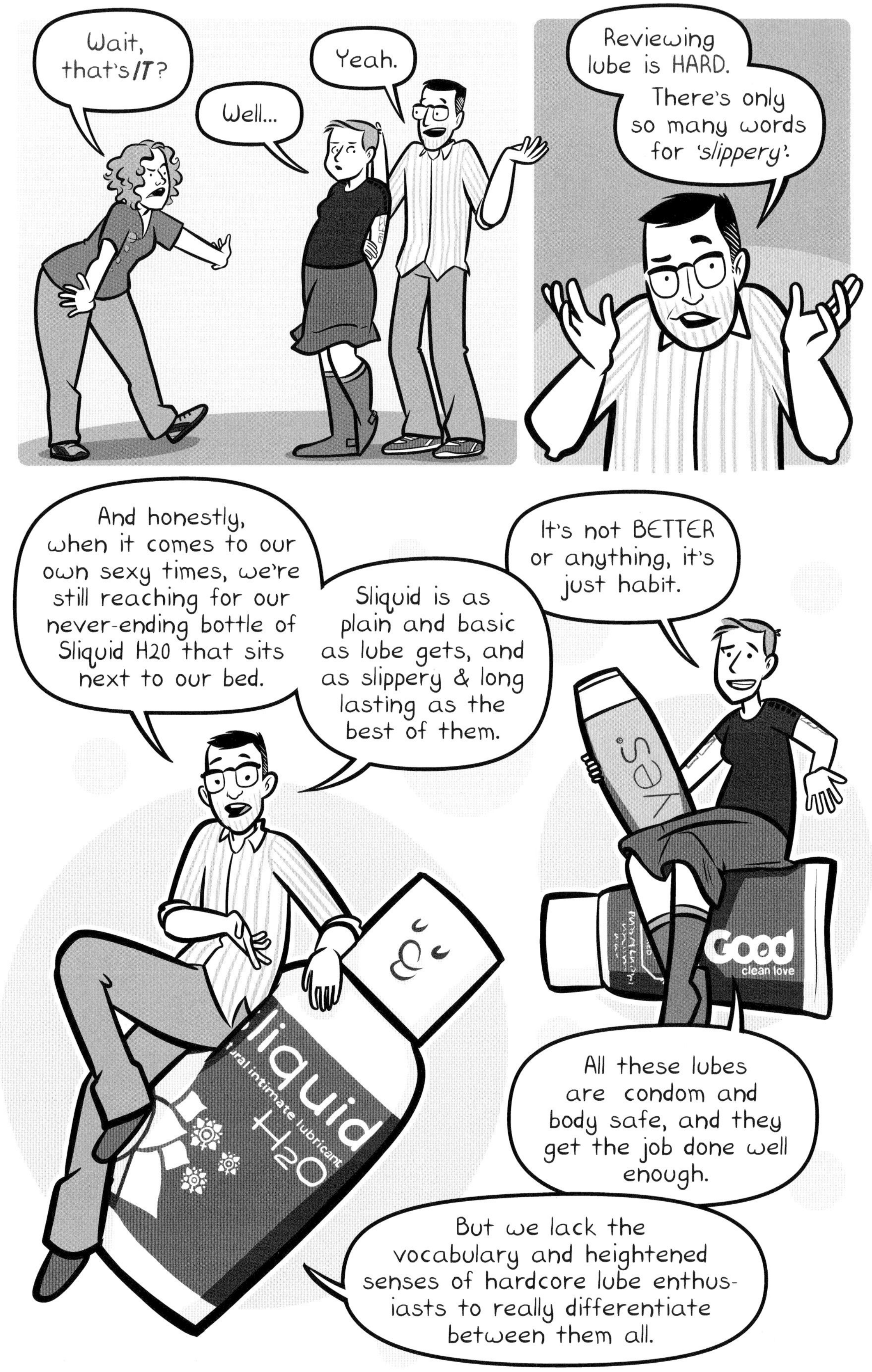
Wait, that's IT?
Well...
Yeah.
Reviewing lube is HARD.
There's only so many words for 'slippery'.
And honestly, when it comes to our own sexy times, we're still reaching for our never-ending bottle of Sliquid H2O that sits next to our bed.
Sliquid is as plain and basic as lube gets, and as slippery & long lasting as the best of them.
It's not BETTER or anything, it's just habit.
sex
Good
clean love
liquid
natural intimate lubricant
H2O
All these lubes are condom and body safe, and they get the job done well enough.
But we lack the vocabulary and heightened senses of hardcore lube enthusiasts to really differentiate between them all.

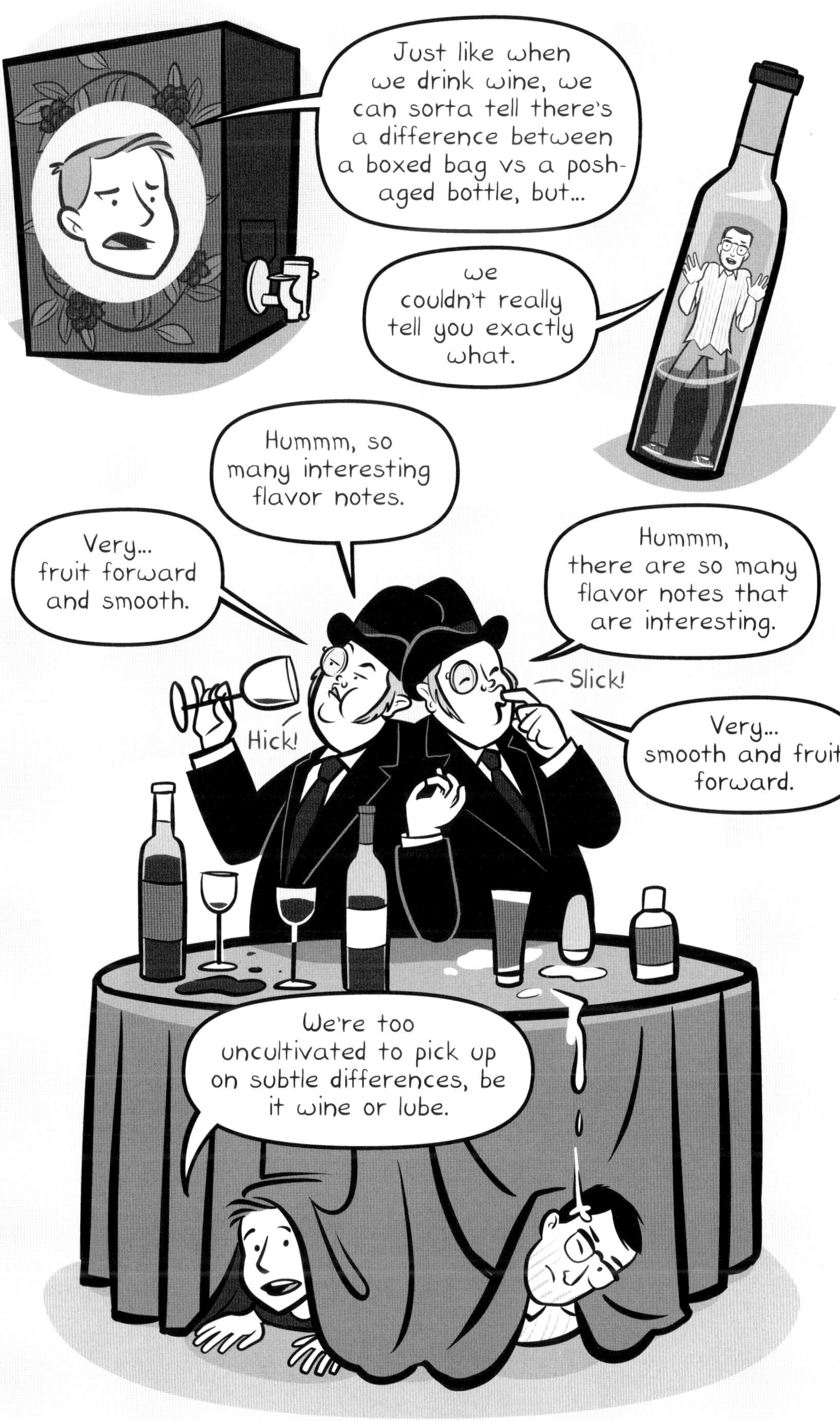

Just like when we drink wine, we can sorta tell there's a difference between a boxed bag vs a posh-aged bottle, but...
we couldn't really tell you exactly what.
Hummm, so many interesting flavor notes.
Very... fruit forward and smooth.
Hummm, there are so many flavor notes that are interesting.
Slick!
Hick!
Very... smooth and fruit forward.
We're too uncultivated to pick up on subtle differences, be it wine or lube.

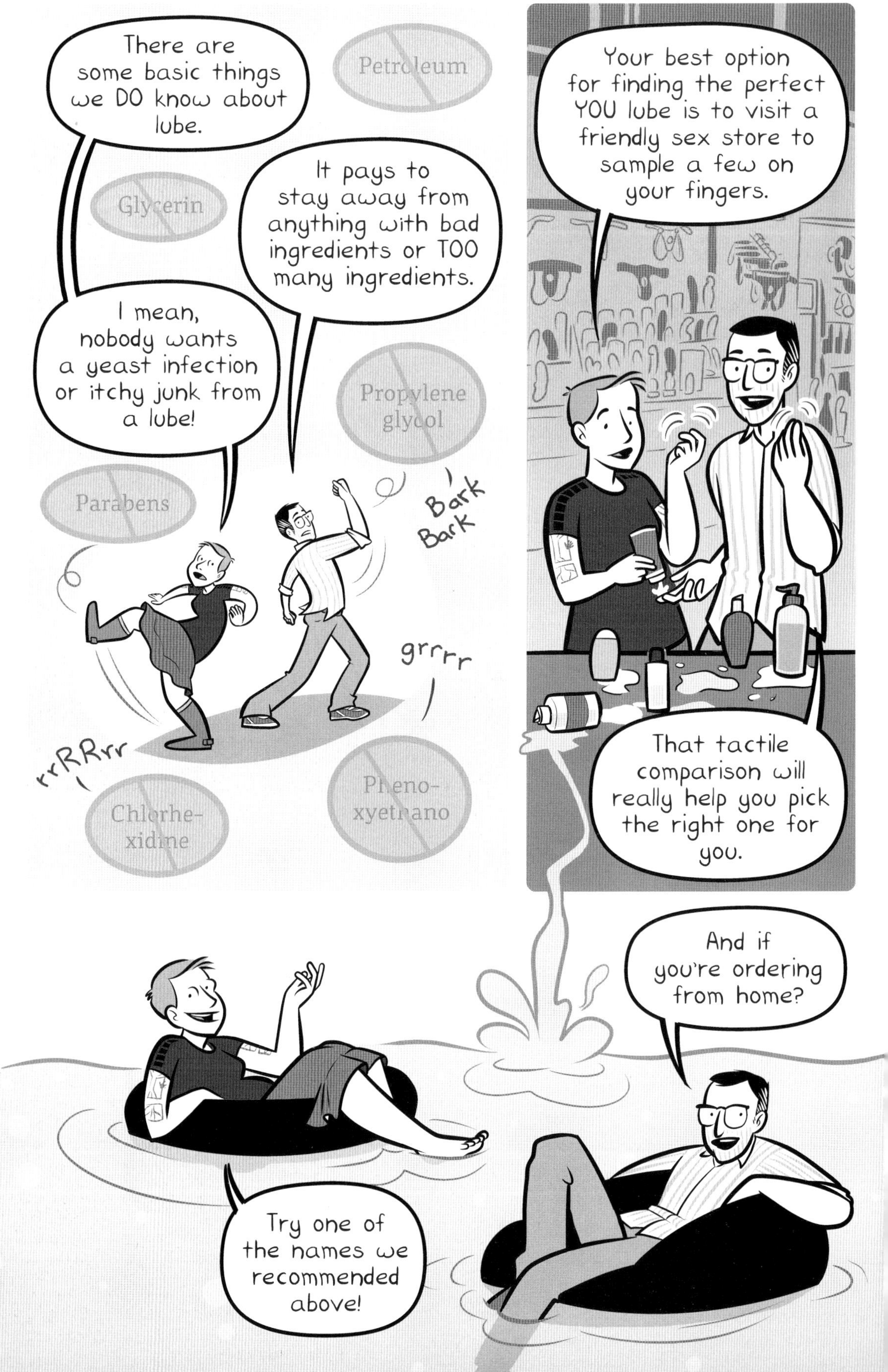
There are some basic things we DO know about lube.
Petroleum
Glycerin
It pays to stay away from anything with bad ingredients or TOO many ingredients.
I mean, nobody wants a yeast infection or itchy junk from a lube!
Propylene glycol
Parabens
Bark Bark
grrrr
rrRRrr
Chlorhexidine
Phenoxyetnano
Your best option for finding the perfect YOU lube is to visit a friendly sex store to sample a few on your fingers.
That tactile comparison will really help you pick the right one for you.
And if you're ordering from home?
Try one of the names we recommended above!

SEX
YOU 101

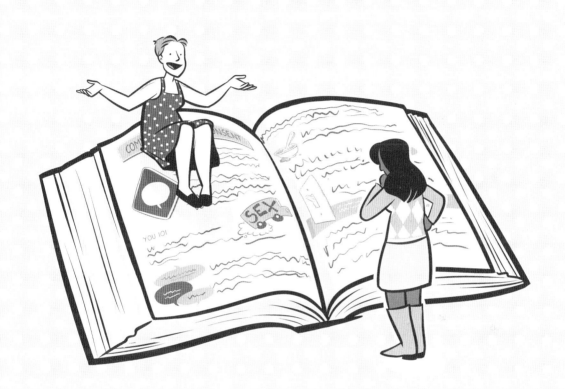

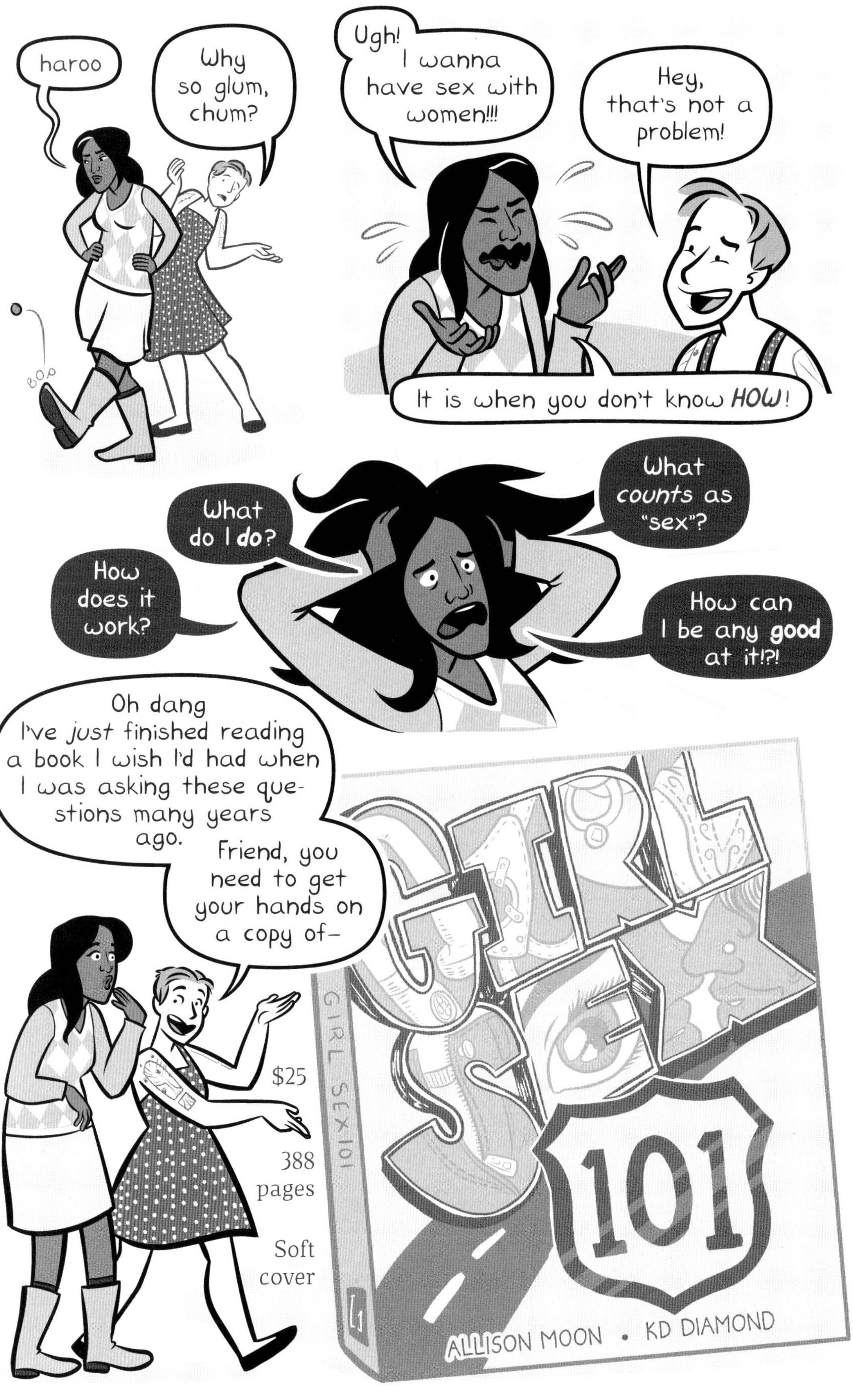
haroo
Why so glum, chum?
BOP
Ugh! I wanna have sex with women!!!
Hey, that's not a problem!
It is when you don't know **HOW**!
What do I **do**?
What *counts* as "sex"?
How does it work?
How can I be any **good** at it!?!
Oh dang I've *just* finished reading a book I wish I'd had when I was asking these questions many years ago.
Friend, you need to get your hands on a copy of–
$25
388 pages
Soft cover
GIRL SEX 101
GIRL SEX 101
ALLISON MOON • KD DIAMOND

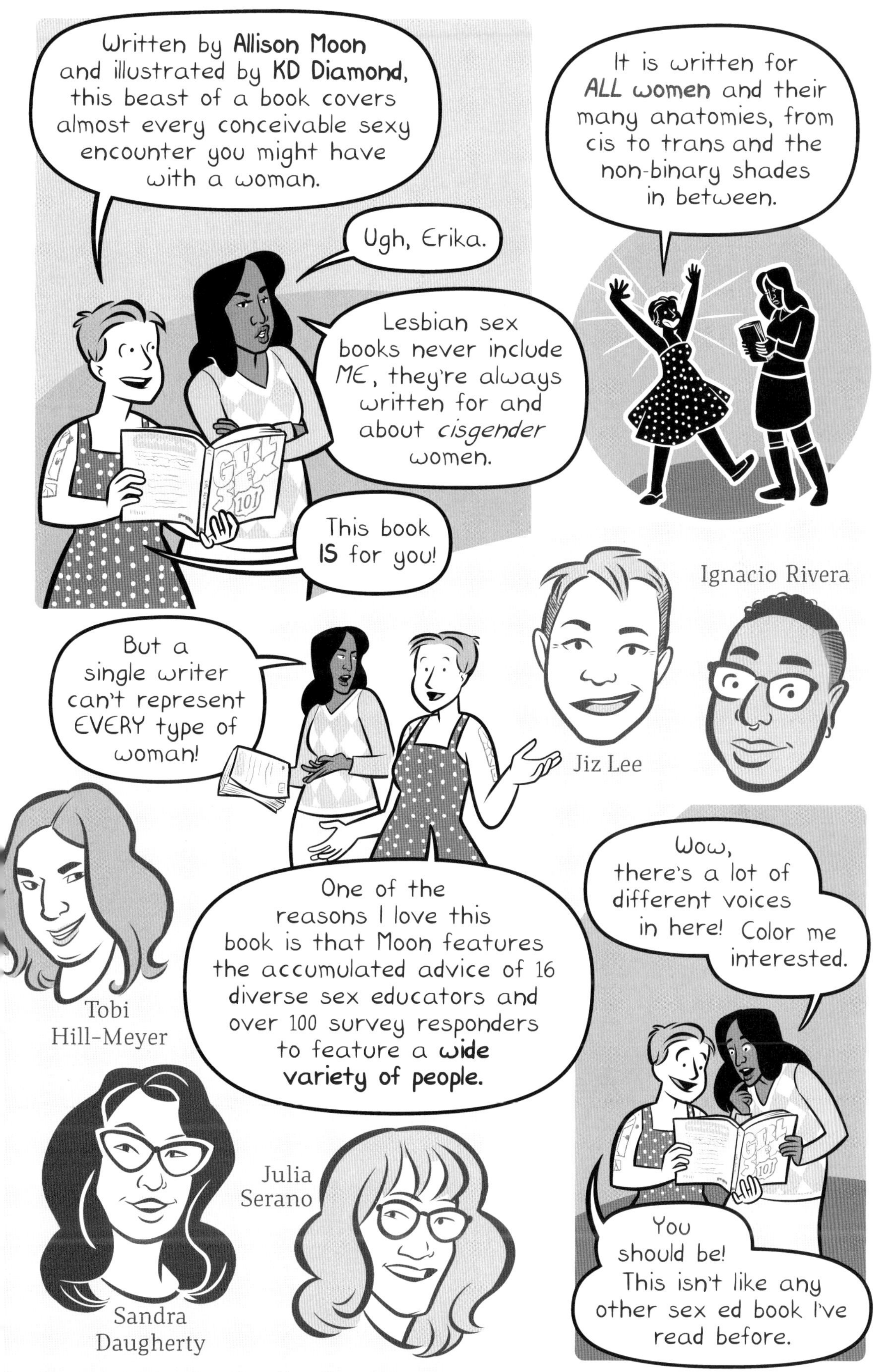
Written by **Allison Moon** and illustrated by **KD Diamond**, this beast of a book covers almost every conceivable sexy encounter you might have with a woman.
Ugh, Erika.
Lesbian sex books never include *ME*, they're always written for and about *cisgender* women.
This book **IS** for you!
It is written for ***ALL* women** and their many anatomies, from cis to trans and the non-binary shades in between.
GIRL SEX 101
Ignacio Rivera
Jiz Lee
But a single writer can't represent EVERY type of woman!
Tobi Hill-Meyer
One of the reasons I love this book is that Moon features the accumulated advice of 16 diverse sex educators and over 100 survey responders to feature a **wide variety of people.**
Wow, there's a lot of different voices in here! Color me interested.
Sandra Daugherty
Julia Serano
You should be! This isn't like any other sex ed book I've read before.

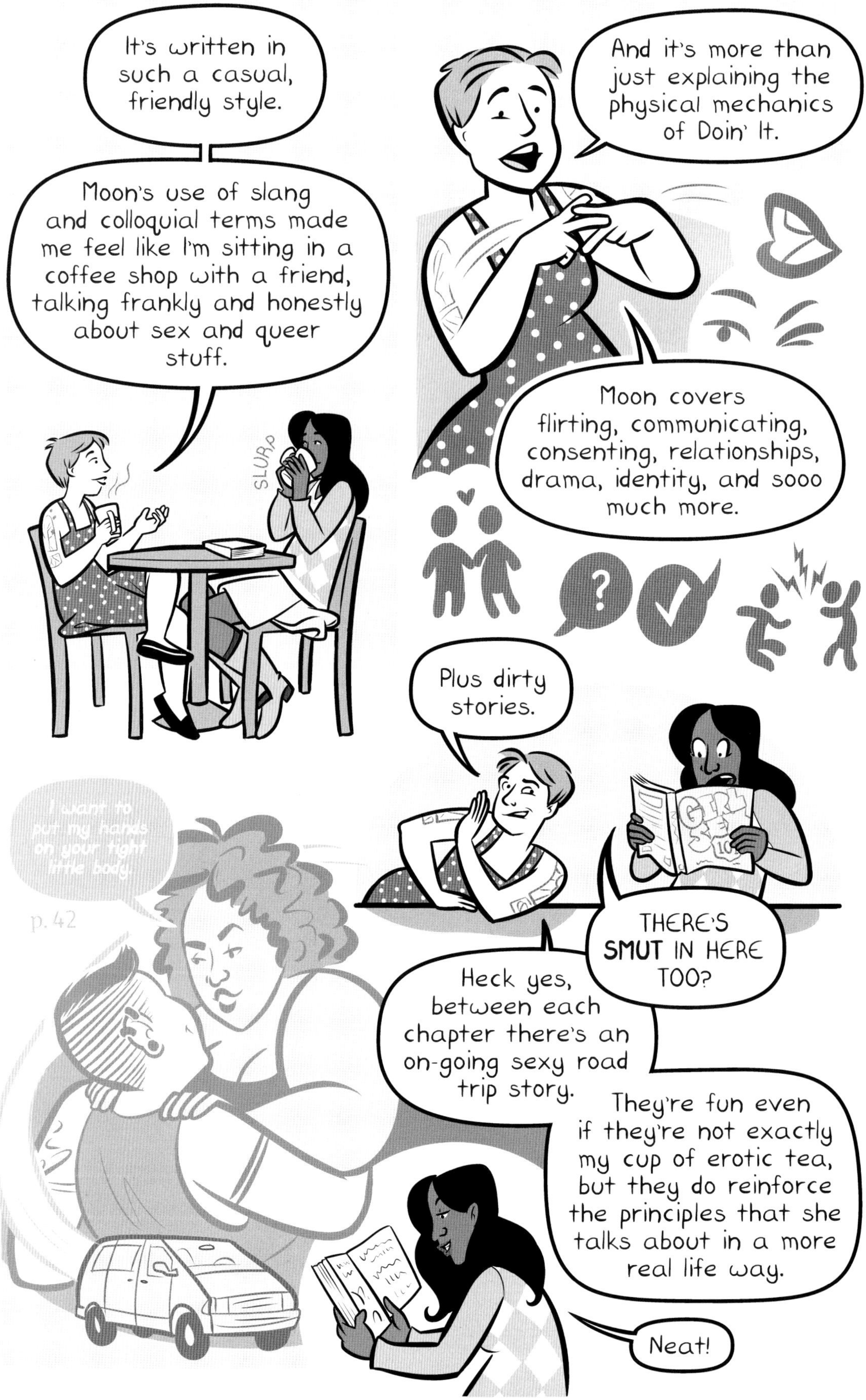
It's written in such a casual, friendly style.
Moon's use of slang and colloquial terms made me feel like I'm sitting in a coffee shop with a friend, talking frankly and honestly about sex and queer stuff.
SLURP
And it's more than just explaining the physical mechanics of Doin' It.
Moon covers flirting, communicating, consenting, relationships, drama, identity, and sooo much more.
?
Plus dirty stories.
I want to put my hands on your tight little body.
p. 42
THERE'S **SMUT** IN HERE TOO?
Heck yes, between each chapter there's an on-going sexy road trip story.
They're fun even if they're not exactly my cup of erotic tea, but they do reinforce the principles that she talks about in a more real life way.
Neat!

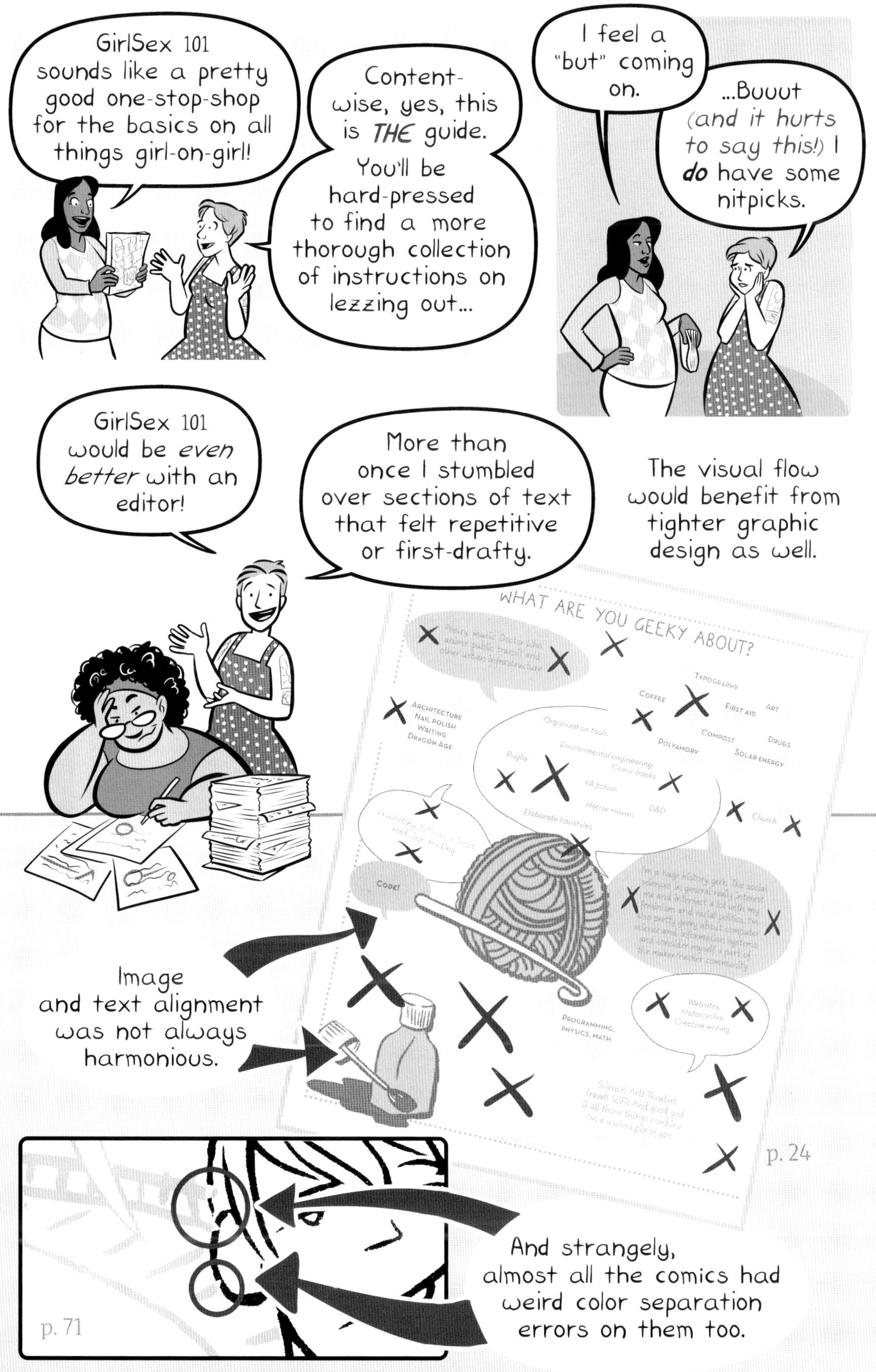

GirlSex 101 sounds like a pretty good one-stop-shop for the basics on all things girl-on-girl!
Content-wise, yes, this is *THE* guide.
You'll be hard-pressed to find a more thorough collection of instructions on lezzing out...
I feel a "but" coming on.
...Buuut (and it hurts to say this!) I **do** have some nitpicks.
GirlSex 101 would be *even better* with an editor!
More than once I stumbled over sections of text that felt repetitive or first-drafty.
The visual flow would benefit from tighter graphic design as well.
WHAT ARE YOU GEEKY ABOUT?
Image and text alignment was not always harmonious.
p. 24
And strangely, almost all the comics had weird color separation errors on them too.
p. 71

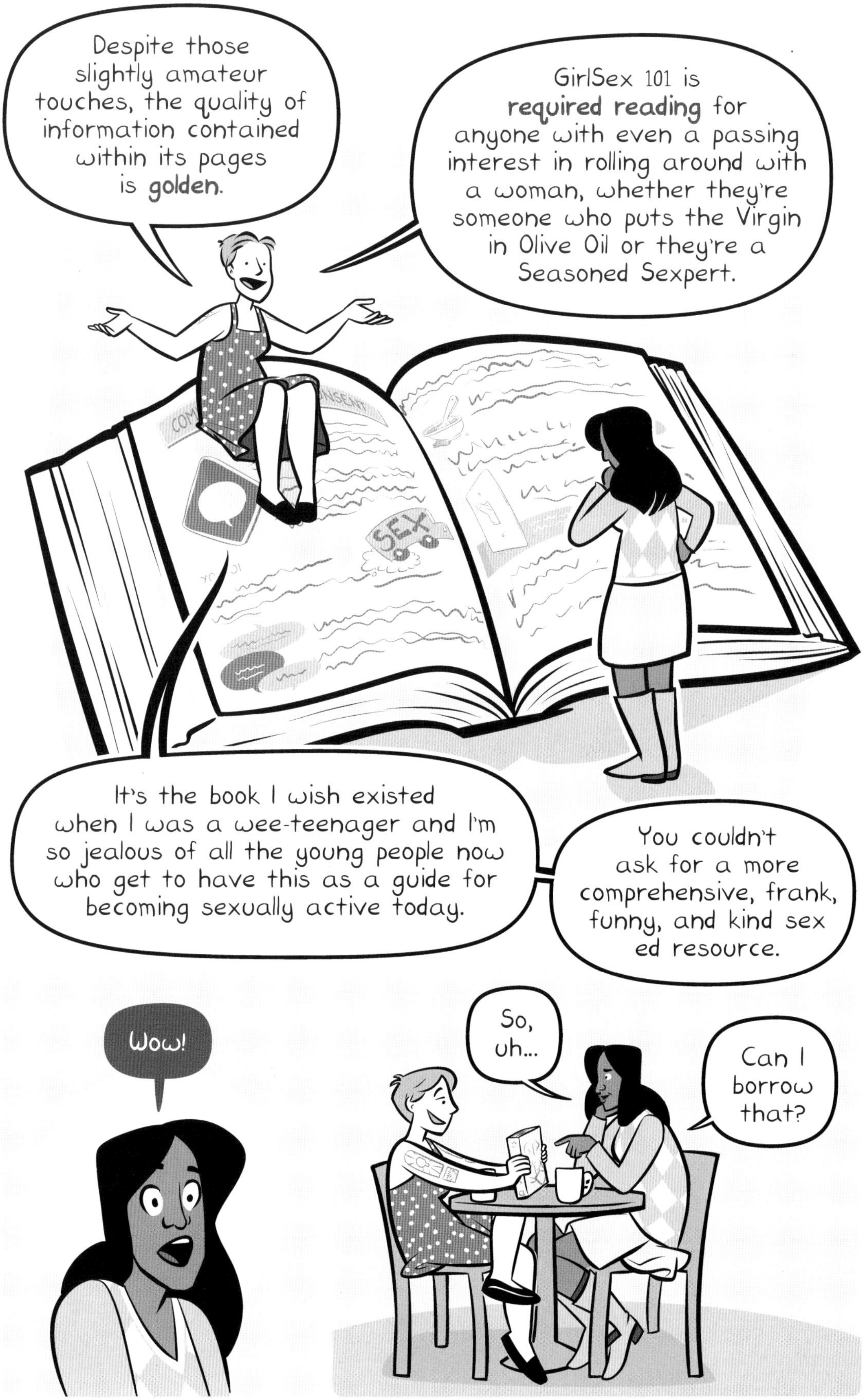

Despite those slightly amateur touches, the quality of information contained within its pages is **golden**.
GirlSex 101 is **required reading** for anyone with even a passing interest in rolling around with a woman, whether they're someone who puts the Virgin in Olive Oil or they're a Seasoned Sexpert.
SEX
It's the book I wish existed when I was a wee-teenager and I'm so jealous of all the young people now who get to have this as a guide for becoming sexually active today.
You couldn't ask for a more comprehensive, frank, funny, and kind sex ed resource.
Wow!
So, uh...
Can I borrow that?

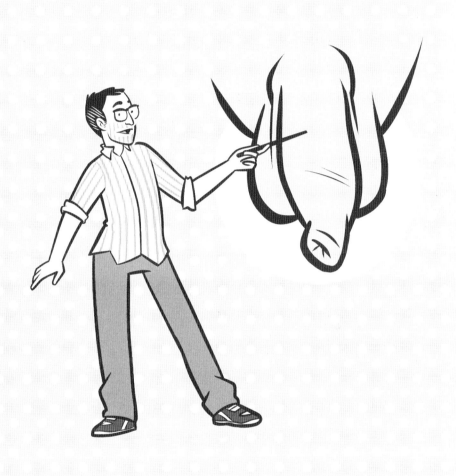

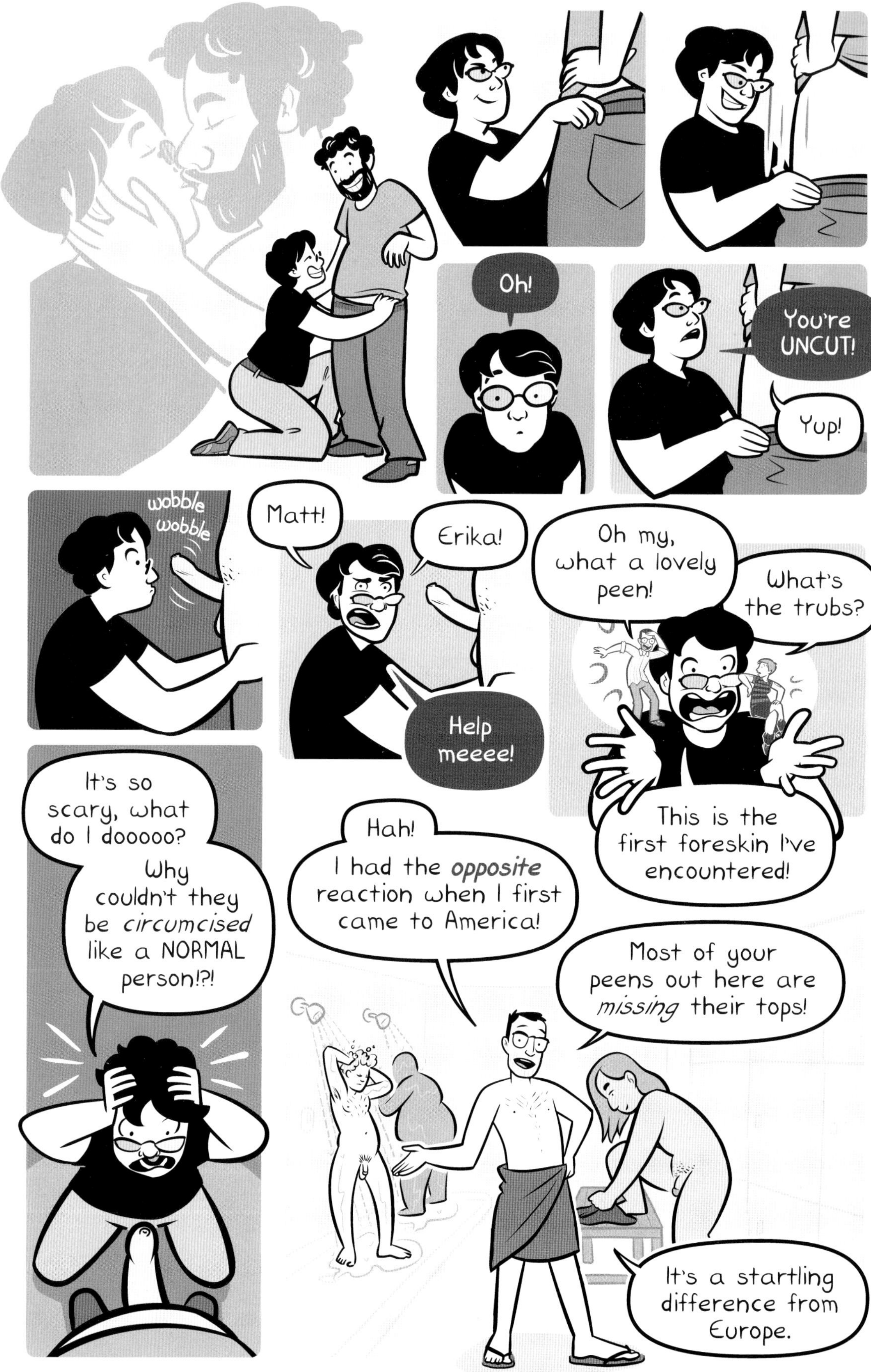
Oh!
You're UNCUT!
Yup!
wobble wobble
Matt!
Erika!
Help meeee!
Oh my, what a lovely peen!
What's the trubs?
This is the first foreskin I've encountered!
It's so scary, what do I dooooo?
Why couldn't they be *circumcised* like a NORMAL person!?!
Hah!
I had the ***opposite*** reaction when I first came to America!
Most of your peens out here are *missing* their tops!
It's a startling difference from Europe.

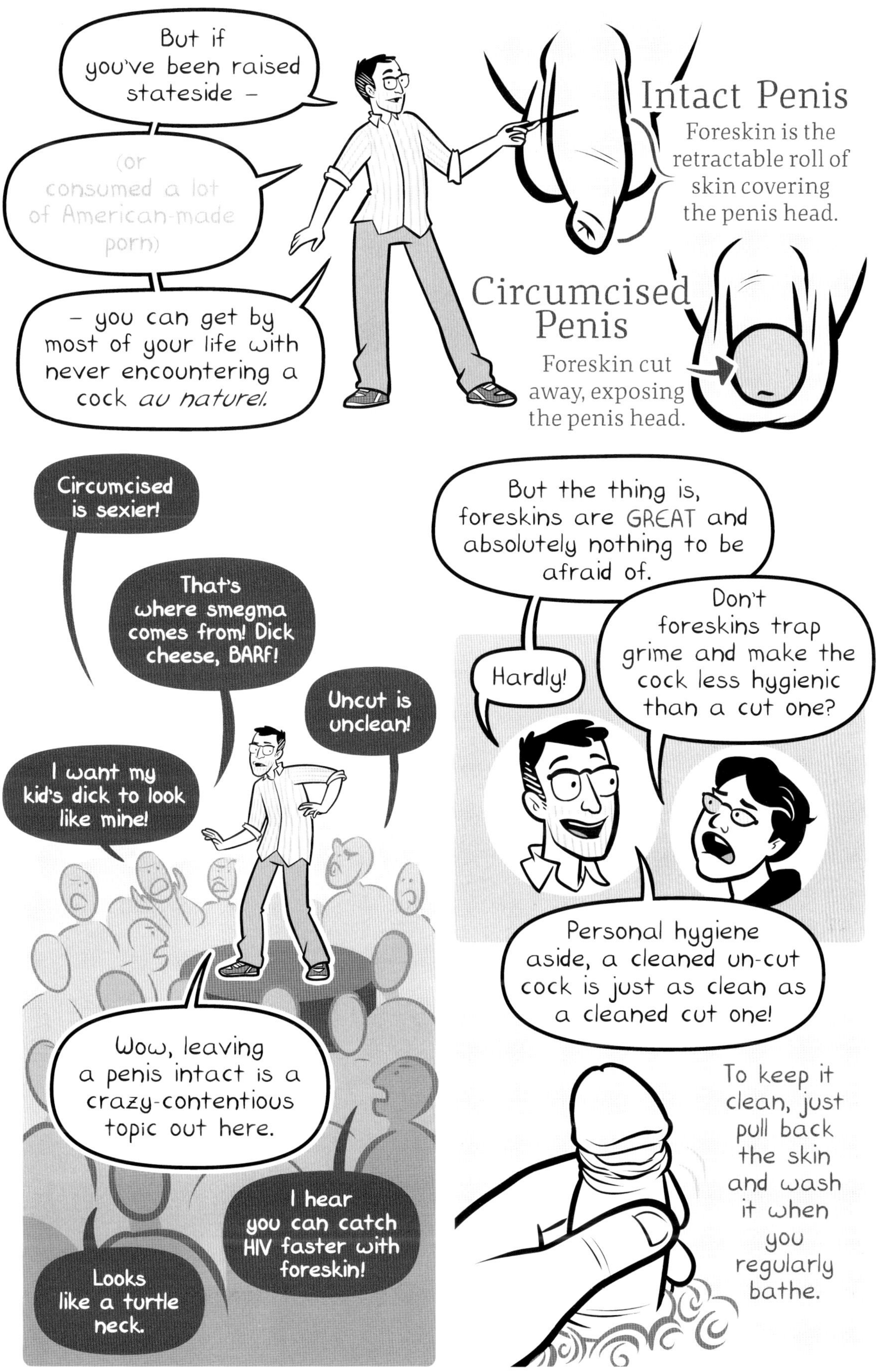

But if you've been raised stateside –
(or consumed a lot of American-made porn)
– you can get by most of your life with never encountering a cock *au naturel.*
Intact Penis
Foreskin is the retractable roll of skin covering the penis head.
Circumcised Penis
Foreskin cut away, exposing the penis head.
Circumcised is sexier!
That's where smegma comes from! Dick cheese, BARF!
Uncut is unclean!
I want my kid's dick to look like mine!
Wow, leaving a penis intact is a crazy-contentious topic out here.
I hear you can catch HIV faster with foreskin!
Looks like a turtle neck.
But the thing is, foreskins are GREAT and absolutely nothing to be afraid of.
Hardly!
Don't foreskins trap grime and make the cock less hygienic than a cut one?
Personal hygiene aside, a cleaned un-cut cock is just as clean as a cleaned cut one!
To keep it clean, just pull back the skin and wash it when you regularly bathe.

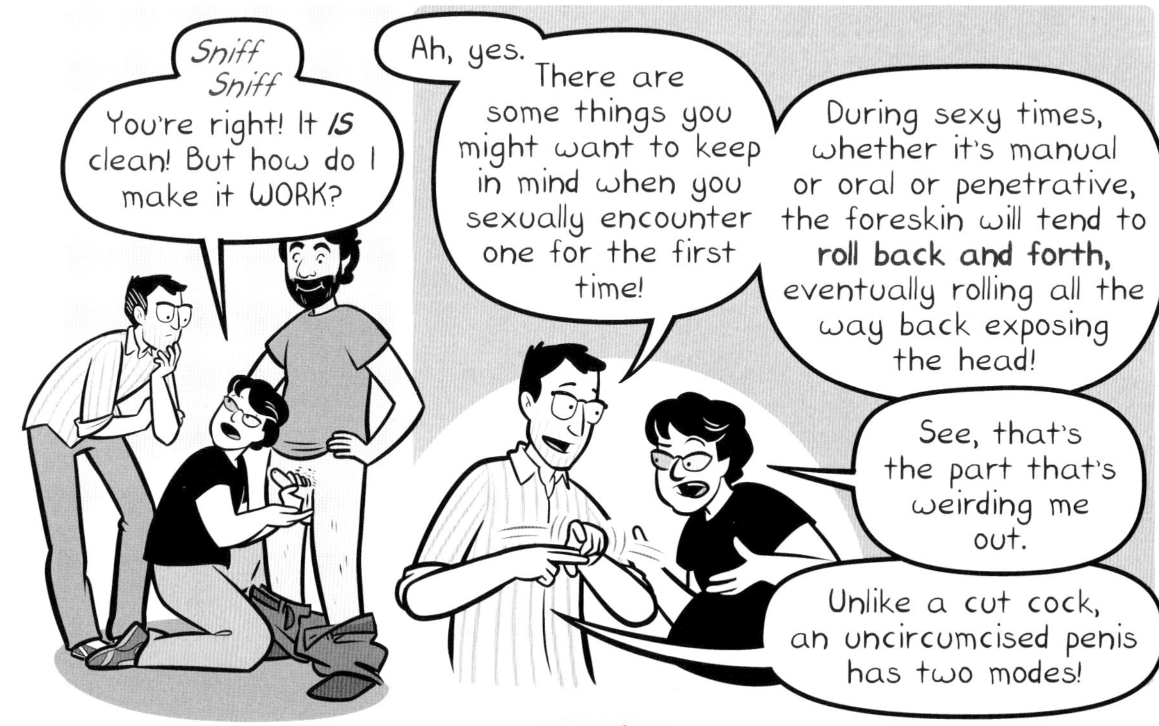
Sniff Sniff
You're right! It IS clean! But how do I make it WORK?
Ah, yes.
There are some things you might want to keep in mind when you sexually encounter one for the first time!
During sexy times, whether it's manual or oral or penetrative, the foreskin will tend to **roll back and forth,** eventually rolling all the way back exposing the head!
See, that's the part that's weirding me out.
Unlike a cut cock, an uncircumcised penis has two modes!

Rolled Up!

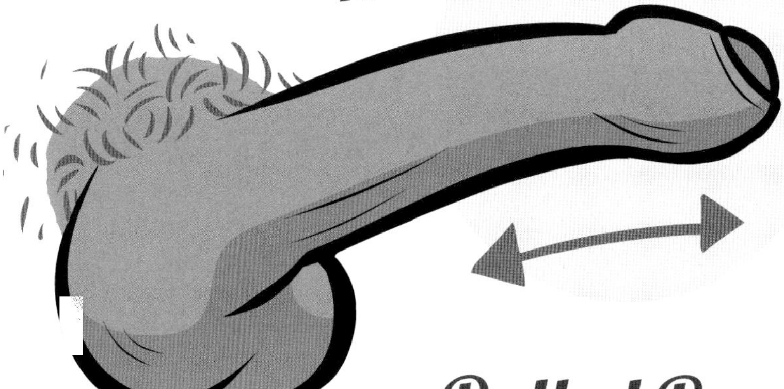

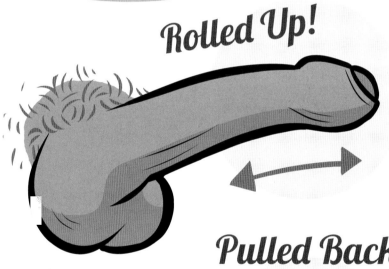

The foreskin will help protect the sensitive head and give it a different, more subdued sensation during sexy times.

That added skin surface area gives you more to play with during handjobs!

Pulled Back!*

*Don't fret if yours can't do this yet, some people's needs stretching that comes with age and some don't ever fully roll back.

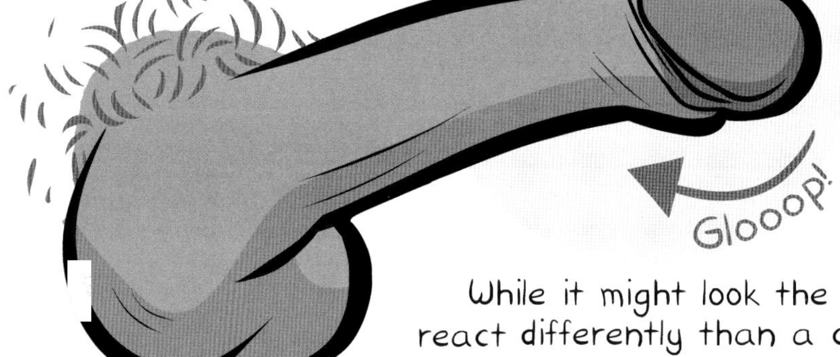
Glooop!

In this state an uncircumcised cock will resemble a circumcised one, but with an added roll of skin behind the head.

While it might look the same, it will probably react differently than a cut one: that head is a lot more sensitive!

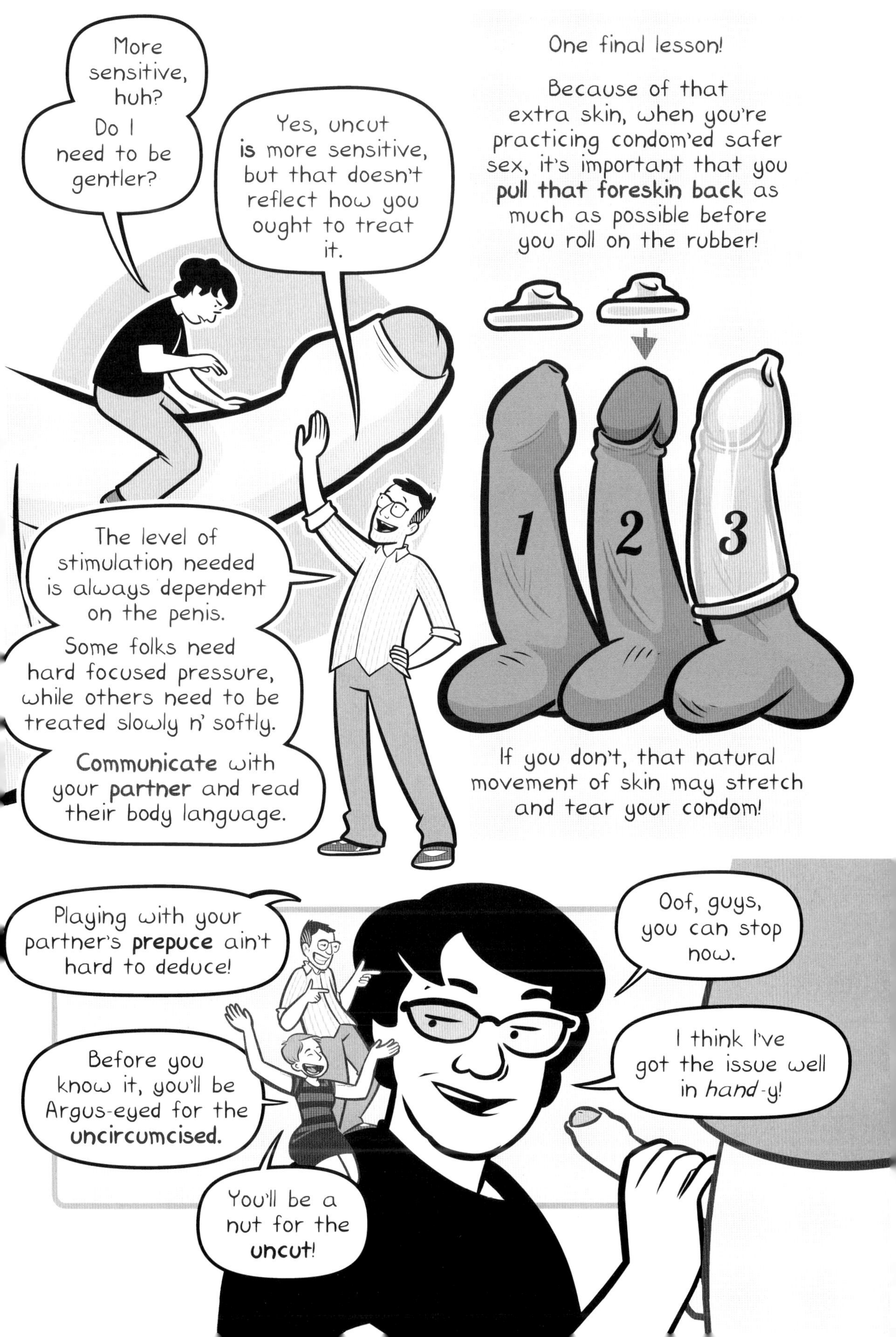
More sensitive, huh?
Do I need to be gentler?
Yes, uncut **is** more sensitive, but that doesn't reflect how you ought to treat it.
The level of stimulation needed is always dependent on the penis.
Some folks need hard focused pressure, while others need to be treated slowly n' softly.
Communicate with your **partner** and read their body language.
One final lesson!
Because of that extra skin, when you're practicing condom'ed safer sex, it's important that you **pull that foreskin back** as much as possible before you roll on the rubber!
1
2
3
If you **don't**, that natural movement of skin may stretch and tear your condom!
Playing with your partner's **prepuce** ain't hard to deduce!
Before you know it, you'll be Argus-eyed for the **uncircumcised.**
You'll be a nut for the **uncut**!
Oof, guys, you can stop now.
I think I've got the issue well in *hand*-y!

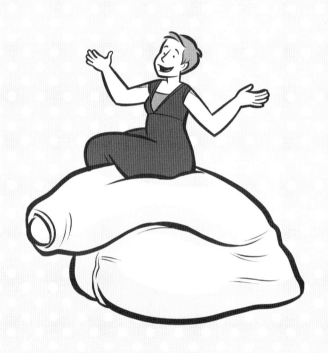

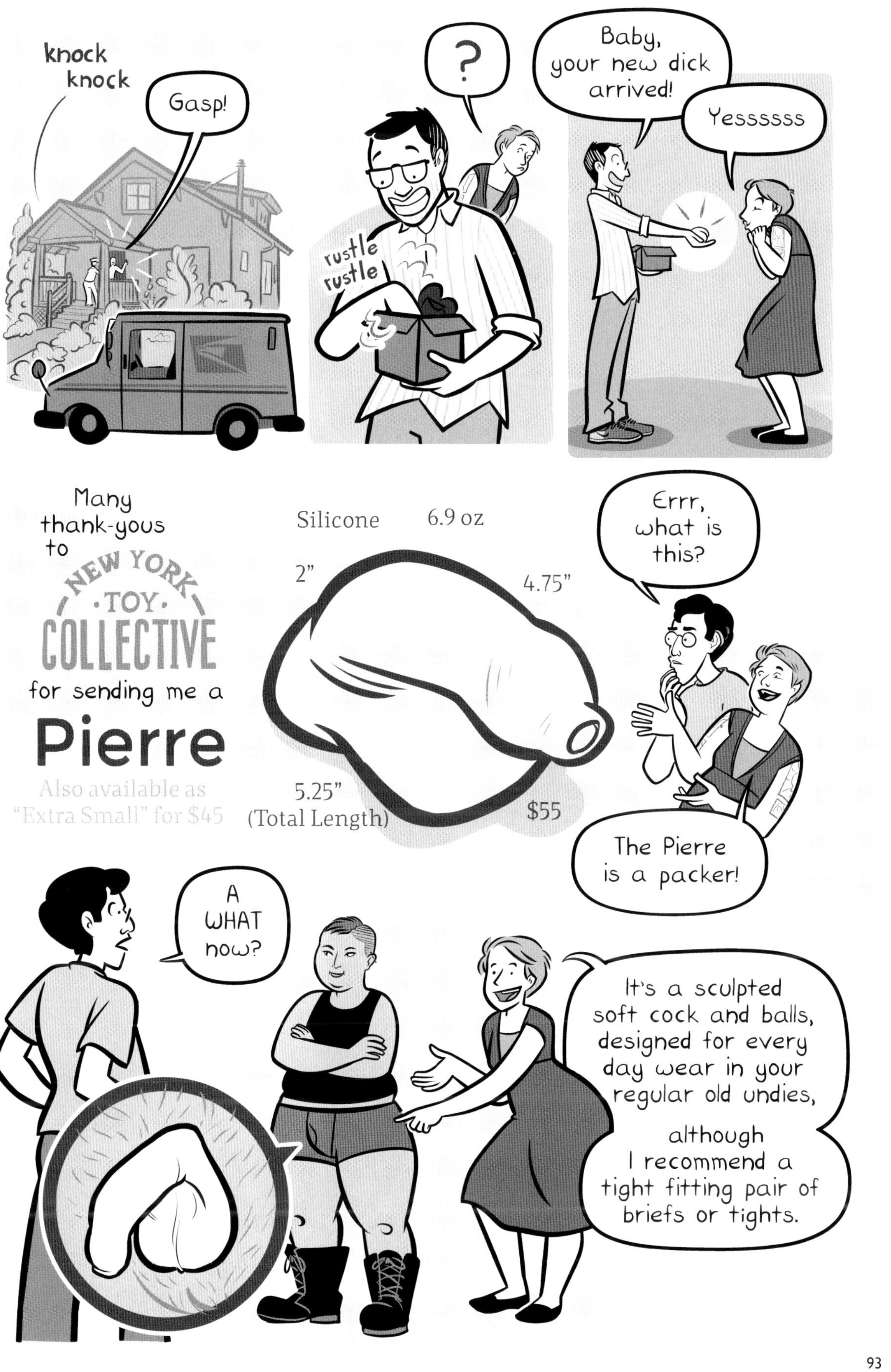
knock knock
Gasp!
?
rustle rustle
Baby, your new dick arrived!
Yessssss
Many thank-yous to
NEW YORK TOY COLLECTIVE
for sending me a
Pierre
Also available as "Extra Small" for $45
Silicone
6.9 oz
2"
4.75"
5.25" (Total Length)
$55
Errr, what is this?
The Pierre is a packer!
A WHAT now?
It's a sculpted soft cock and balls, designed for every day wear in your regular old undies,
although I recommend a tight fitting pair of briefs or tights.

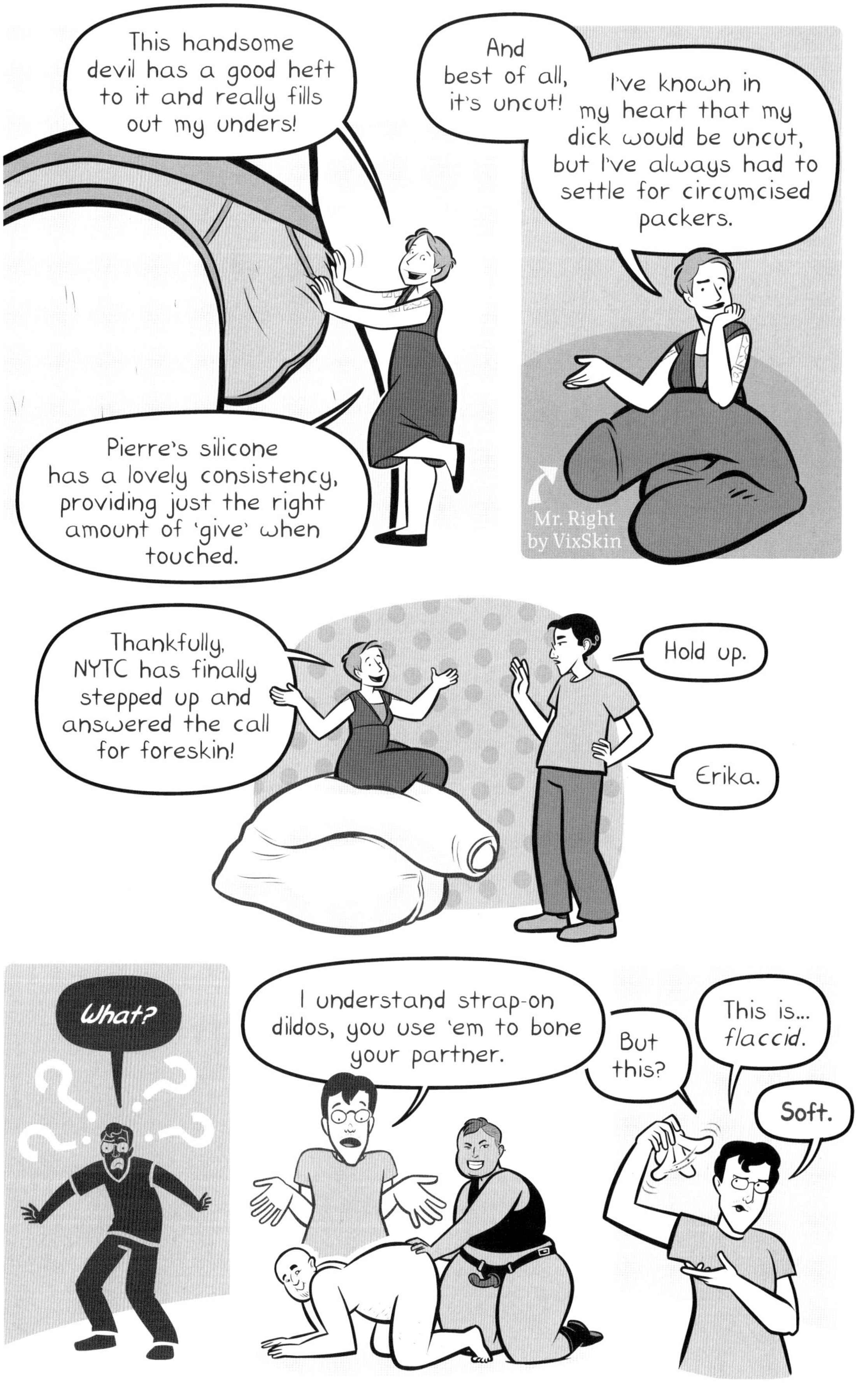
This handsome devil has a good heft to it and really fills out my unders!
Pierre's silicone has a lovely consistency, providing just the right amount of 'give' when touched.
And best of all, it's uncut!
I've known in my heart that my dick would be uncut, but I've always had to settle for circumcised packers.
Mr. Right by VixSkin
Thankfully, NYTC has finally stepped up and answered the call for foreskin!
Hold up.
Erika.
What?
I understand strap-on dildos, you use 'em to bone your partner.
But this?
This is... *flaccid*.
Soft.

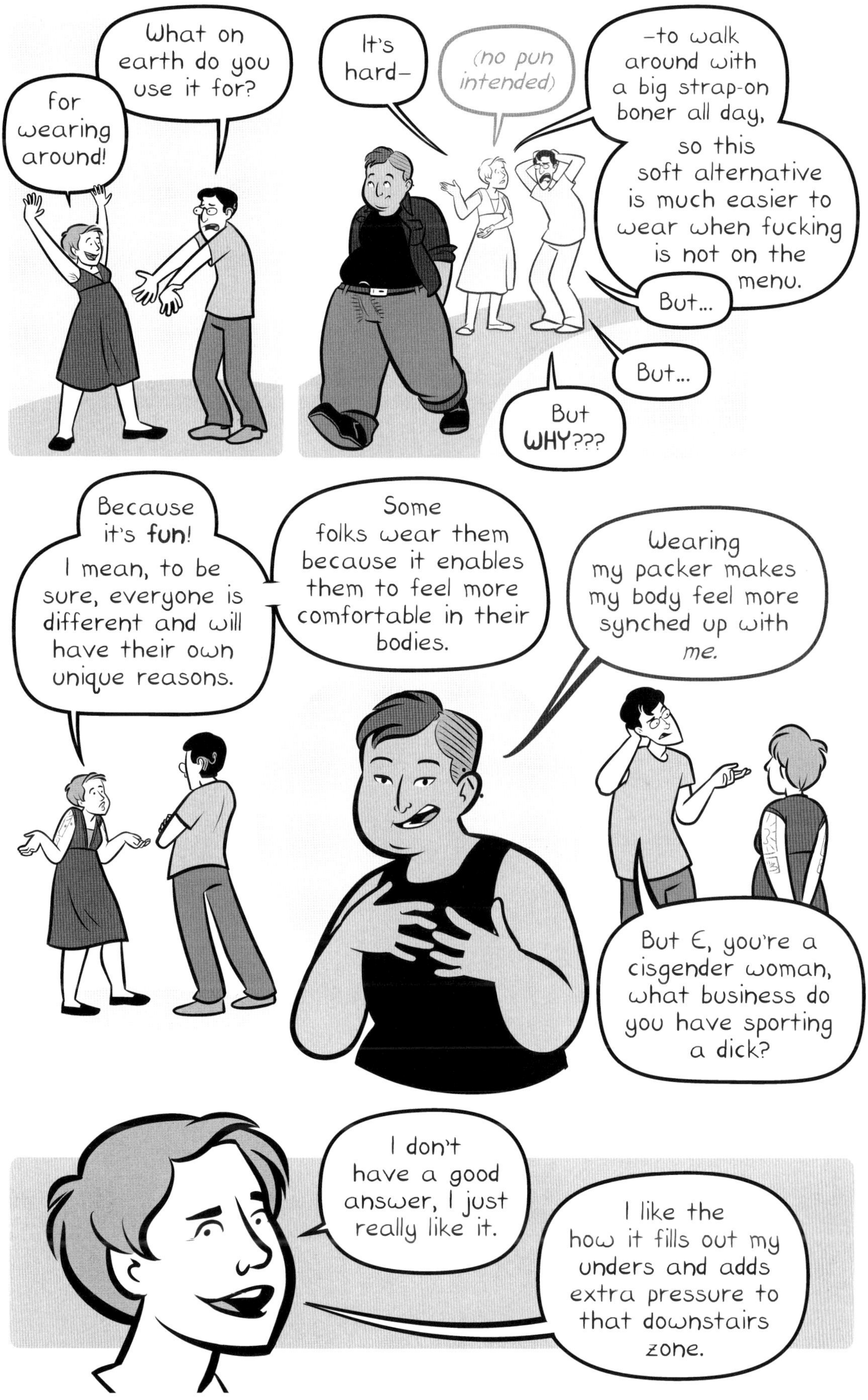
What on earth do you use it for?
for wearing around!
It's hard–
(no pun intended)
–to walk around with a big strap-on boner all day,
so this soft alternative is much easier to wear when fucking is not on the menu.
But...
But...
But WHY???
Because it's fun!
I mean, to be sure, everyone is different and will have their own unique reasons.
Some folks wear them because it enables them to feel more comfortable in their bodies.
Wearing my packer makes my body feel more synched up with me.
But E, you're a cisgender woman, what business do you have sporting a dick?
I don't have a good answer, I just really like it.
I like the how it fills out my unders and adds extra pressure to that downstairs zone.

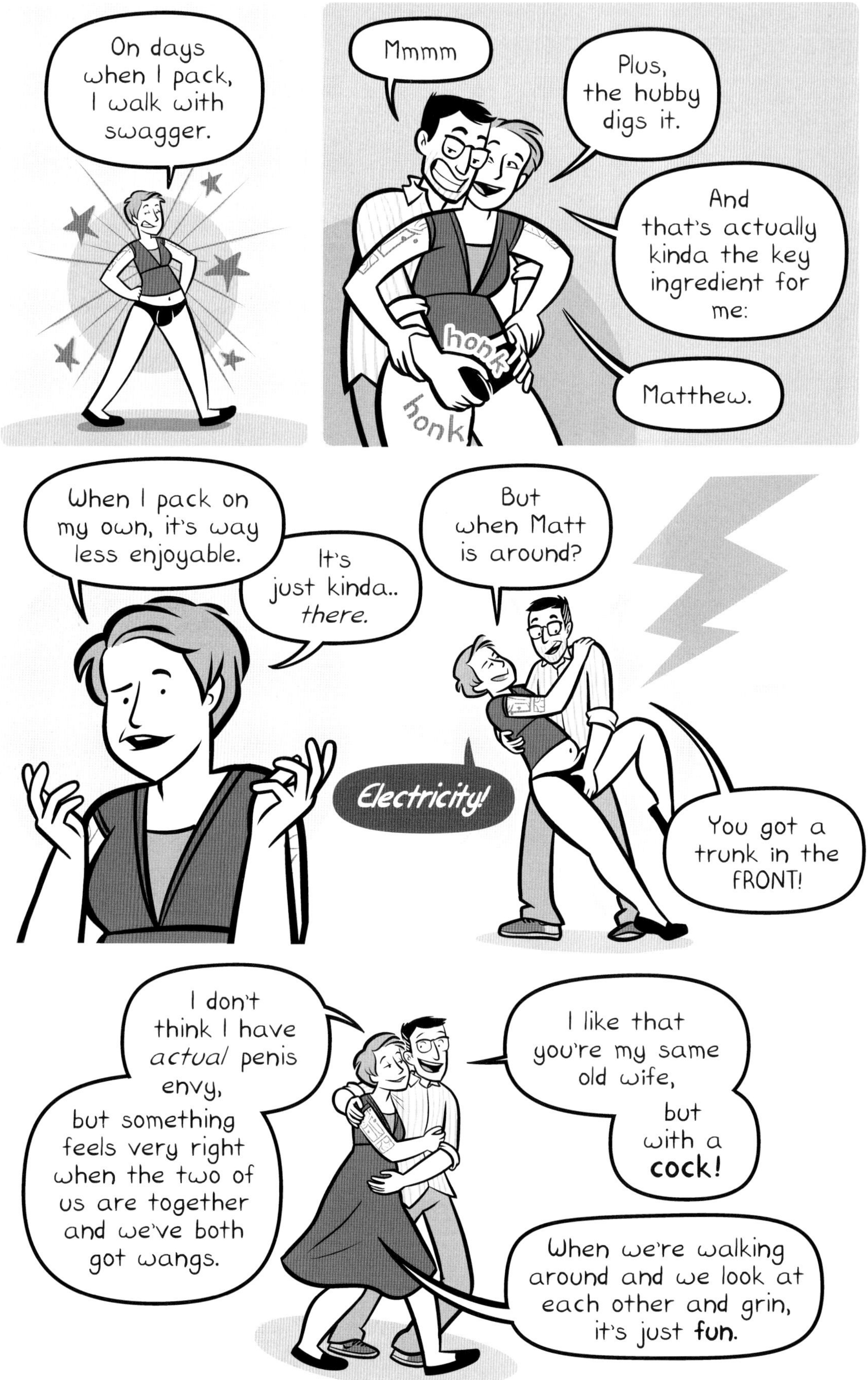
On days when I pack, I walk with swagger.
Mmmm
Plus, the hubby digs it.
And that's actually kinda the key ingredient for me:
Matthew.
honk
honk
When I pack on my own, it's way less enjoyable.
It's just kinda.. *there.*
But when Matt is around?
Electricity!
You got a trunk in the FRONT!
I don't think I have *actual* penis envy,
but something feels very right when the two of us are together and we've both got wangs.
I like that you're my same old wife,
but with a **cock!**
When we're walking around and we look at each other and grin, it's just **fun.**

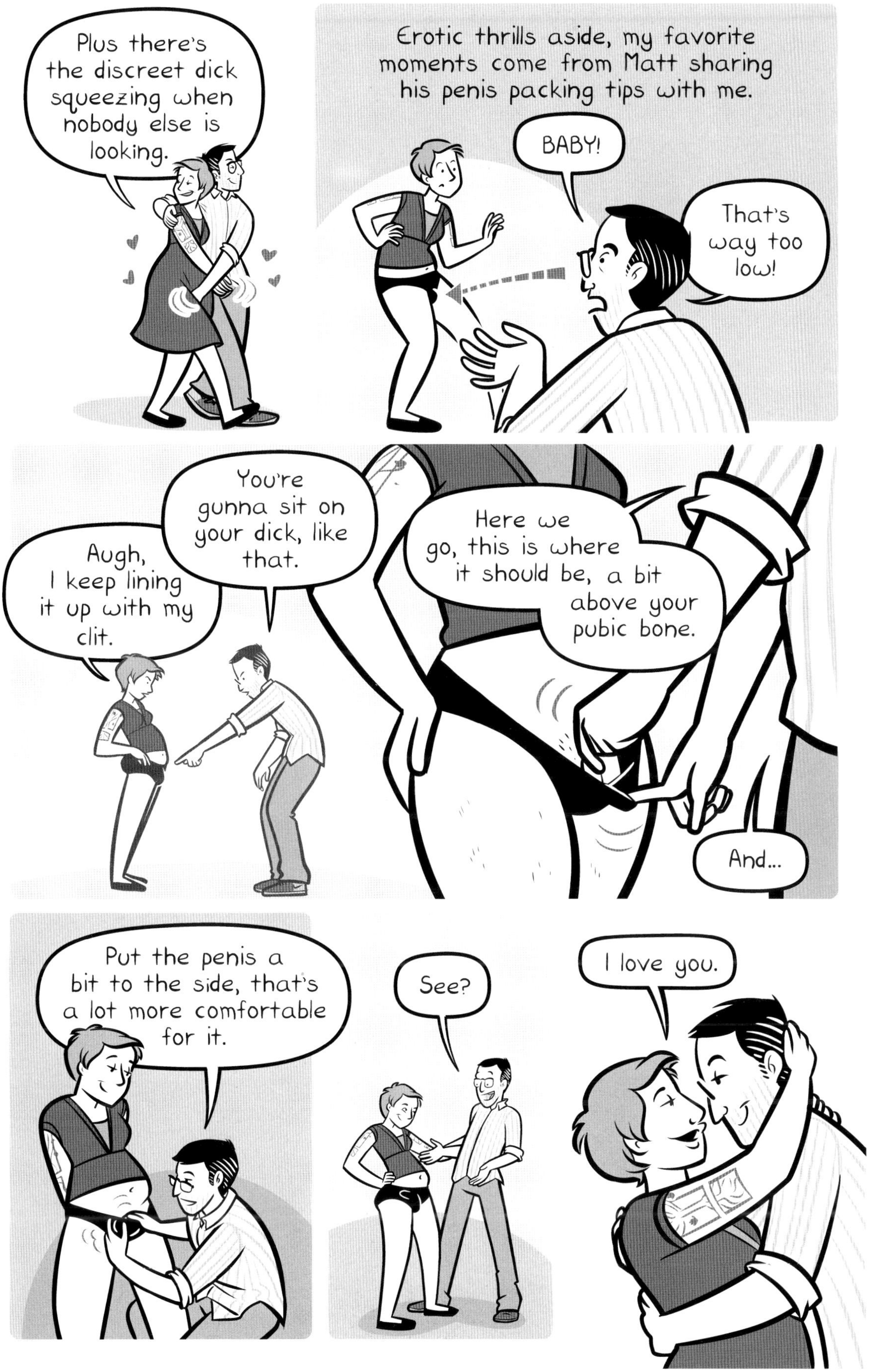

Plus there's the discreet dick squeezing when nobody else is looking.
Erotic thrills aside, my favorite moments come from Matt sharing his penis packing tips with me.
BABY!
That's way too low!
Augh, I keep lining it up with my clit.
You're gunna sit on your dick, like that.
Here we go, this is where it should be, a bit above your pubic bone.
And...
Put the penis a bit to the side, that's a lot more comfortable for it.
See?
I love you.

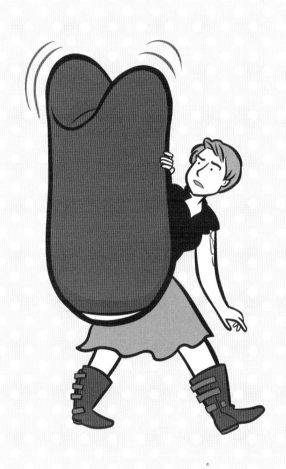

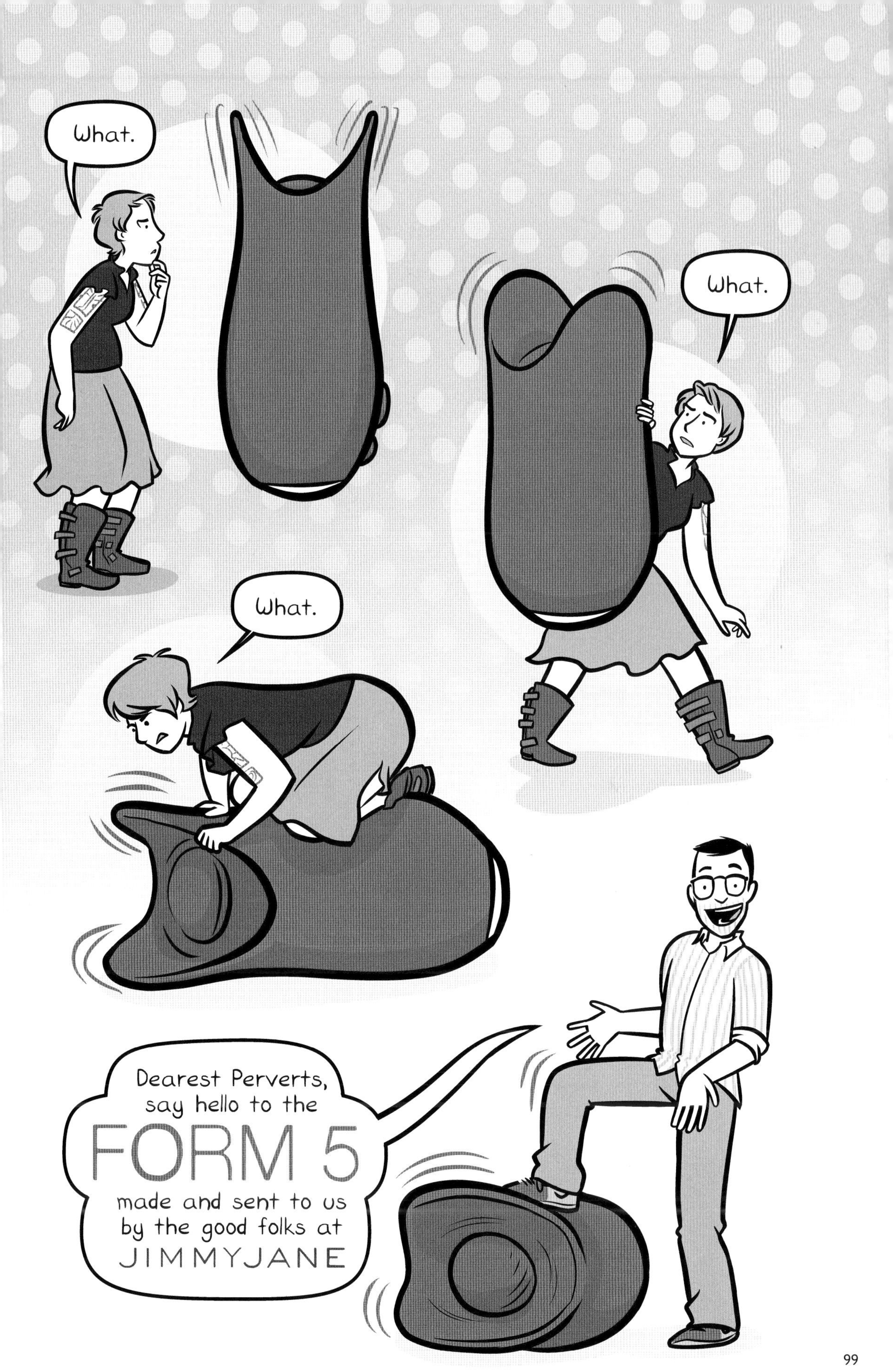
What.
What.
What.
Dearest Perverts, say hello to the FORM 5 made and sent to us by the good folks at JIMMYJANE

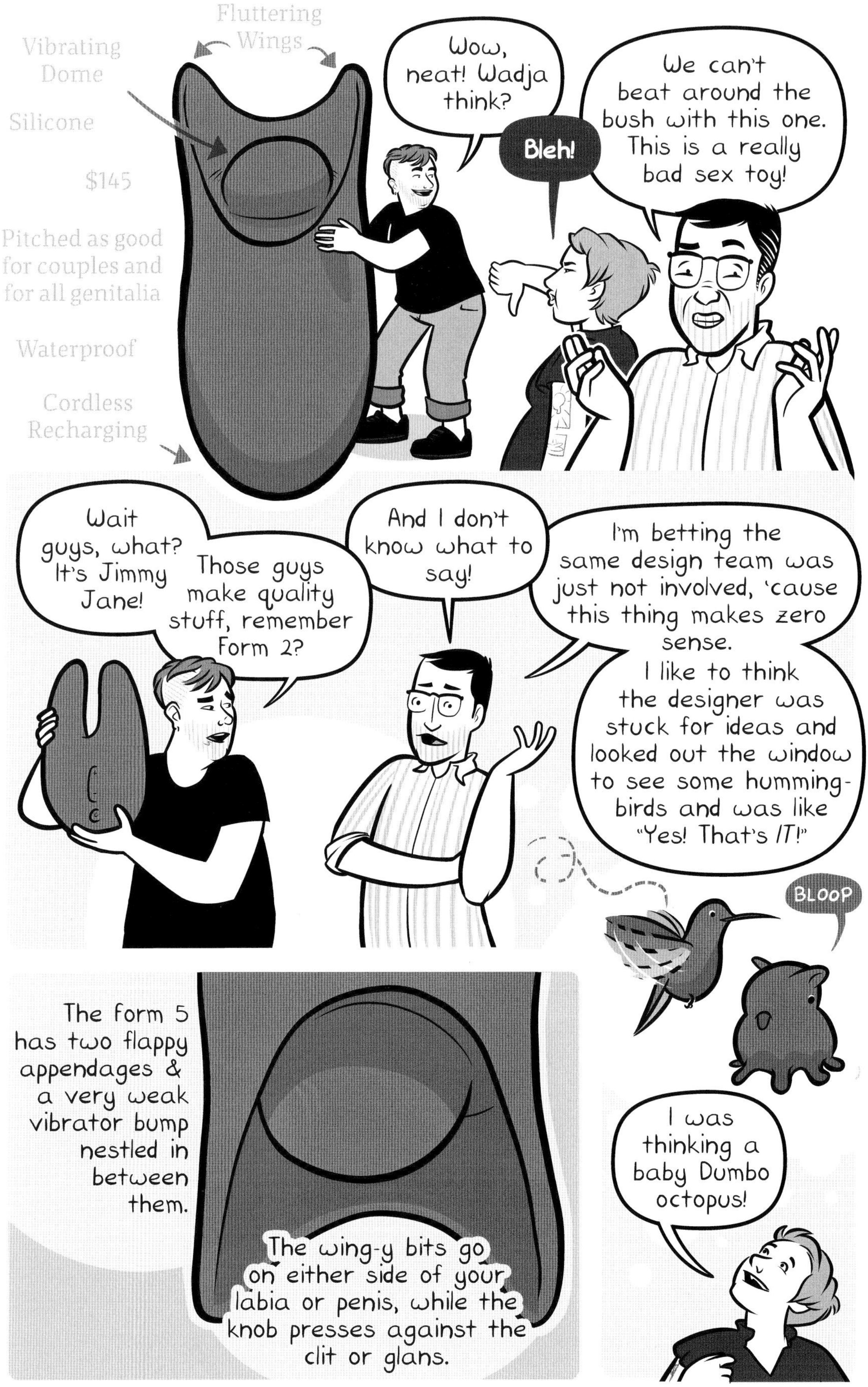
Fluttering Wings
Vibrating Dome
Silicone
$145
Pitched as good for couples and for all genitalia
Waterproof
Cordless Recharging
Wow, neat! Wadja think?
Bleh!
We can't beat around the bush with this one. This is a really bad sex toy!
Wait guys, what? It's Jimmy Jane!
Those guys make quality stuff, remember Form 2?
And I don't know what to say!
I'm betting the same design team was just not involved, 'cause this thing makes zero sense.
I like to think the designer was stuck for ideas and looked out the window to see some humming-birds and was like "Yes! That's IT!"
BLOOP
The form 5 has two flappy appendages & a very weak vibrator bump nestled in between them.
The wing-y bits go on either side of your labia or penis, while the knob presses against the clit or glans.
I was thinking a baby Dumbo octopus!

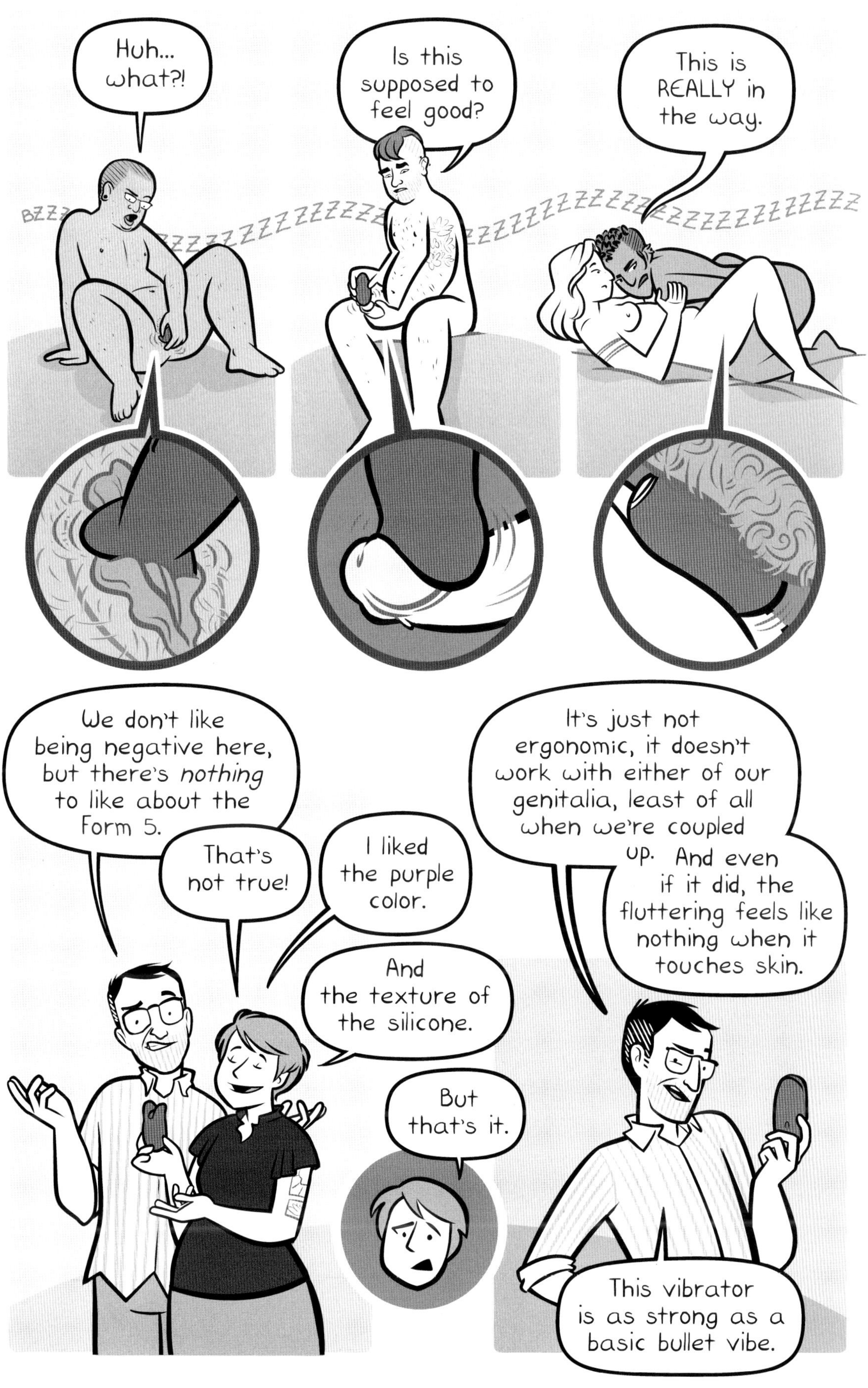
Huh... what?!
Is this supposed to feel good?
This is REALLY in the way.
BZZZZZZZZZZZZZZZZZZZZZZZZZZZZZZZZZZZZZZZZZZZZZZZZ
We don't like being negative here, but there's *nothing* to like about the Form 5.
That's not true!
I liked the purple color.
And the texture of the silicone.
But that's it.
It's just not ergonomic, it doesn't work with either of our genitalia, least of all when we're coupled up.
And even if it did, the fluttering feels like nothing when it touches skin.
This vibrator is as strong as a basic bullet vibe.

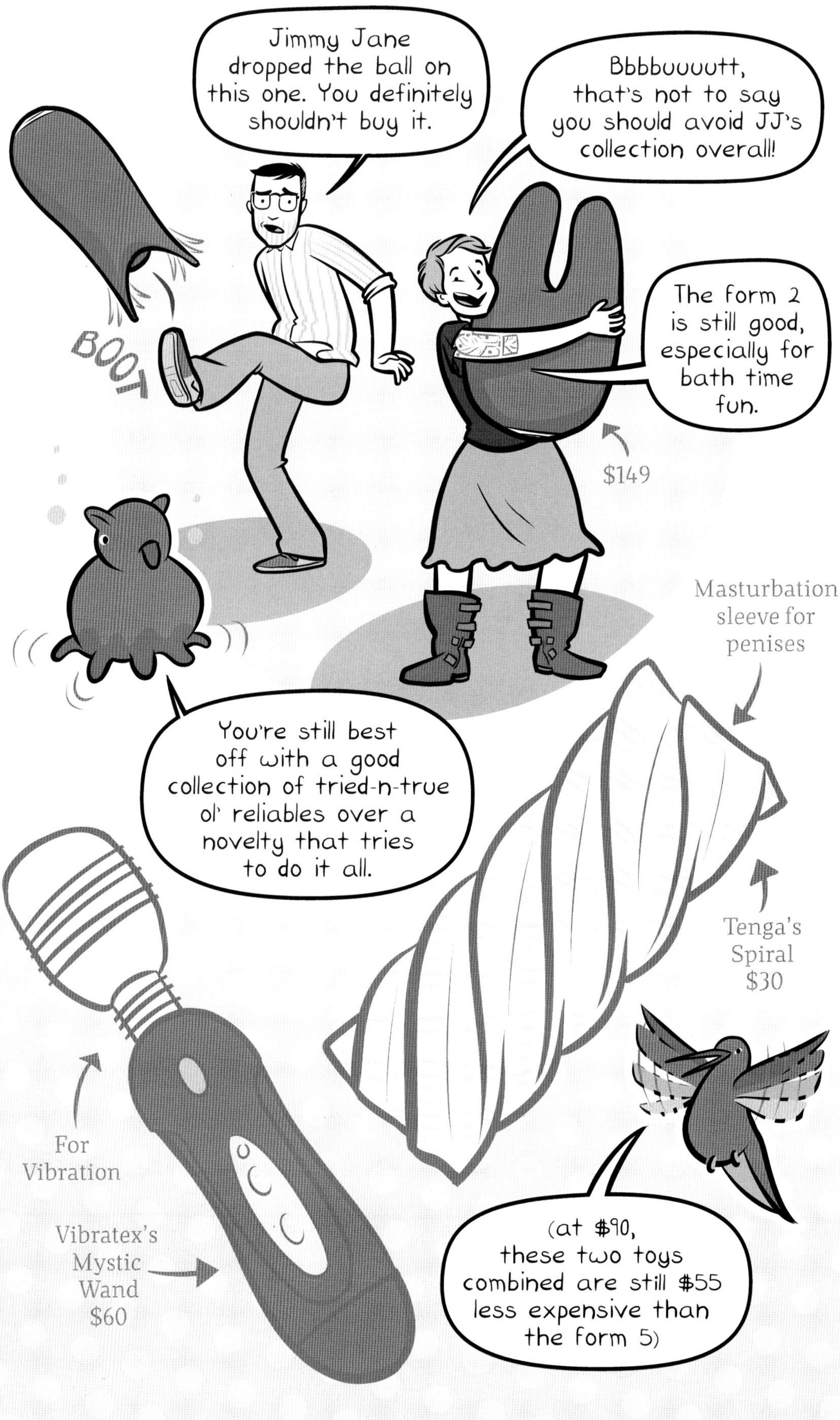
Jimmy Jane dropped the ball on this one. You definitely shouldn't buy it.
BOOT
Bbbbuuuutt, that's not to say you should avoid JJ's collection overall!
The form 2 is still good, especially for bath time fun.
$149
Masturbation sleeve for penises
You're still best off with a good collection of tried-n-true ol' reliables over a novelty that tries to do it all.
Tenga's Spiral $30
For Vibration
Vibratex's Mystic Wand $60
(at $90, these two toys combined are still $55 less expensive than the form 5)

FLESHLIGHT GO

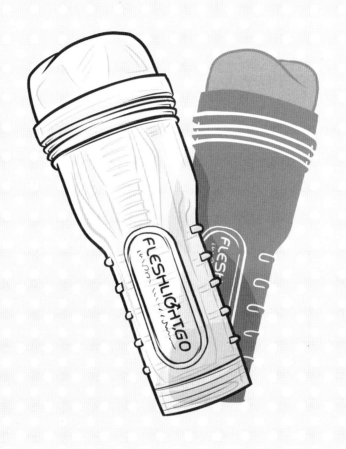

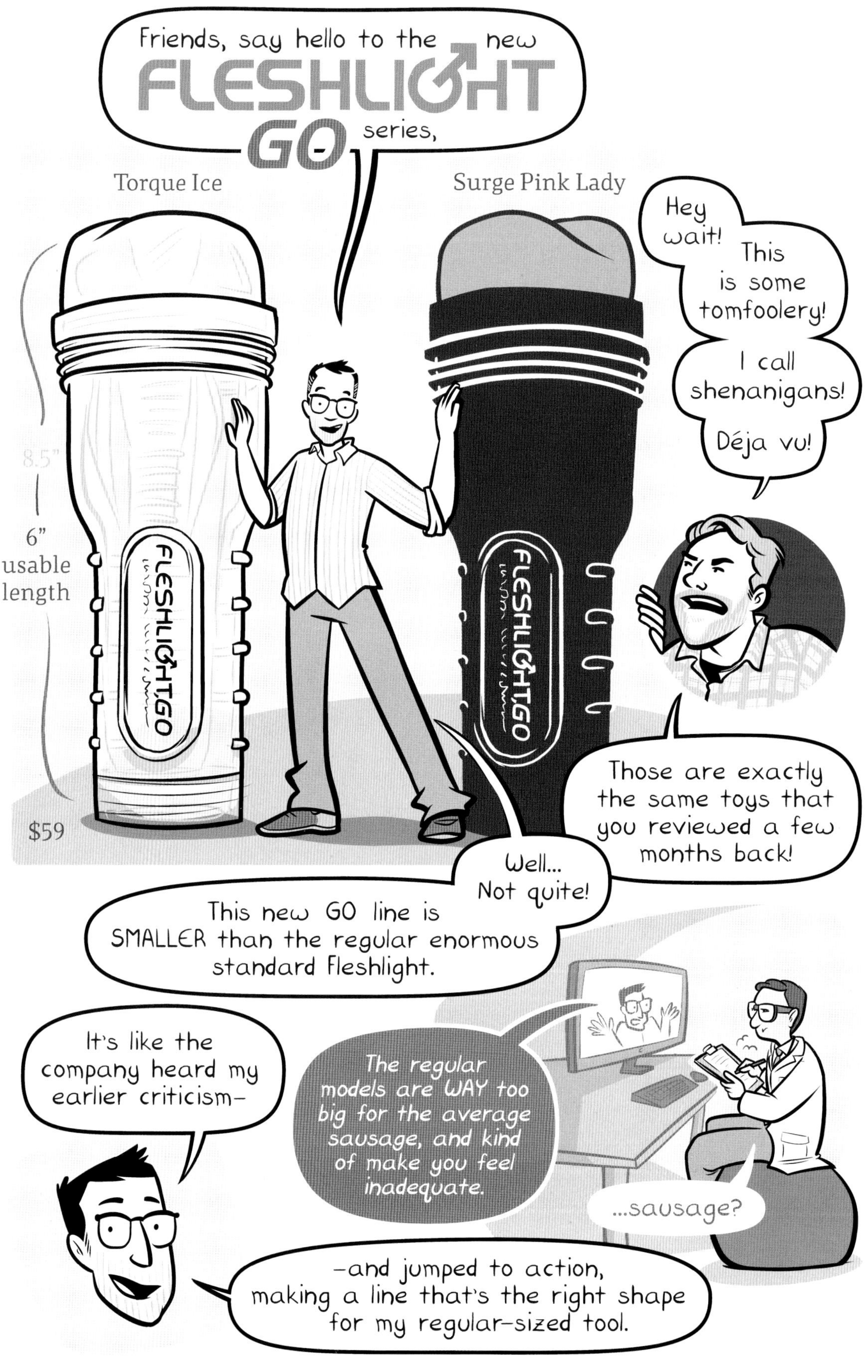
Friends, say hello to the new FLESHLIGHT GO series,
Torque Ice
Surge Pink Lady
8.5"
6" usable length
$59
FLESHLIGHT GO
FLESHLIGHT GO
Hey wait! This is some tomfoolery!
I call shenanigans!
Déja vu!
Those are exactly the same toys that you reviewed a few months back!
Well... Not quite!
This new GO line is SMALLER than the regular enormous standard Fleshlight.
It's like the company heard my earlier criticism–
The regular models are WAY too big for the average sausage, and kind of make you feel inadequate.
...sausage?
–and jumped to action, making a line that's the right shape for my regular-sized tool.

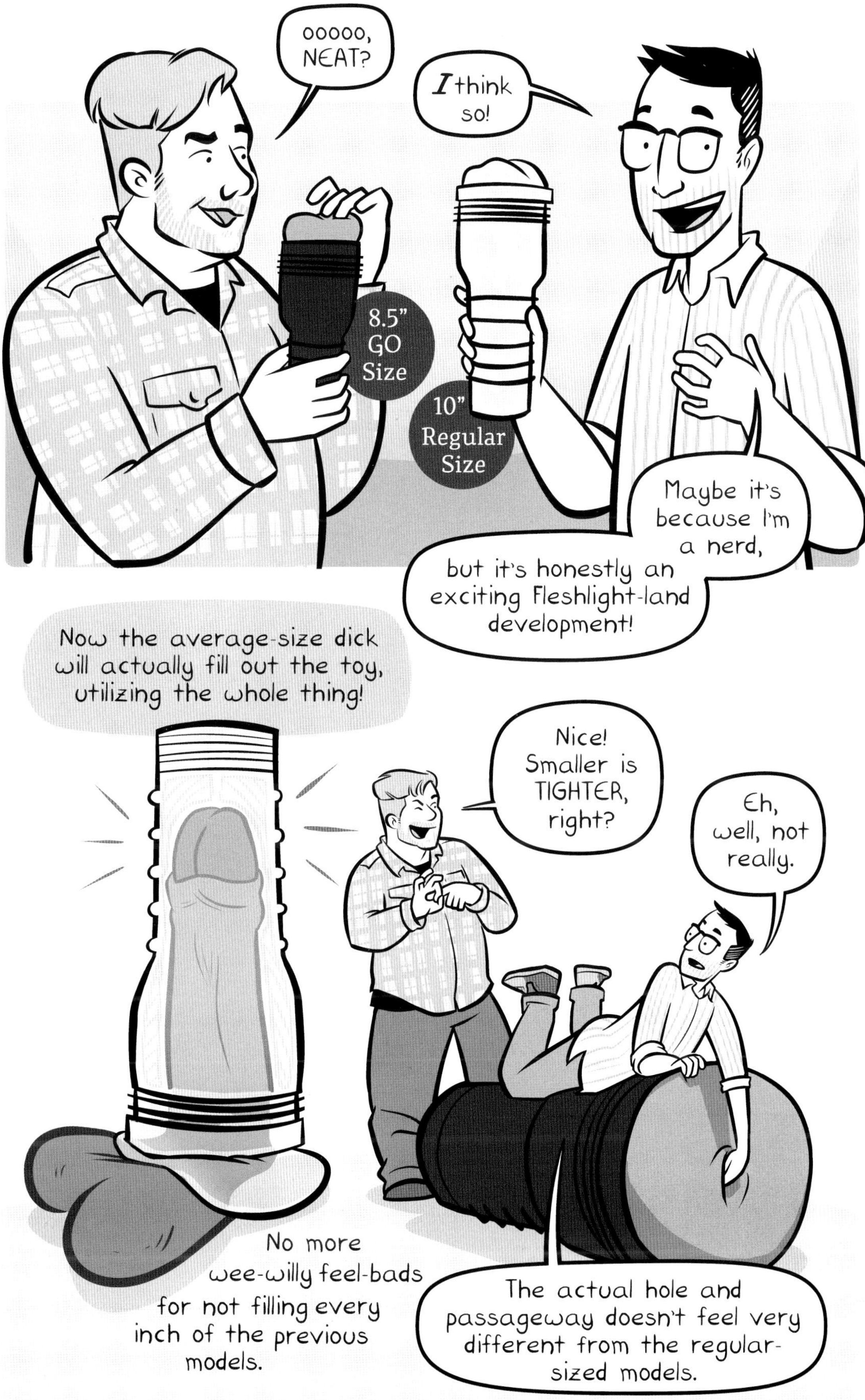
ooooo, NEAT?
I think so!
8.5" GO Size
10" Regular Size
Maybe it's because I'm a nerd,
but it's honestly an exciting Fleshlight-land development!
Now the average-size dick will actually fill out the toy, utilizing the whole thing!
Nice! Smaller is TIGHTER, right?
Eh, well, not really.
No more wee-willy feel-bads for not filling every inch of the previous models.
The actual hole and passageway doesn't feel very different from the regular-sized models.

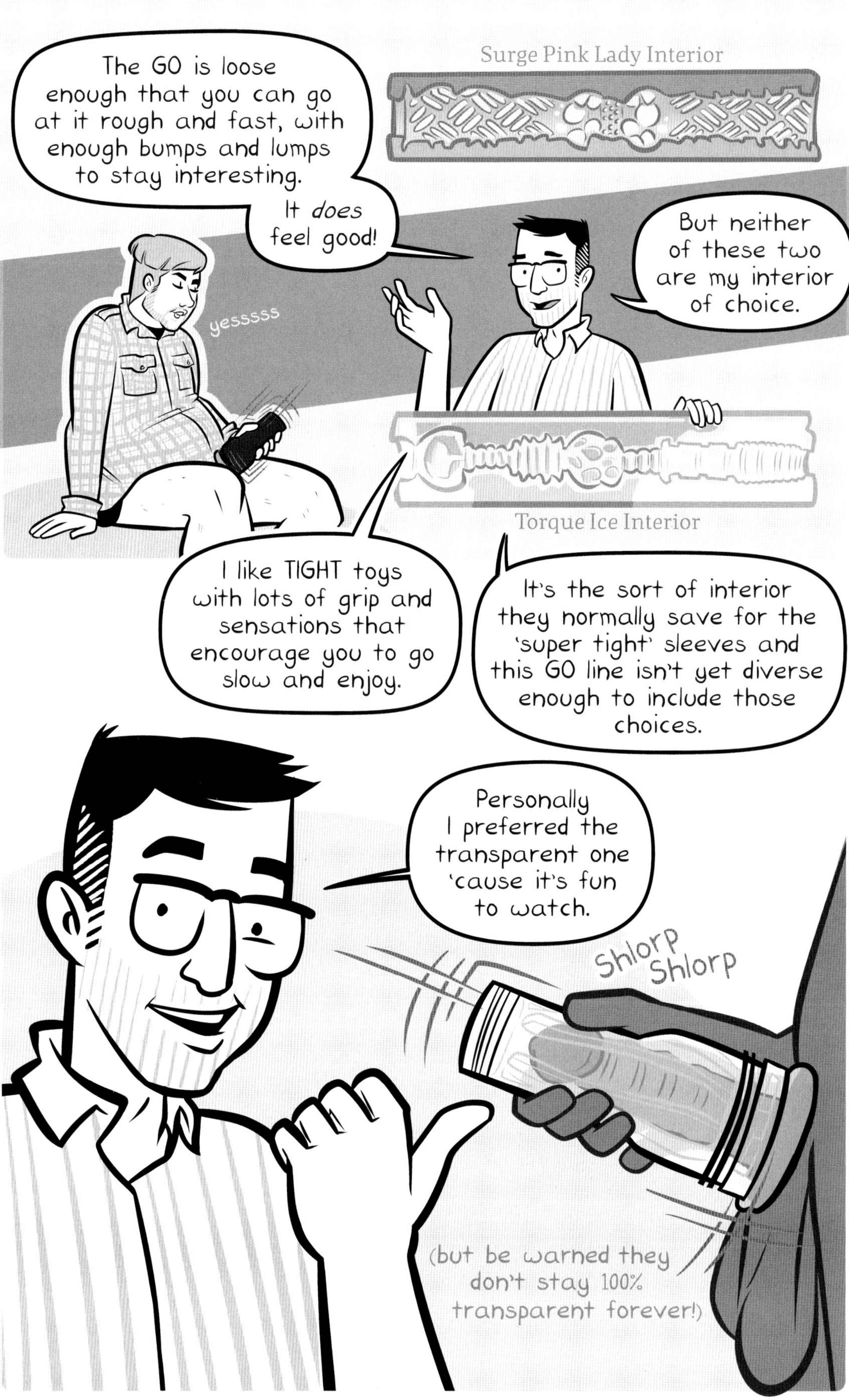
The GO is loose enough that you can go at it rough and fast, with enough bumps and lumps to stay interesting.
Surge Pink Lady Interior
It *does* feel good!
But neither of these two are my interior of choice.
yessssss
Torque Ice Interior
I like TIGHT toys with lots of grip and sensations that encourage you to go slow and enjoy.
It's the sort of interior they normally save for the 'super tight' sleeves and this GO line isn't yet diverse enough to include those choices.
Personally I preferred the transparent one 'cause it's fun to watch.
Shlorp Shlorp
(but be warned they don't stay 100% transparent forever!)

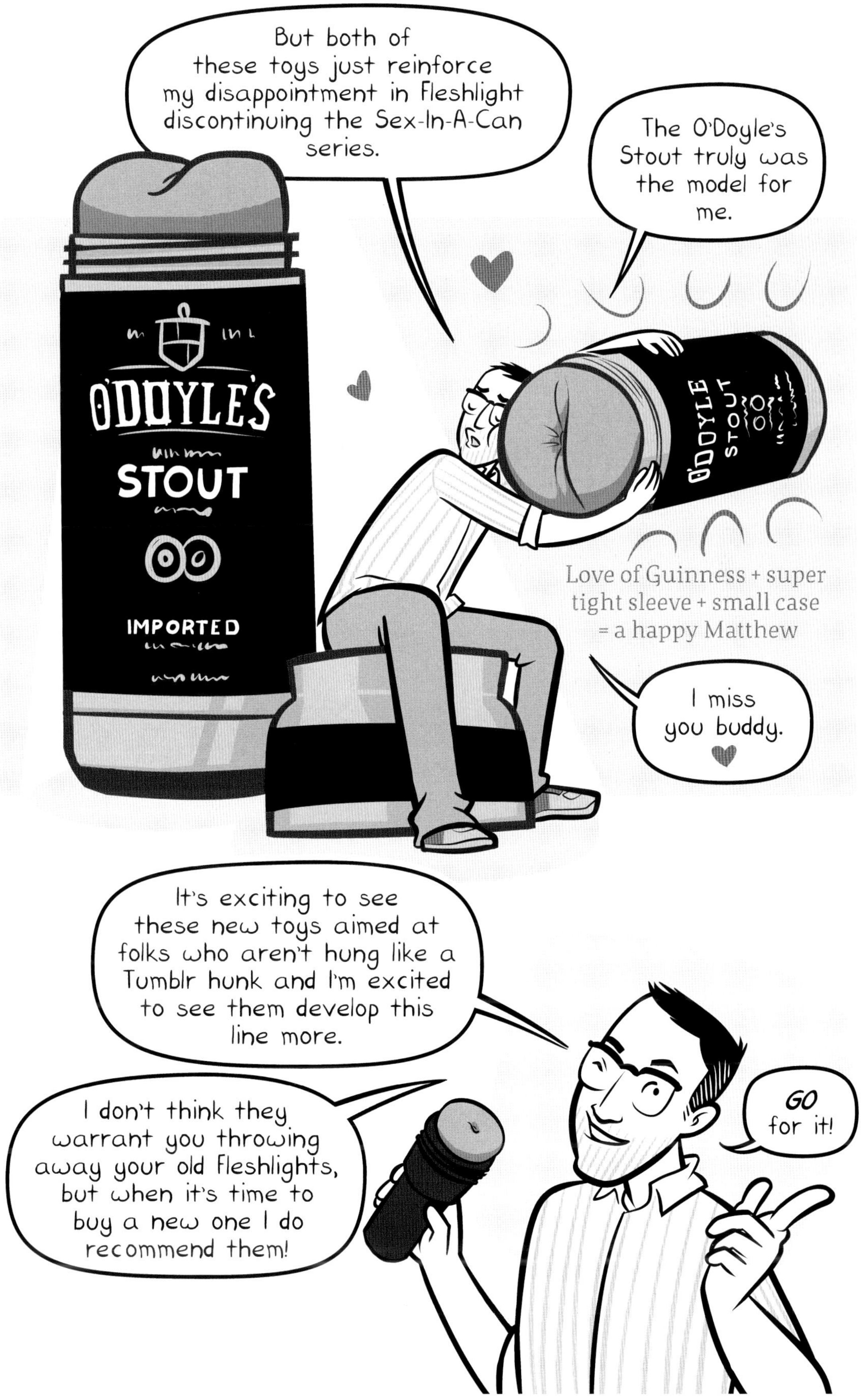
But both of these toys just reinforce my disappointment in Fleshlight discontinuing the Sex-In-A-Can series.
The O'Doyle's Stout truly was the model for me.
O'DOYLE'S
STOUT
IMPORTED
O'DOYLE
STOUT
Love of Guinness + super tight sleeve + small case = a happy Matthew
I miss you buddy.
It's exciting to see these new toys aimed at folks who aren't hung like a Tumblr hunk and I'm excited to see them develop this line more.
I don't think they warrant you throwing away your old Fleshlights, but when it's time to buy a new one I do recommend them!
GO for it!

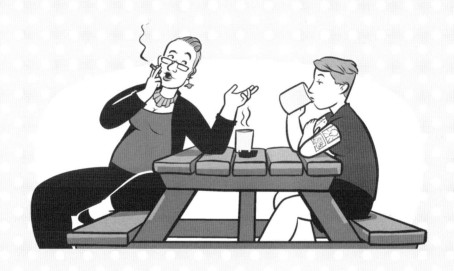

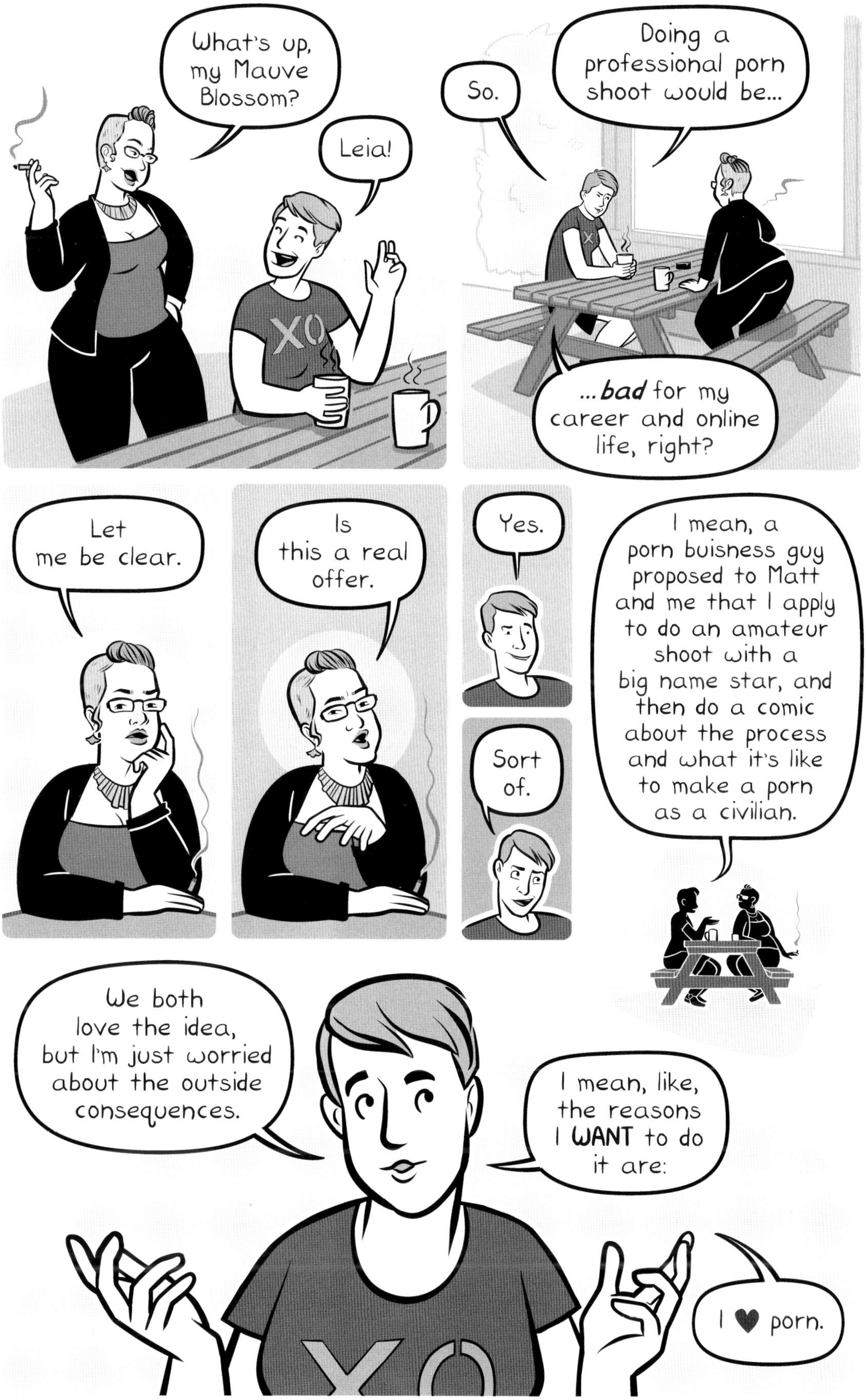
What's up, my Mauve Blossom?
Leia!
So.
Doing a professional porn shoot would be...
...**bad** for my career and online life, right?
Let me be clear.
Is this a real offer.
Yes.
Sort of.
I mean, a porn buisness guy proposed to Matt and me that I apply to do an amateur shoot with a big name star, and then do a comic about the process and what it's like to make a porn as a civilian.
We both love the idea, but I'm just worried about the outside consequences.
I mean, like, the reasons I **WANT** to do it are:
I ♥ porn.

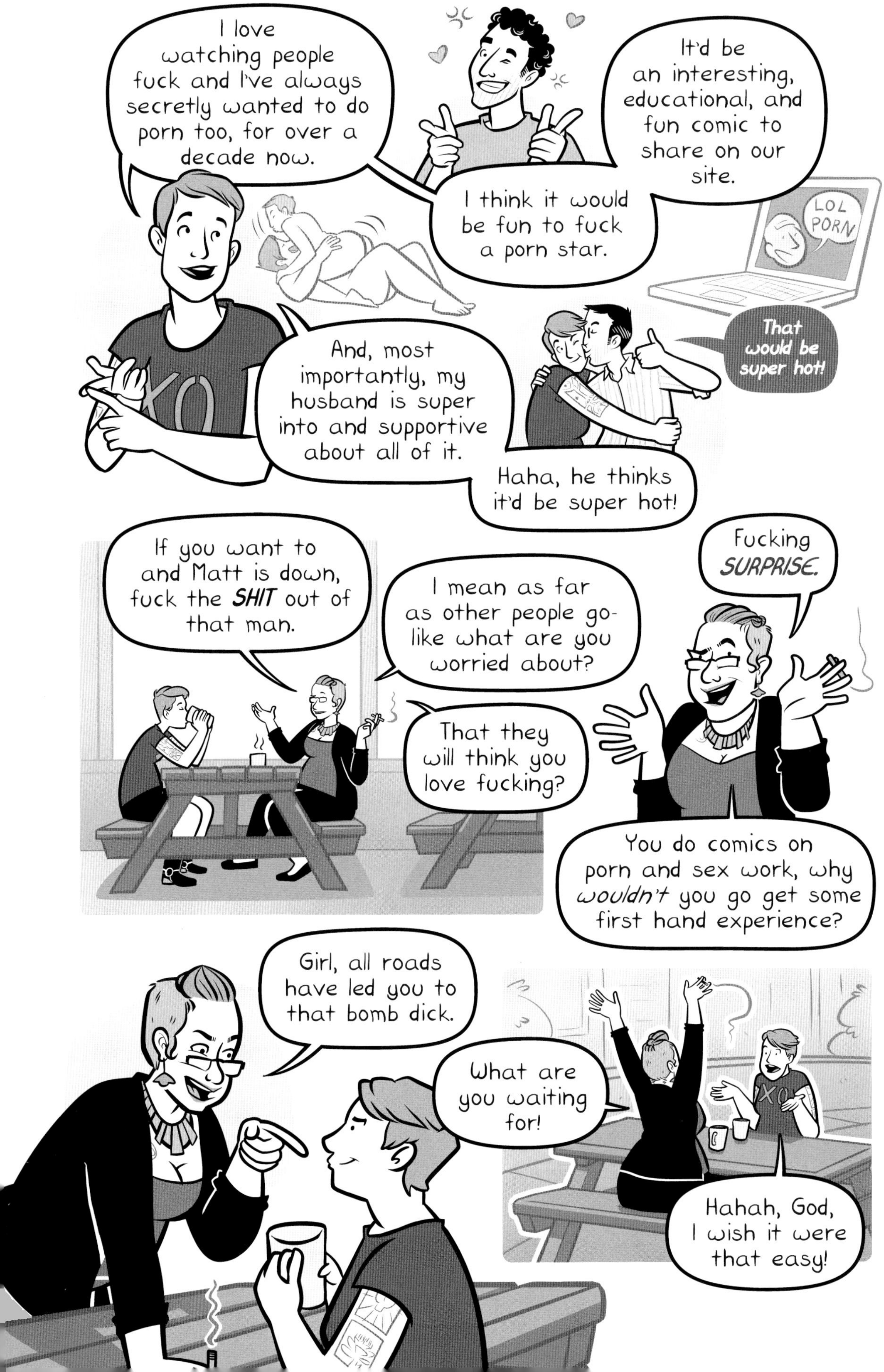
I love watching people fuck and I've always secretly wanted to do porn too, for over a decade now.
It'd be an interesting, educational, and fun comic to share on our site.
I think it would be fun to fuck a porn star.
LOL PORN
And, most importantly, my husband is super into and supportive about all of it.
That would be super hot!
Haha, he thinks it'd be super hot!
If you want to and Matt is down, fuck the SHIT out of that man.
I mean as far as other people go- like what are you worried about?
That they will think you love fucking?
Fucking SURPRISE.
You do comics on porn and sex work, why wouldn't you go get some first hand experience?
Girl, all roads have led you to that bomb dick.
What are you waiting for!
Hahah, God, I wish it were that easy!

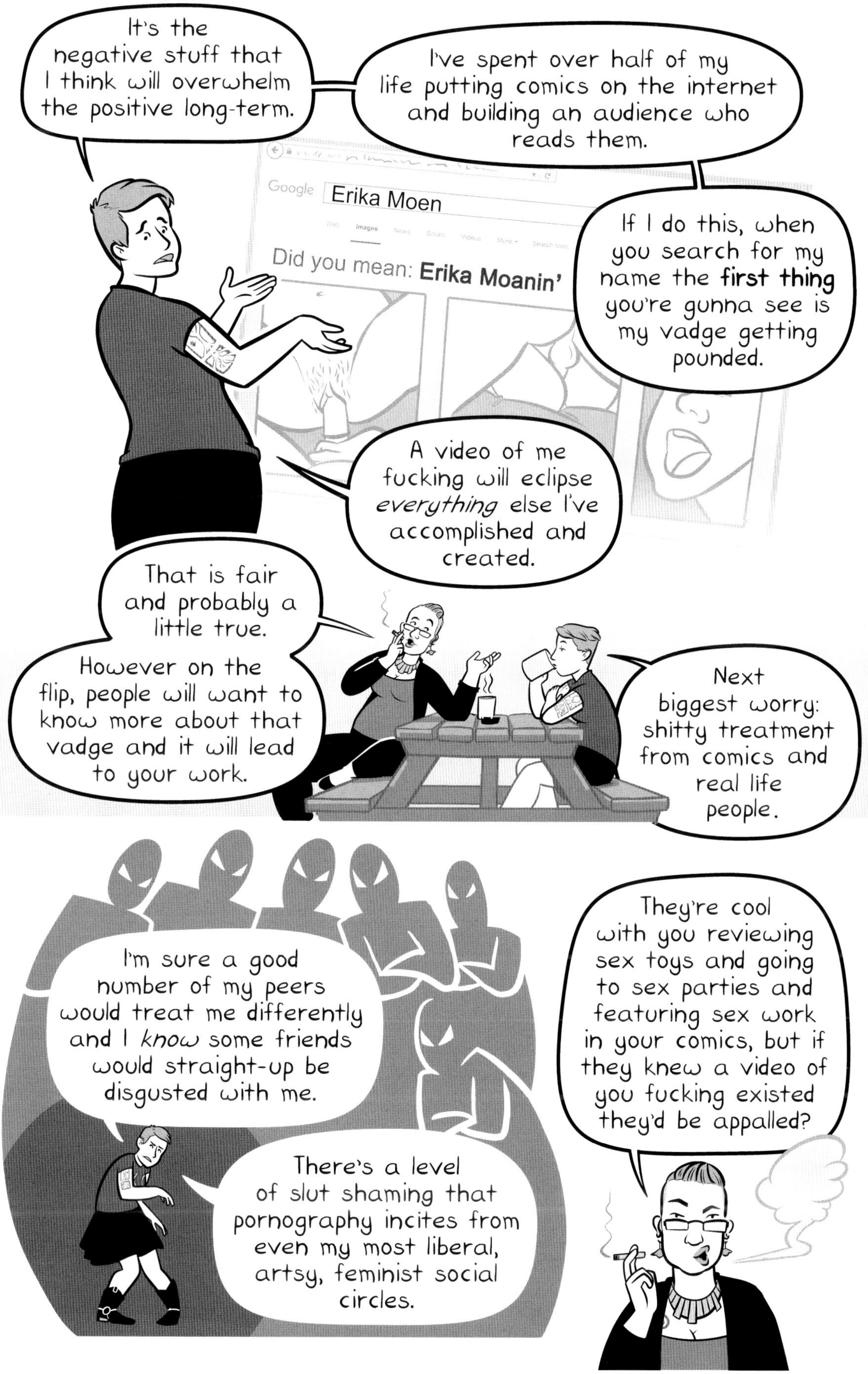
It's the negative stuff that I think will overwhelm the positive long-term.
I've spent over half of my life putting comics on the internet and building an audience who reads them.
Google
Erika Moen
Did you mean: Erika Moanin'
If I do this, when you search for my name the first thing you're gunna see is my vadge getting pounded.
A video of me fucking will eclipse everything else I've accomplished and created.
That is fair and probably a little true.
However on the flip, people will want to know more about that vadge and it will lead to your work.
Next biggest worry: shitty treatment from comics and real life people.
I'm sure a good number of my peers would treat me differently and I know some friends would straight-up be disgusted with me.
There's a level of slut shaming that pornography incites from even my most liberal, artsy, feminist social circles.
They're cool with you reviewing sex toys and going to sex parties and featuring sex work in your comics, but if they knew a video of you fucking existed they'd be appalled?

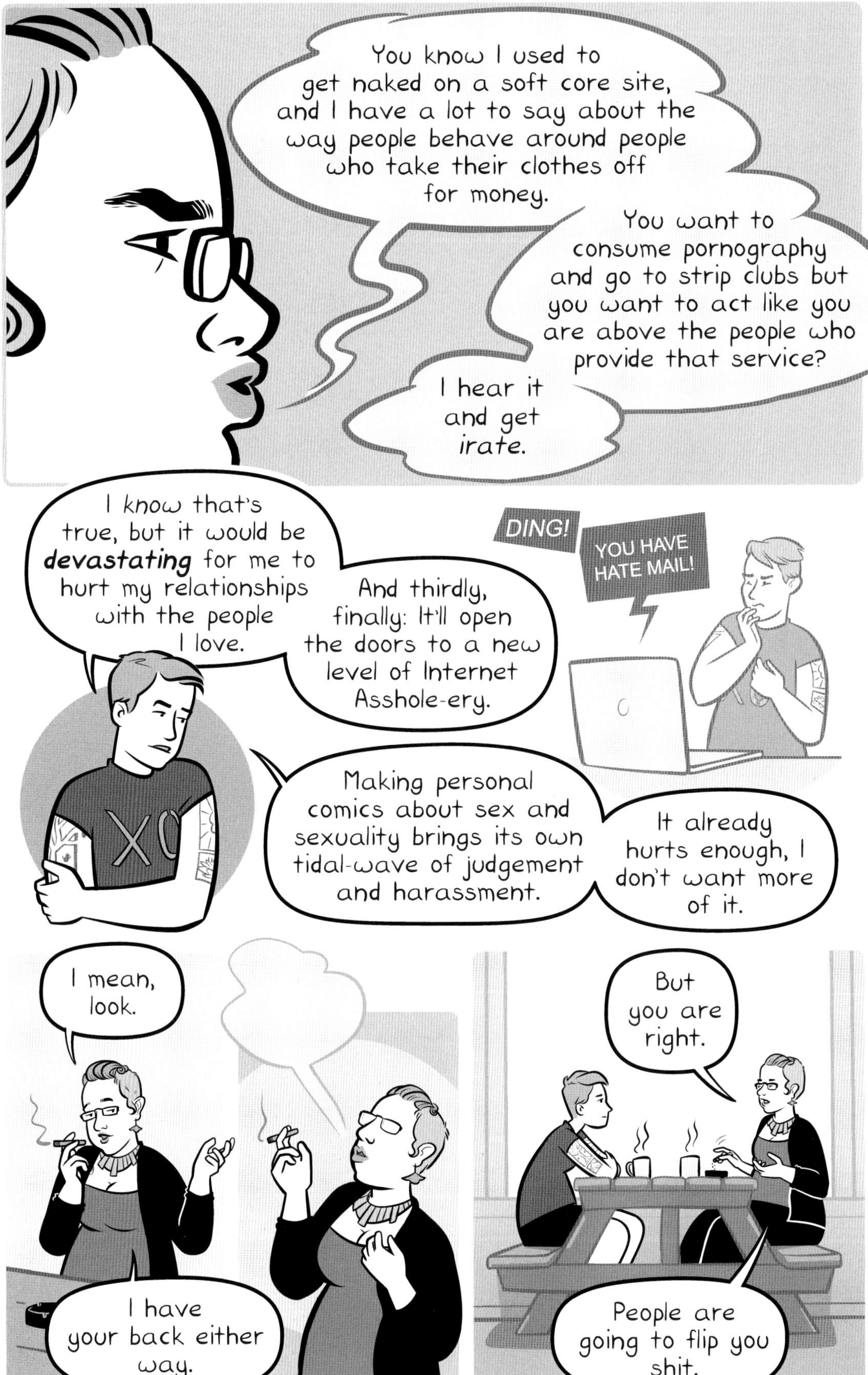
You know I used to get naked on a soft core site, and I have a lot to say about the way people behave around people who take their clothes off for money.
You want to consume pornography and go to strip clubs but you want to act like you are above the people who provide that service?
I hear it and get irate.
I know that's true, but it would be devastating for me to hurt my relationships with the people I love.
And thirdly, finally: It'll open the doors to a new level of Internet Asshole-ery.
DING!
YOU HAVE HATE MAIL!
Making personal comics about sex and sexuality brings its own tidal-wave of judgement and harassment.
It already hurts enough, I don't want more of it.
I mean, look.
I have your back either way.
But you are right.
People are going to flip you shit.

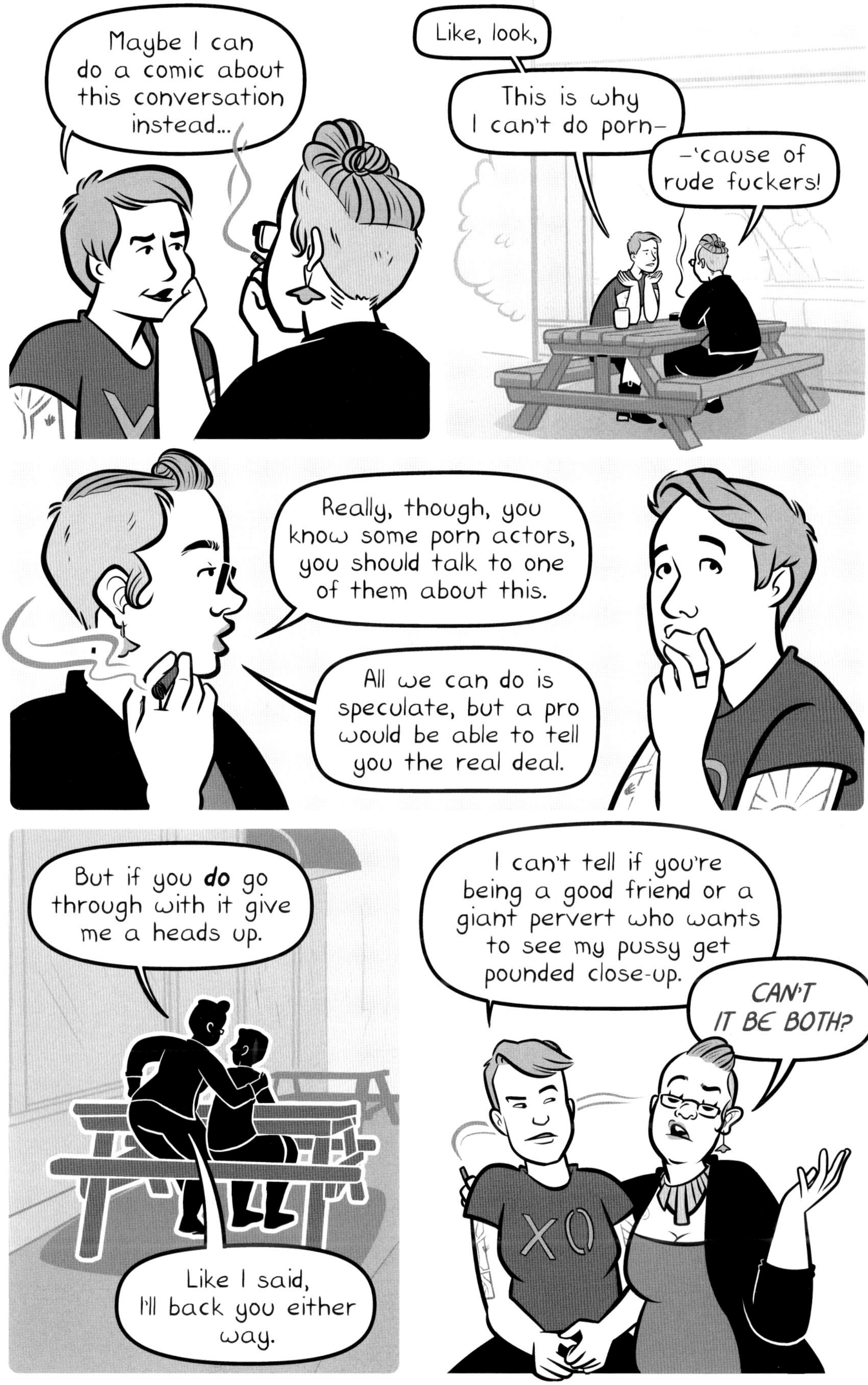

Maybe I can do a comic about this conversation instead...
Like, look,
This is why I can't do porn–
–'cause of rude fuckers!
Really, though, you know some porn actors, you should talk to one of them about this.
All we can do is speculate, but a pro would be able to tell you the real deal.
But if you **do** go through with it give me a heads up.
Like I said, I'll back you either way.
I can't tell if you're being a good friend or a giant pervert who wants to see my pussy get pounded close-up.
CAN'T IT BE BOTH?

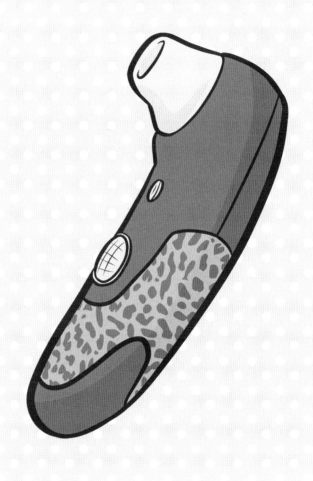

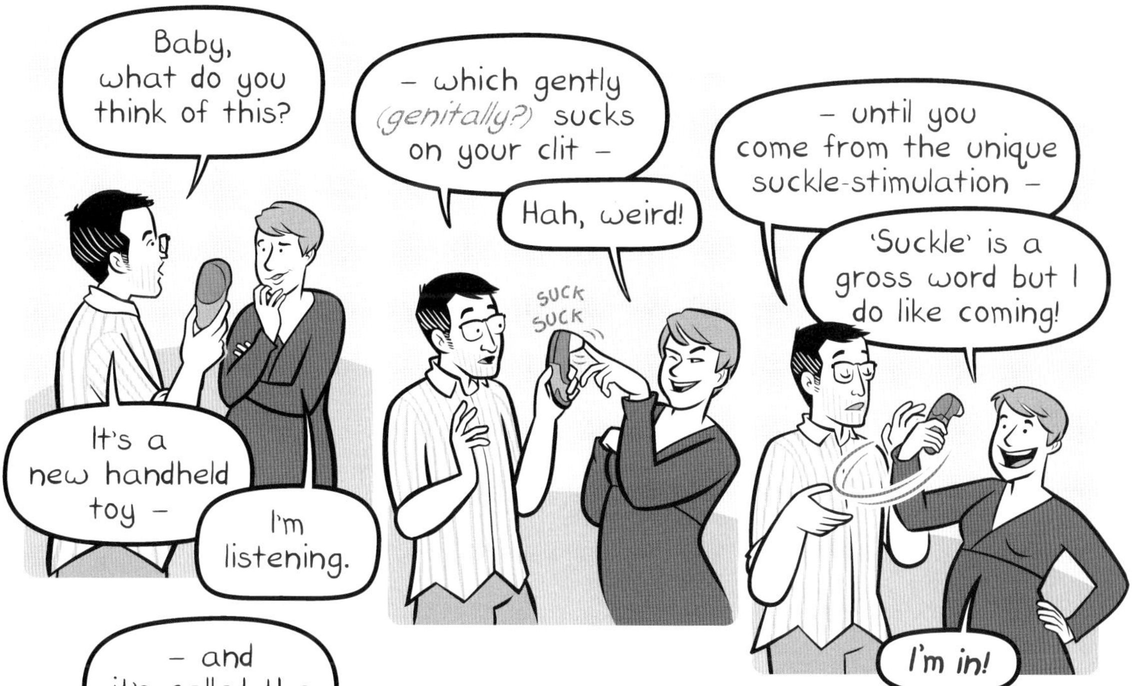
Baby, what do you think of this?
It's a new handheld toy –
I'm listening.
– which gently (genitally?) sucks on your clit –
Hah, weird!
SUCK SUCK
– until you come from the unique suckle-stimulation –
'Suckle' is a gross word but I do like coming!
I'm in!

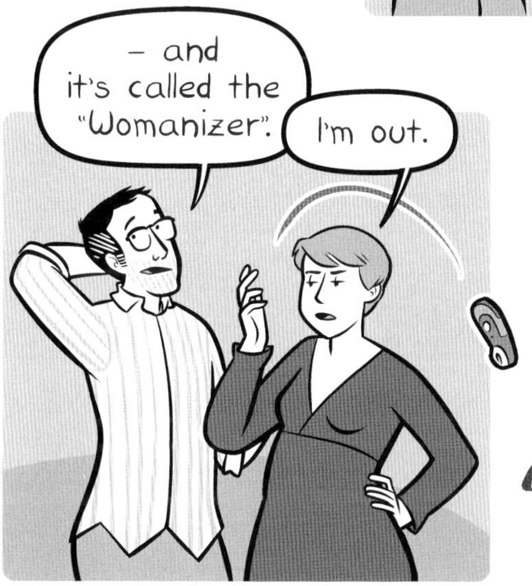
– and it's called the "Womanizer".
I'm out.

In the end we did have our friends-with-benefits at

GOOD VIBRATIONS®

send me a

womanizer

Thanks, guys!

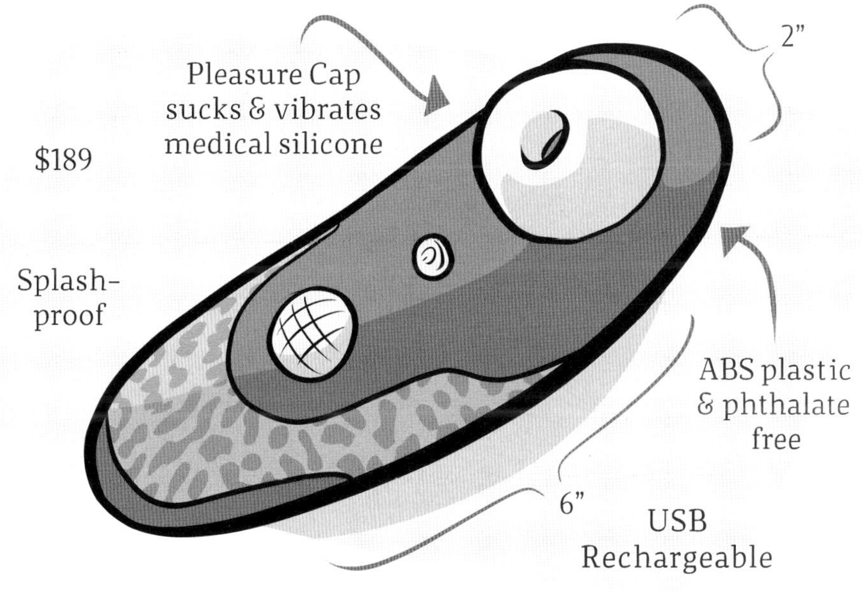
Pleasure Cap sucks & vibrates medical silicone
2"
$189
Splash-proof
ABS plastic & phthalate free
6"
USB Rechargeable

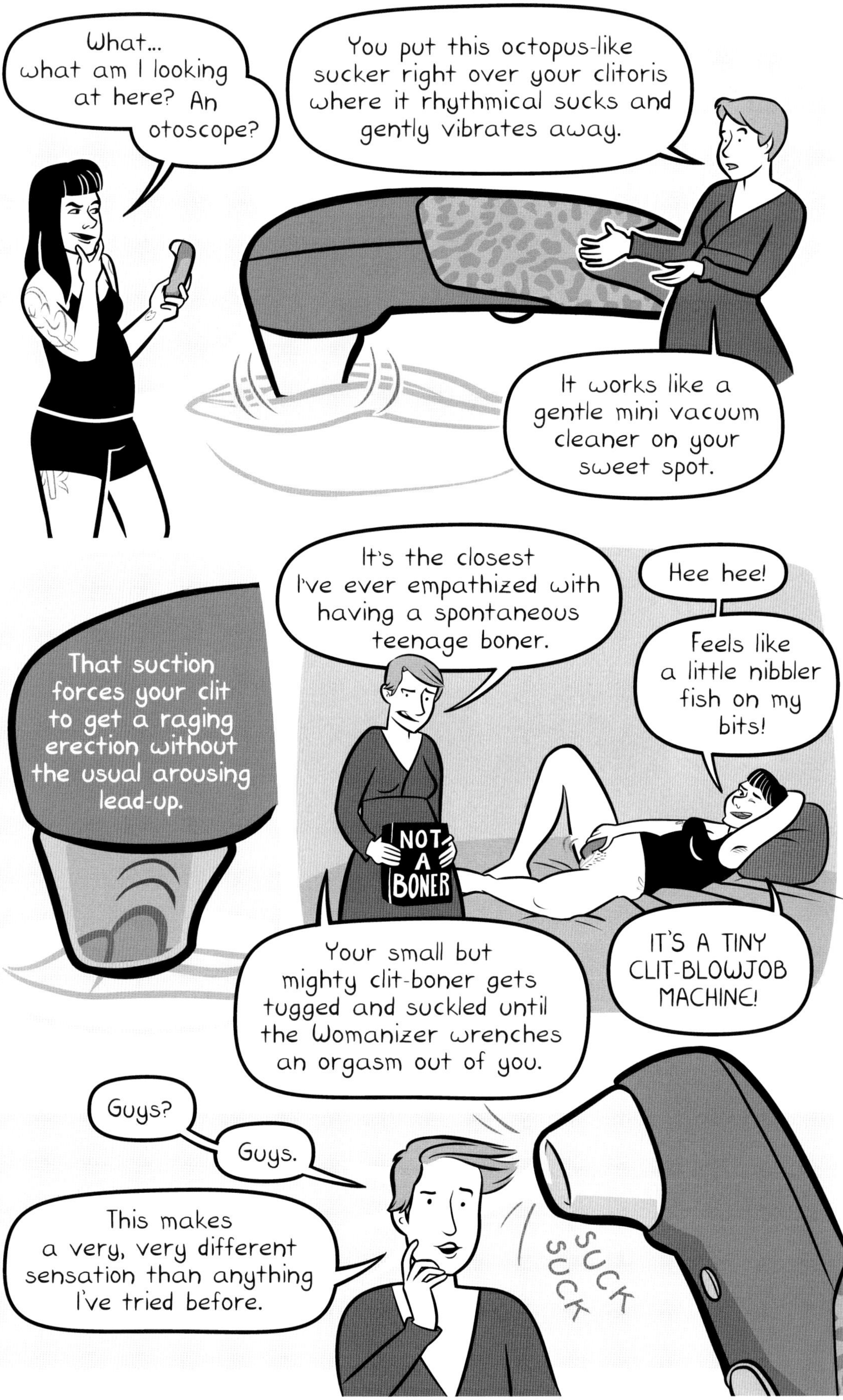

What... what am I looking at here? An otoscope?
You put this octopus-like sucker right over your clitoris where it rhythmical sucks and gently vibrates away.
It works like a gentle mini vacuum cleaner on your sweet spot.
That suction forces your clit to get a raging erection without the usual arousing lead-up.
It's the closest I've ever empathized with having a spontaneous teenage boner.
Hee hee!
Feels like a little nibbler fish on my bits!
NOT A BONER
Your small but mighty clit-boner gets tugged and suckled until the Womanizer wrenches an orgasm out of you.
IT'S A TINY CLIT-BLOWJOB MACHINE!
Guys?
Guys.
This makes a very, very different sensation than anything I've tried before.
SUCK SUCK

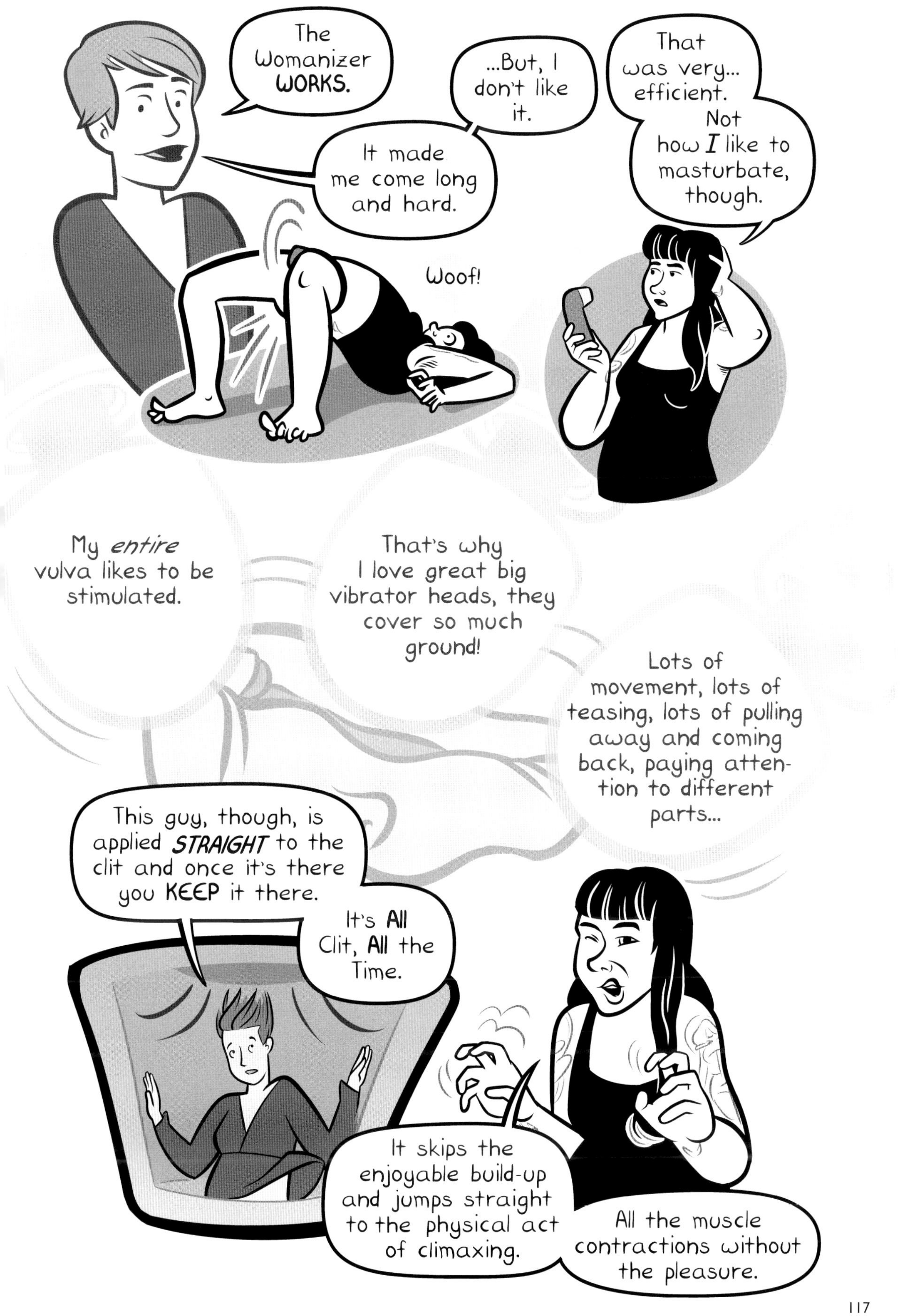
The Womanizer **WORKS.**
It made me come long and hard.
...But, I don't like it.
Woof!
That was very... efficient.
Not how *I* like to masturbate, though.
My *entire* vulva likes to be stimulated.
That's why I love great big vibrator heads, they cover so much ground!
Lots of movement, lots of teasing, lots of pulling away and coming back, paying atten-tion to different parts...
This guy, though, is applied ***STRAIGHT*** to the clit and once it's there you **KEEP** it there.
It's **All** Clit, **All** the Time.
It skips the enjoyable build-up and jumps straight to the physical act of climaxing.
All the muscle contractions without the pleasure.

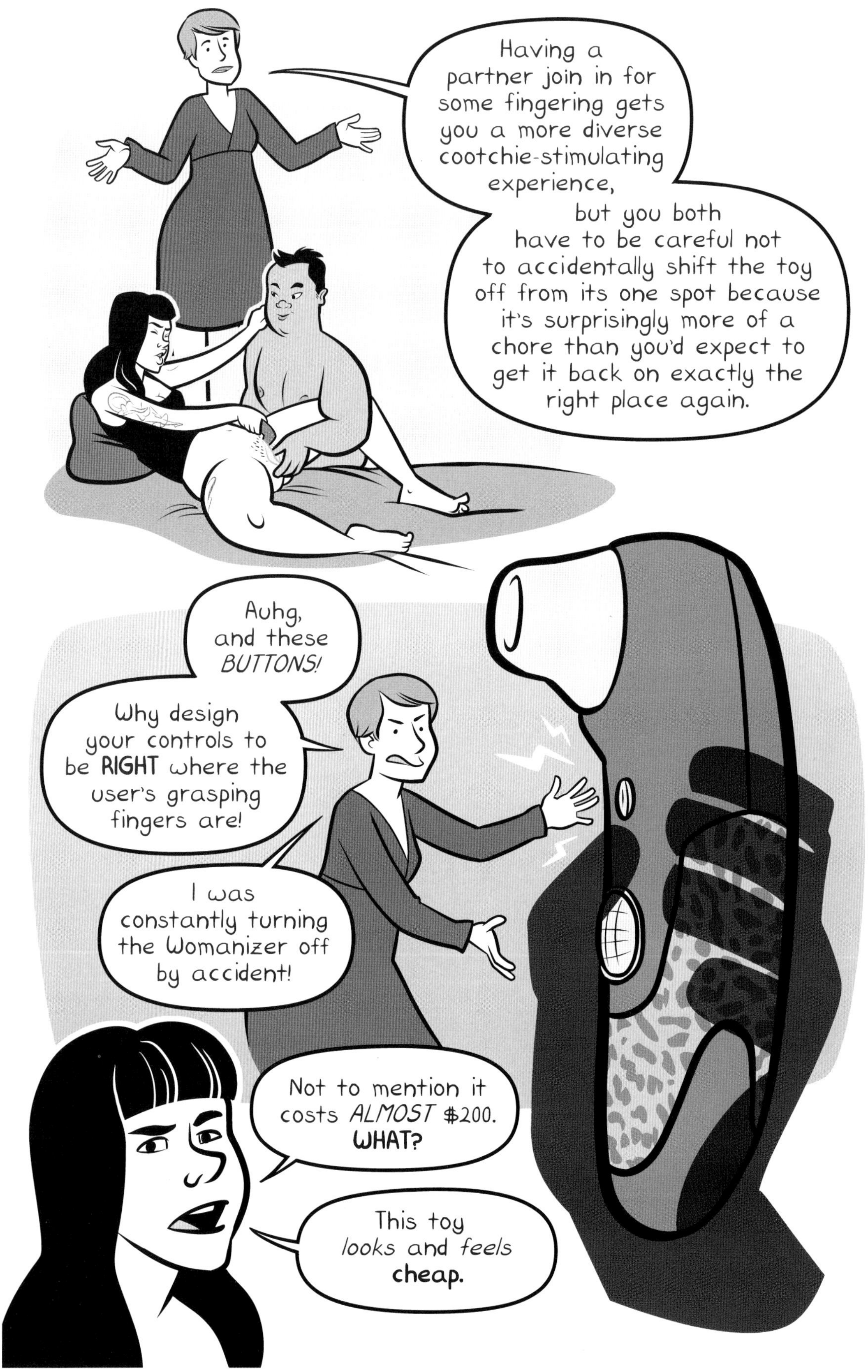
Having a partner join in for some fingering gets you a more diverse cootchie-stimulating experience,
but you both have to be careful not to accidentally shift the toy off from its one spot because it's surprisingly more of a chore than you'd expect to get it back on exactly the right place again.
Auhg, and these *BUTTONS!*
Why design your controls to be **RIGHT** where the user's grasping fingers are!
I was constantly turning the Womanizer off by accident!
Not to mention it costs *ALMOST* $200. **WHAT?**
This toy *looks* and *feels* **cheap.**

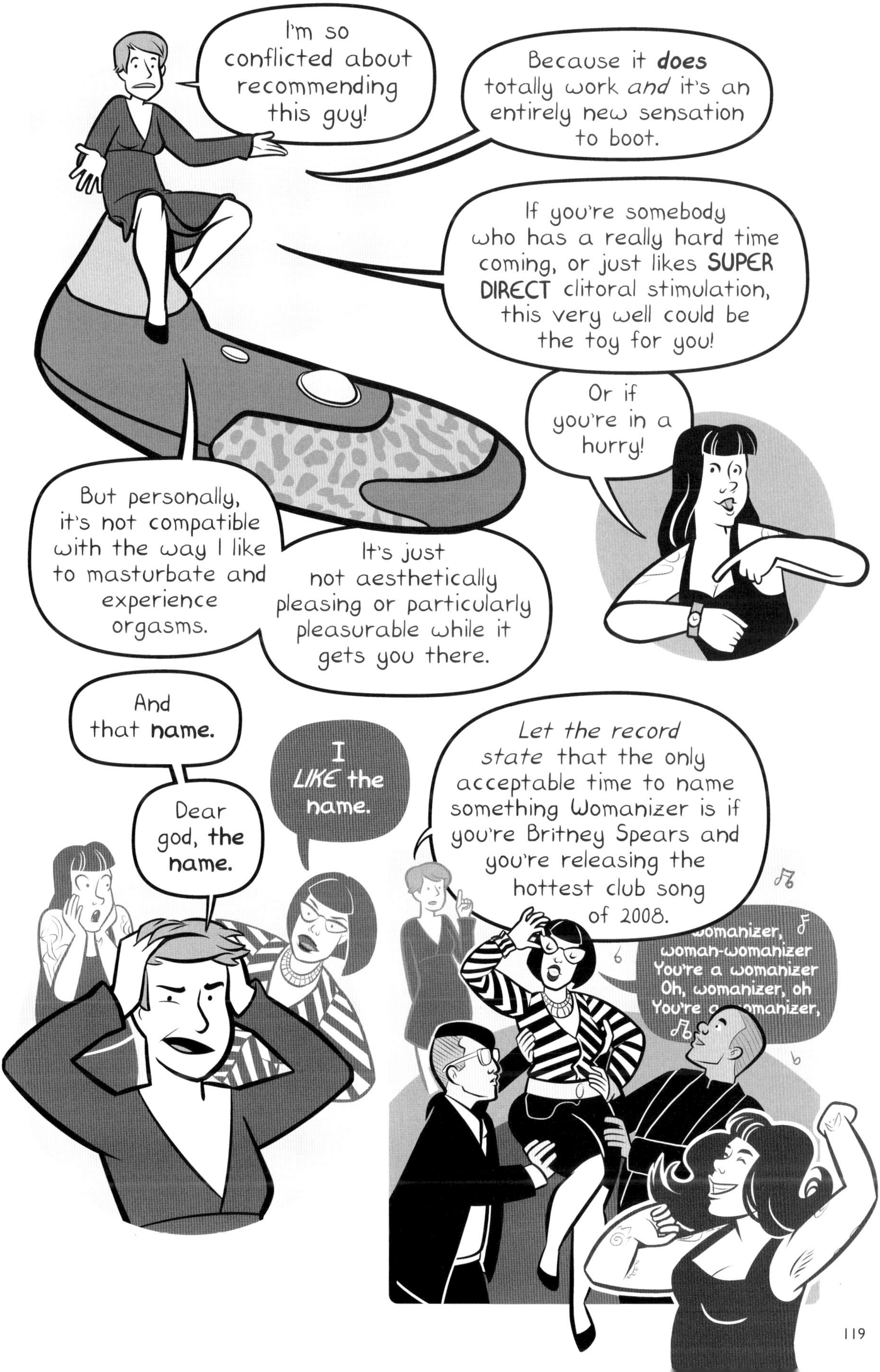

I'm so conflicted about recommending this guy!
Because it **does** totally work *and* it's an entirely new sensation to boot.
If you're somebody who has a really hard time coming, or just likes **SUPER DIRECT** clitoral stimulation, this very well could be the toy for you!
Or if you're in a hurry!
But personally, it's not compatible with the way I like to masturbate and experience orgasms.
It's just not aesthetically pleasing or particularly pleasurable while it gets you there.
And that **name.**
Dear god, **the name.**
I *LIKE* the name.
Let the record state that the only acceptable time to name something Womanizer is if you're Britney Spears and you're releasing the hottest club song of 2008.
womanizer,
woman-womanizer
You're a womanizer
Oh, womanizer, oh
You're omanizer,

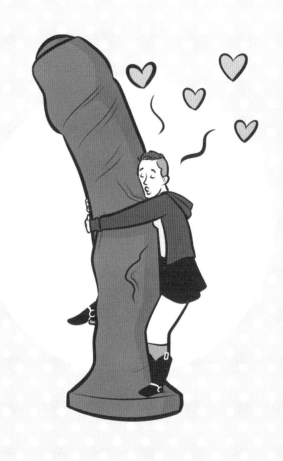

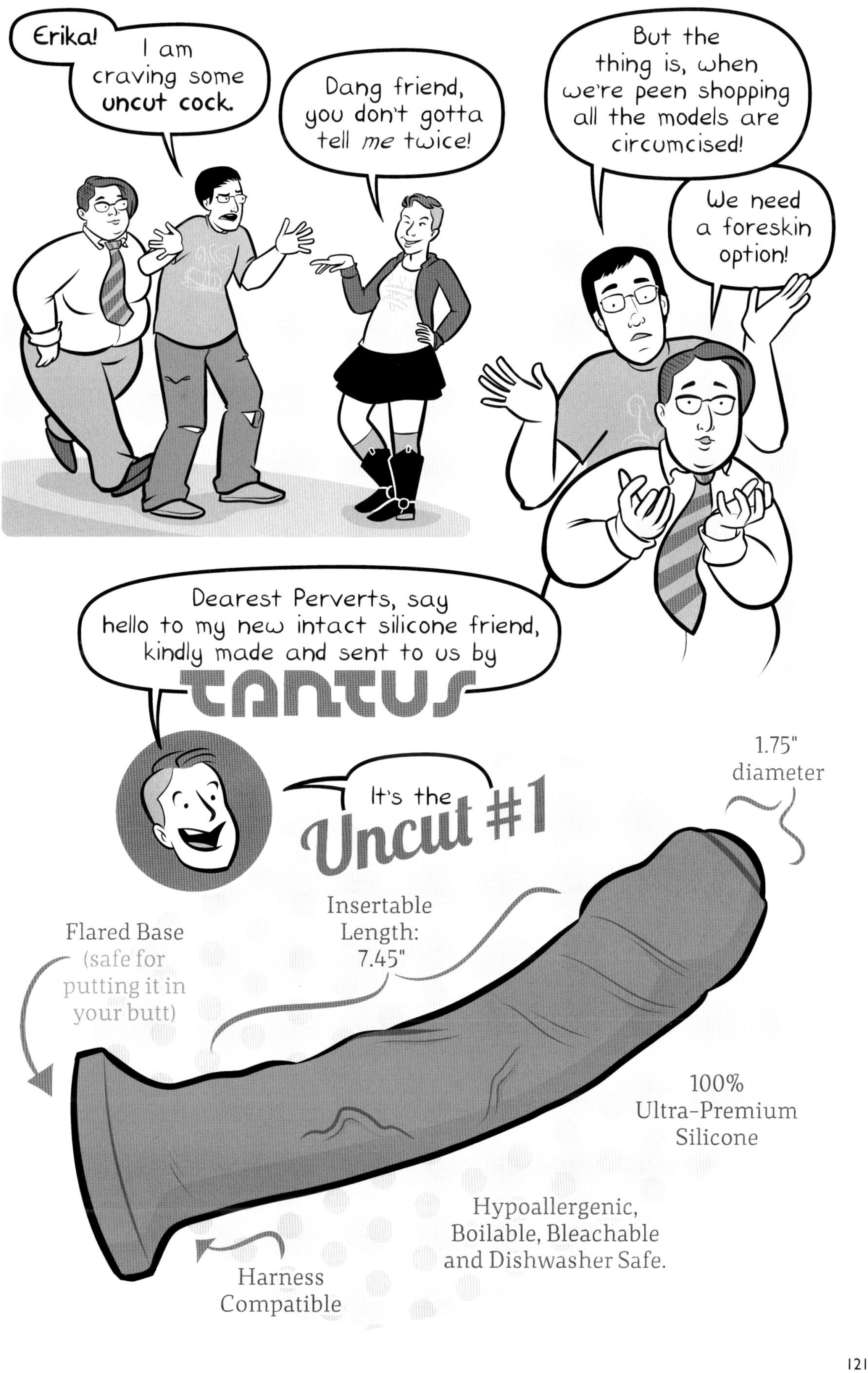

Erika!
I am craving some **uncut cock.**
Dang friend, you don't gotta tell *me* twice!
But the thing is, when we're peen shopping all the models are circumcised!
We need a foreskin option!
Dearest Perverts, say hello to my new intact silicone friend, kindly made and sent to us by
TANTUS
It's the
Uncut #1
1.75" diameter
Insertable Length: 7.45"
Flared Base (safe for putting it in your butt)
100% Ultra-Premium Silicone
Hypoallergenic, Boilable, Bleachable and Dishwasher Safe.
Harness Compatible

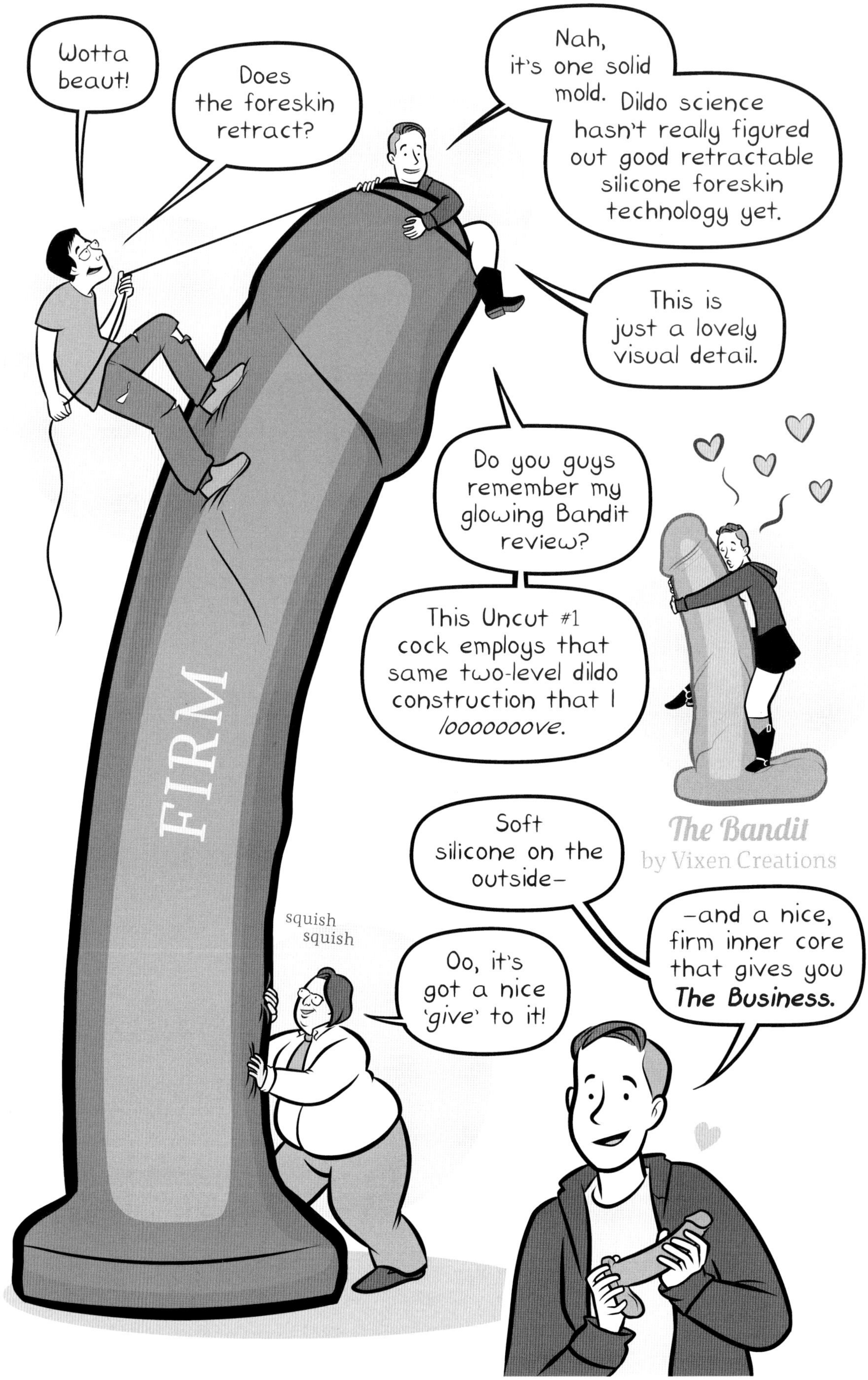
Wotta beaut!
Does the foreskin retract?
Nah, it's one solid mold.
Dildo science hasn't really figured out good retractable silicone foreskin technology yet.
This is just a lovely visual detail.
Do you guys remember my glowing Bandit review?
This Uncut #1 cock employs that same two-level dildo construction that I *looooooove*.
The Bandit
by Vixen Creations
FIRM
Soft silicone on the outside–
–and a nice, firm inner core that gives you **The Business.**
squish squish
Oo, it's got a nice 'give' to it!

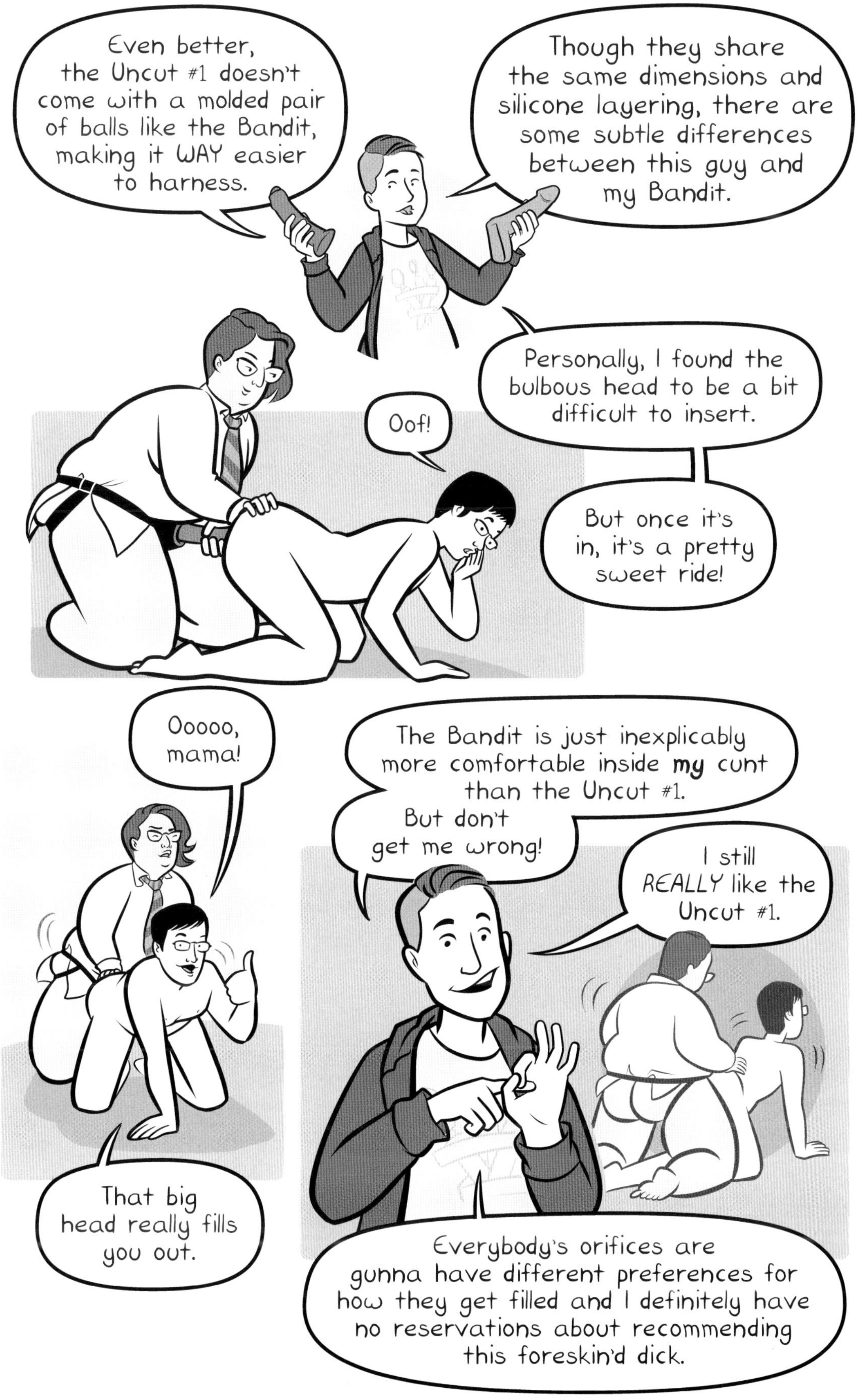
Even better, the Uncut #1 doesn't come with a molded pair of balls like the Bandit, making it WAY easier to harness.
Though they share the same dimensions and silicone layering, there are some subtle differences between this guy and my Bandit.
Personally, I found the bulbous head to be a bit difficult to insert.
Oof!
But once it's in, it's a pretty sweet ride!
Ooooo, mama!
That big head really fills you out.
The Bandit is just inexplicably more comfortable inside my cunt than the Uncut #1.
But don't get me wrong!
I still REALLY like the Uncut #1.
Everybody's orifices are gunna have different preferences for how they get filled and I definitely have no reservations about recommending this foreskin'd dick.

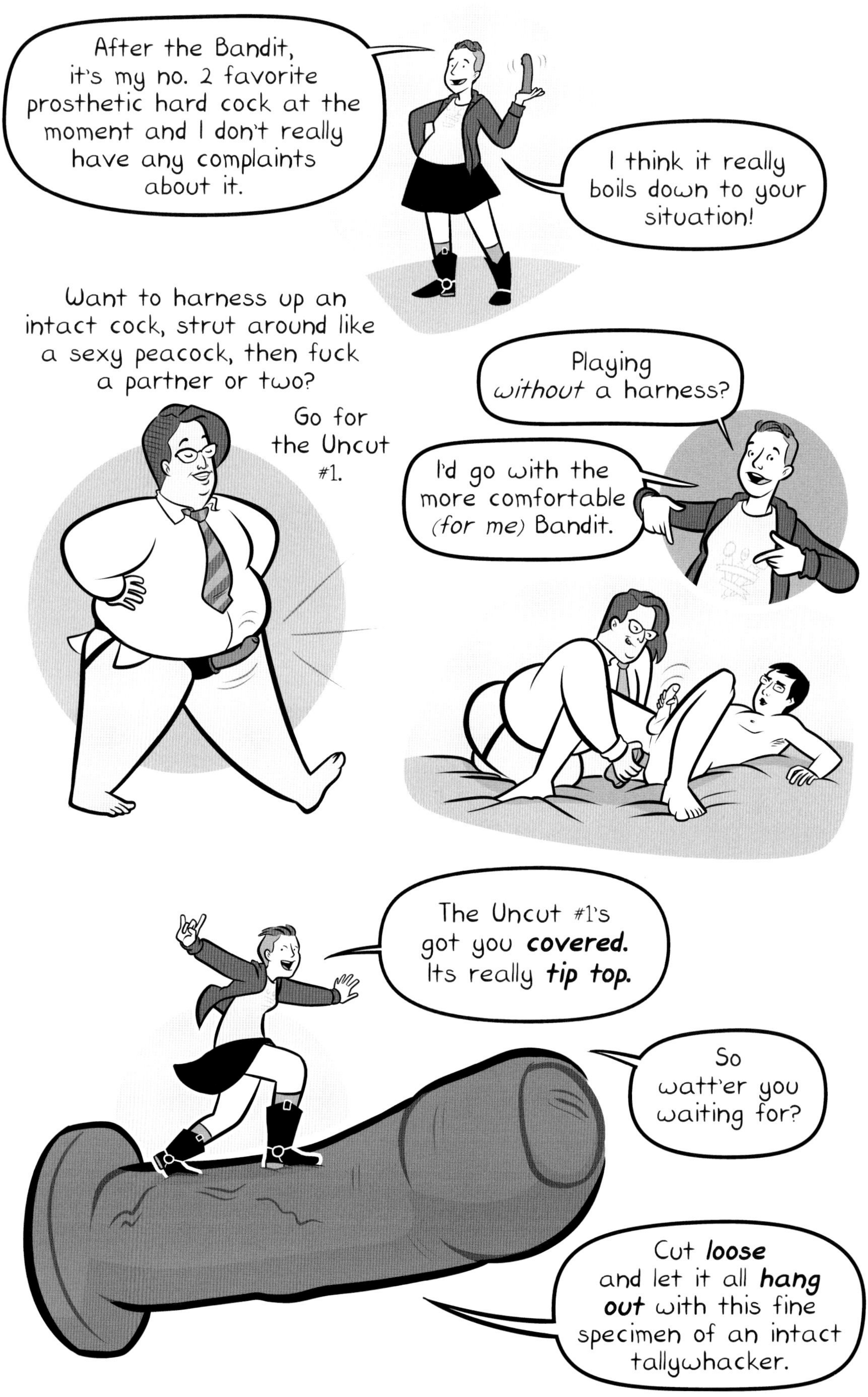
After the Bandit, it's my no. 2 favorite prosthetic hard cock at the moment and I don't really have any complaints about it.
I think it really boils down to your situation!
Want to harness up an intact cock, strut around like a sexy peacock, then fuck a partner or two?
Go for the Uncut #1.
Playing *without* a harness?
I'd go with the more comfortable *(for me)* Bandit.
The Uncut #1's got you **covered.** Its really **tip top.**
So watt'er you waiting for?
Cut **loose** and let it all **hang out** with this fine specimen of an intact tallywhacker.

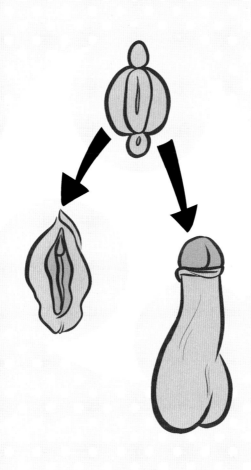

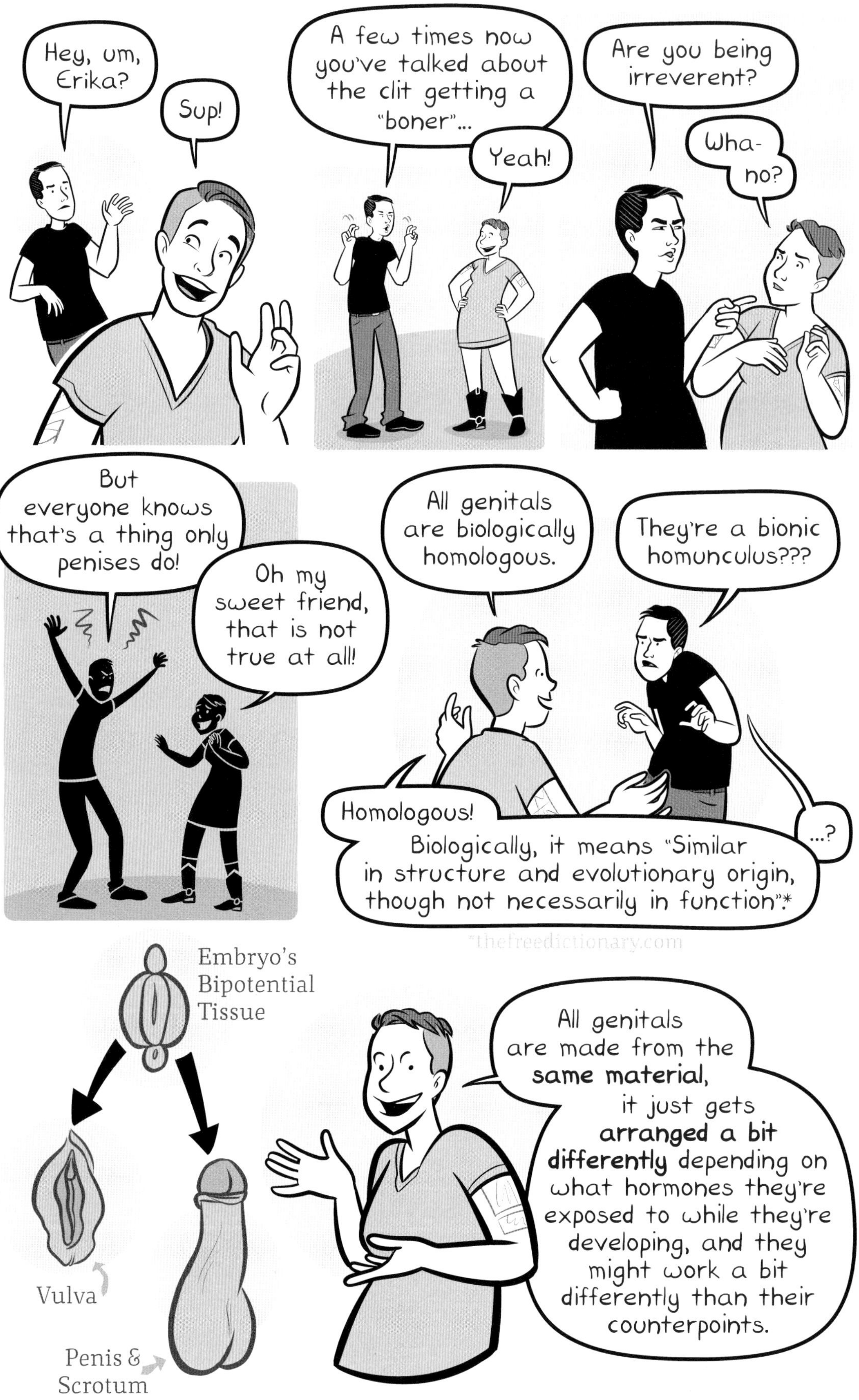

Hey, um, Erika?
Sup!
A few times now you've talked about the clit getting a "boner"...
Yeah!
Are you being irreverent?
Wha- no?
But everyone knows that's a thing only penises do!
Oh my sweet friend, that is not true at all!
All genitals are biologically homologous.
They're a bionic homunculus???
Homologous! Biologically, it means "Similar in structure and evolutionary origin, though not necessarily in function".*
...?
*thefreedictionary.com
Embryo's Bipotential Tissue
Vulva
Penis & Scrotum
All genitals are made from the **same material**, it just gets **arranged a bit differently** depending on what hormones they're exposed to while they're developing, and they might work a bit differently than their counterpoints.

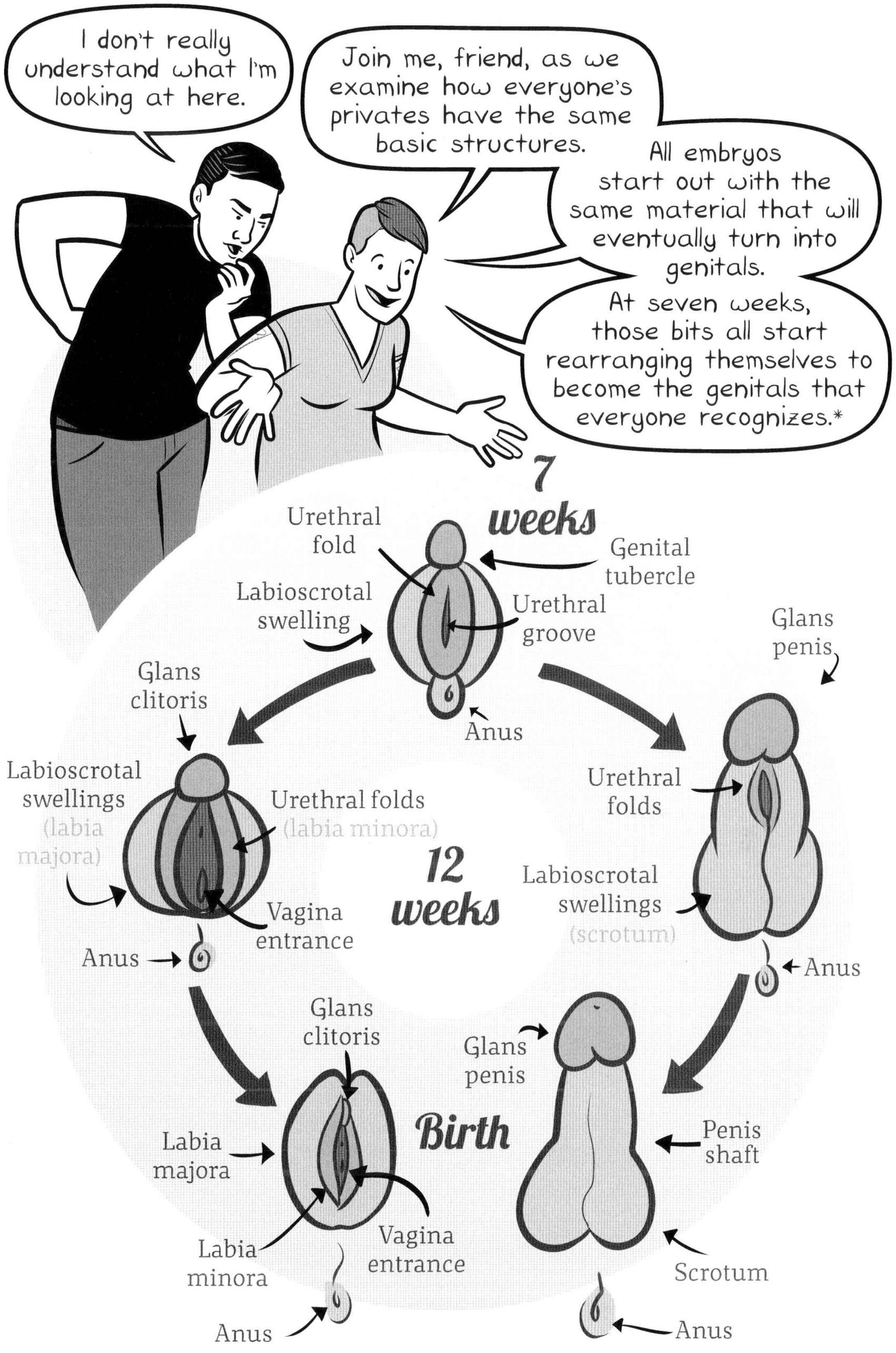
I don't really understand what I'm looking at here.
Join me, friend, as we examine how everyone's privates have the same basic structures.
All embryos start out with the same material that will eventually turn into genitals.
At seven weeks, those bits all start rearranging themselves to become the genitals that everyone recognizes.*
7 weeks
Urethral fold
Genital tubercle
Labioscrotal swelling
Urethral groove
Anus
Glans clitoris
Labioscrotal swellings (labia majora)
Urethral folds (labia minora)
Vagina entrance
Anus
12 weeks
Glans penis
Urethral folds
Labioscrotal swellings (scrotum)
Anus
Glans clitoris
Labia majora
Labia minora
Vagina entrance
Anus
Birth
Glans penis
Penis shaft
Scrotum
Anus

*Some intersex folks can have genitalia that includes a combination of characteristics attributed to typical vulvas and penises/testicles, though being intersex definitely does not always show up in an externally visible way.

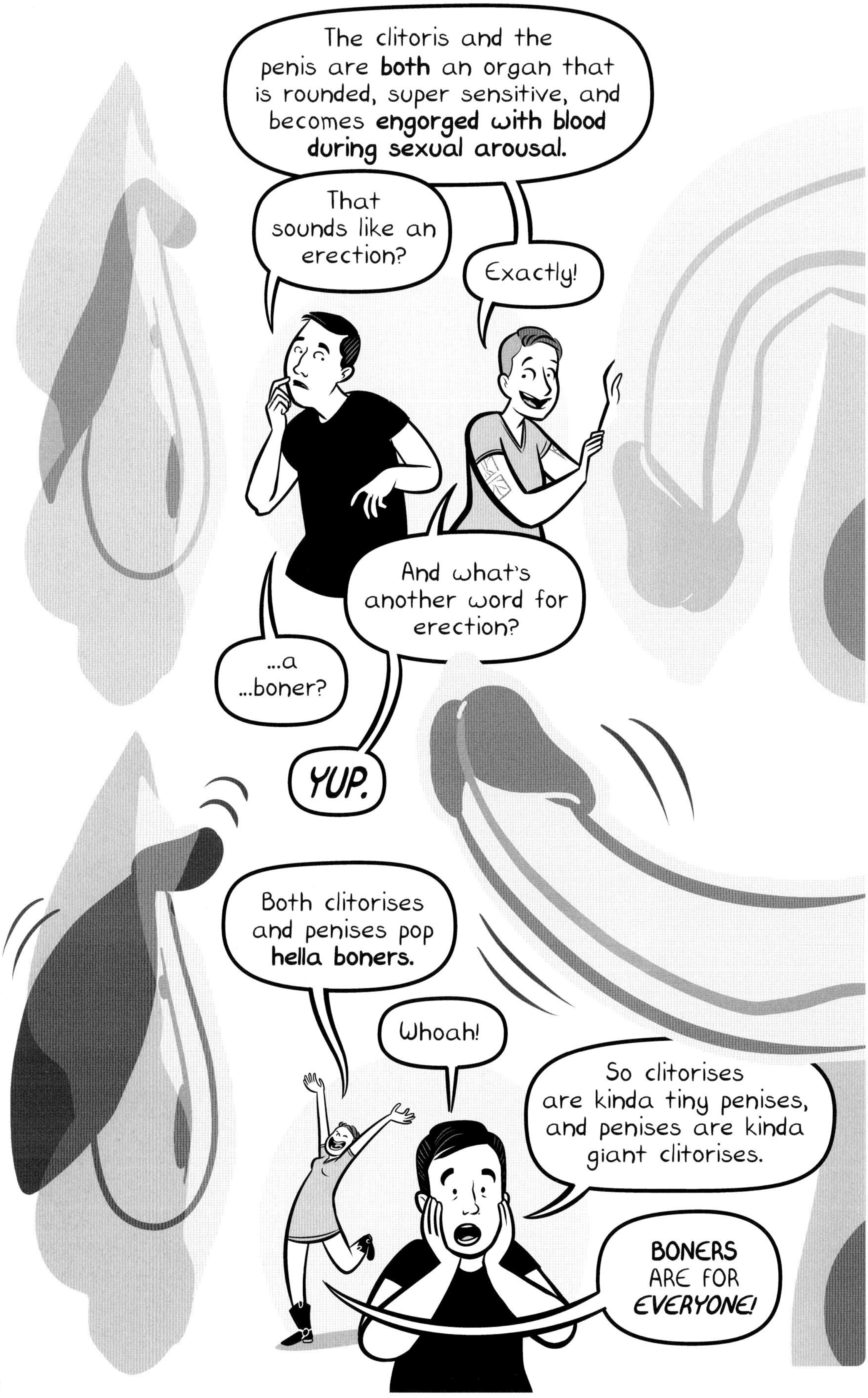
The clitoris and the penis are **both** an organ that is rounded, super sensitive, and becomes **engorged with blood during sexual arousal.**
That sounds like an erection?
Exactly!
And what's another word for erection?
...a ...boner?
YUP.
Both clitorises and penises pop **hella boners.**
Whoah!
So clitorises are kinda tiny penises, and penises are kinda giant clitorises.
BONERS ARE FOR *EVERYONE!*

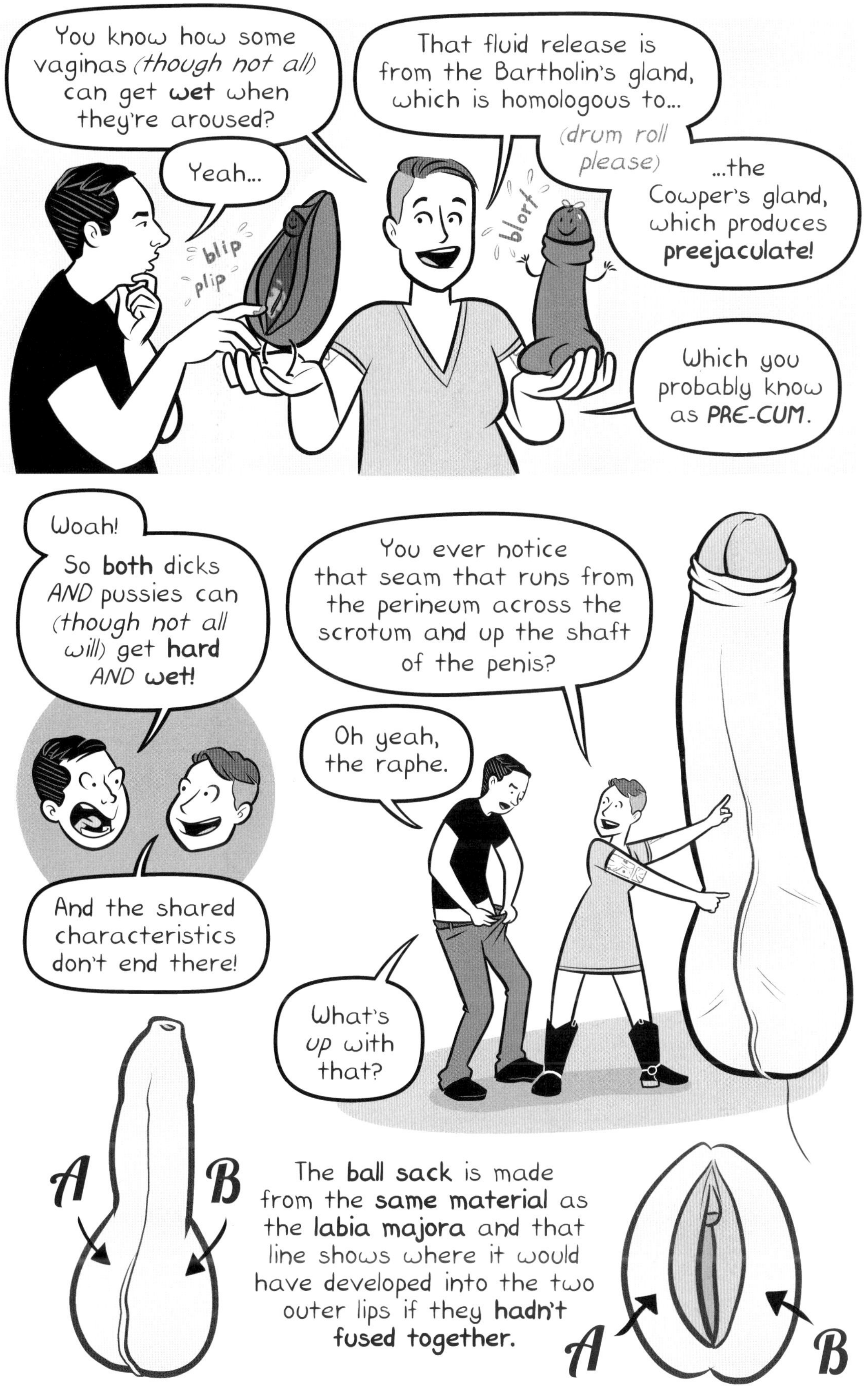
You know how some vaginas (though not all) can get wet when they're aroused?
Yeah...
blip
plip
That fluid release is from the Bartholin's gland, which is homologous to...
(drum roll please)
...the Cowper's gland, which produces preejaculate!
blorf
Which you probably know as PRE-CUM.
Woah! So both dicks AND pussies can (though not all will) get hard AND wet!
And the shared characteristics don't end there!
You ever notice that seam that runs from the perineum across the scrotum and up the shaft of the penis?
Oh yeah, the raphe.
What's up with that?
A
B
The ball sack is made from the same material as the labia majora and that line shows where it would have developed into the two outer lips if they hadn't fused together.
A
B

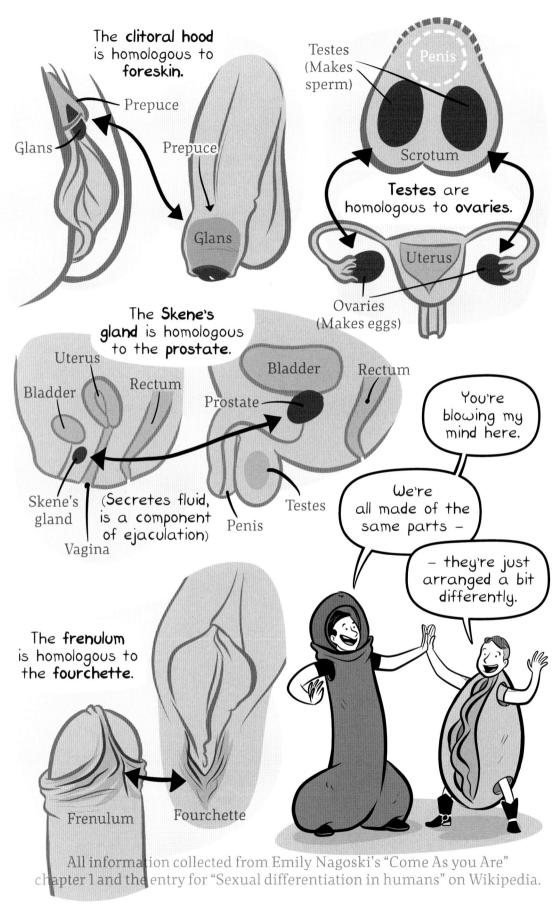

The **clitoral hood** is homologous to **foreskin**.

Prepuce

Glans

Prepuce

Glans

Testes (Makes sperm)

Penis

Scrotum

Testes are homologous to **ovaries**.

Uterus

Ovaries (Makes eggs)

The **Skene's gland** is homologous to the **prostate**.

Uterus

Bladder

Rectum

Bladder

Rectum

Prostate

Skene's gland

(Secretes fluid, is a component of ejaculation)

Testes

Penis

Vagina

You're blowing my mind here.

We're all made of the same parts —

— they're just arranged a bit differently.

The **frenulum** is homologous to the **fourchette**.

Frenulum

Fourchette

All information collected from Emily Nagoski's "Come As you Are" chapter 1 and the entry for "Sexual differentiation in humans" on Wikipedia.

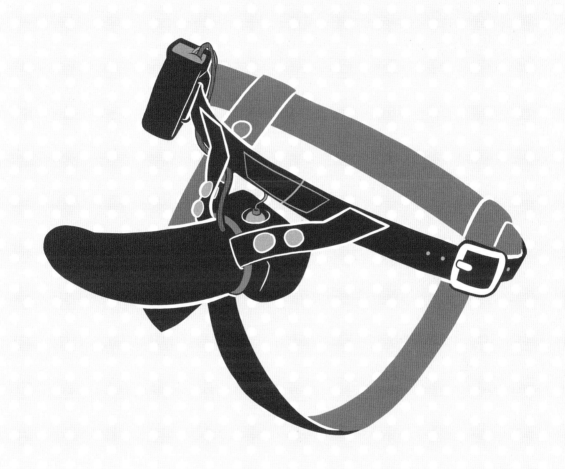

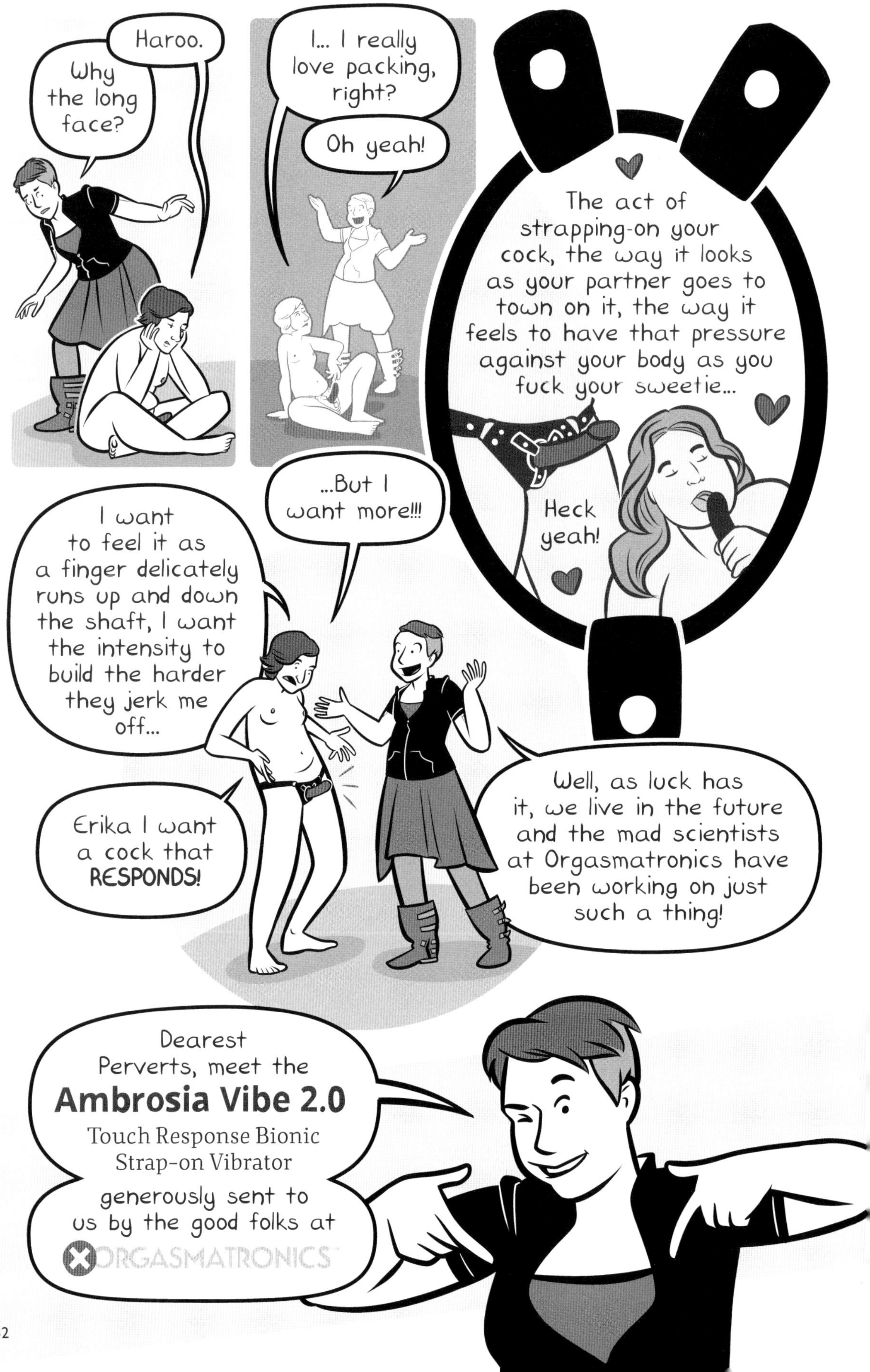
Why the long face?
Haroo.
I... I really love packing, right?
Oh yeah!
The act of strapping-on your cock, the way it looks as your partner goes to town on it, the way it feels to have that pressure against your body as you fuck your sweetie...
Heck yeah!
I want to feel it as a finger delicately runs up and down the shaft, I want the intensity to build the harder they jerk me off...
...But I want more!!!
Erika I want a cock that **RESPONDS!**
Well, as luck has it, we live in the future and the mad scientists at Orgasmatronics have been working on just such a thing!
Dearest Perverts, meet the
Ambrosia Vibe 2.0
Touch Response Bionic Strap-on Vibrator
generously sent to us by the good folks at
ORGASMATRONICS

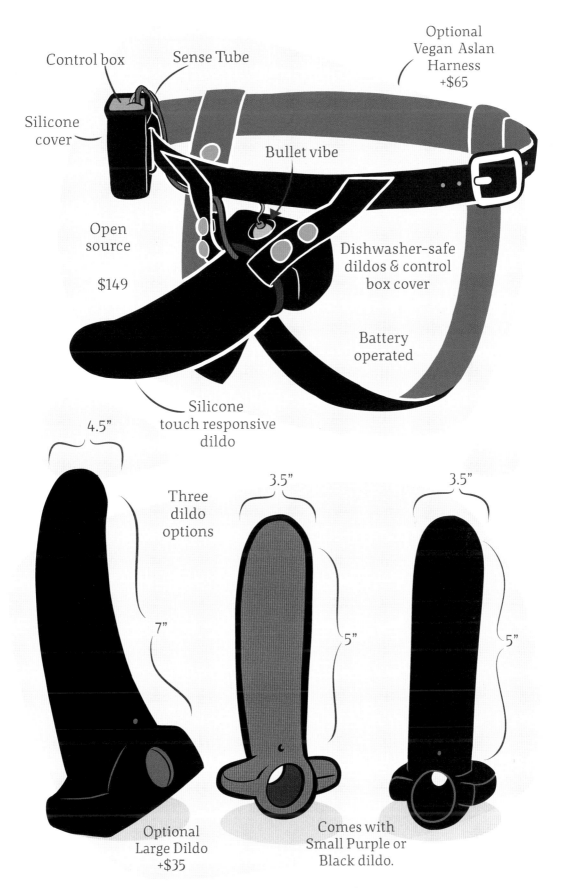

Control box

Sense Tube

Optional
Vegan Aslan
Harness
+$65

Silicone
cover

Bullet vibe

Open
source

$149

Dishwasher-safe
dildos & control
box cover

Battery
operated

Silicone
touch responsive
dildo

4.5"

Three
dildo
options

3.5"

3.5"

7"

5"

5"

Optional
Large Dildo
+$35

Comes with
Small Purple or
Black dildo.

All silicone medical-grade.

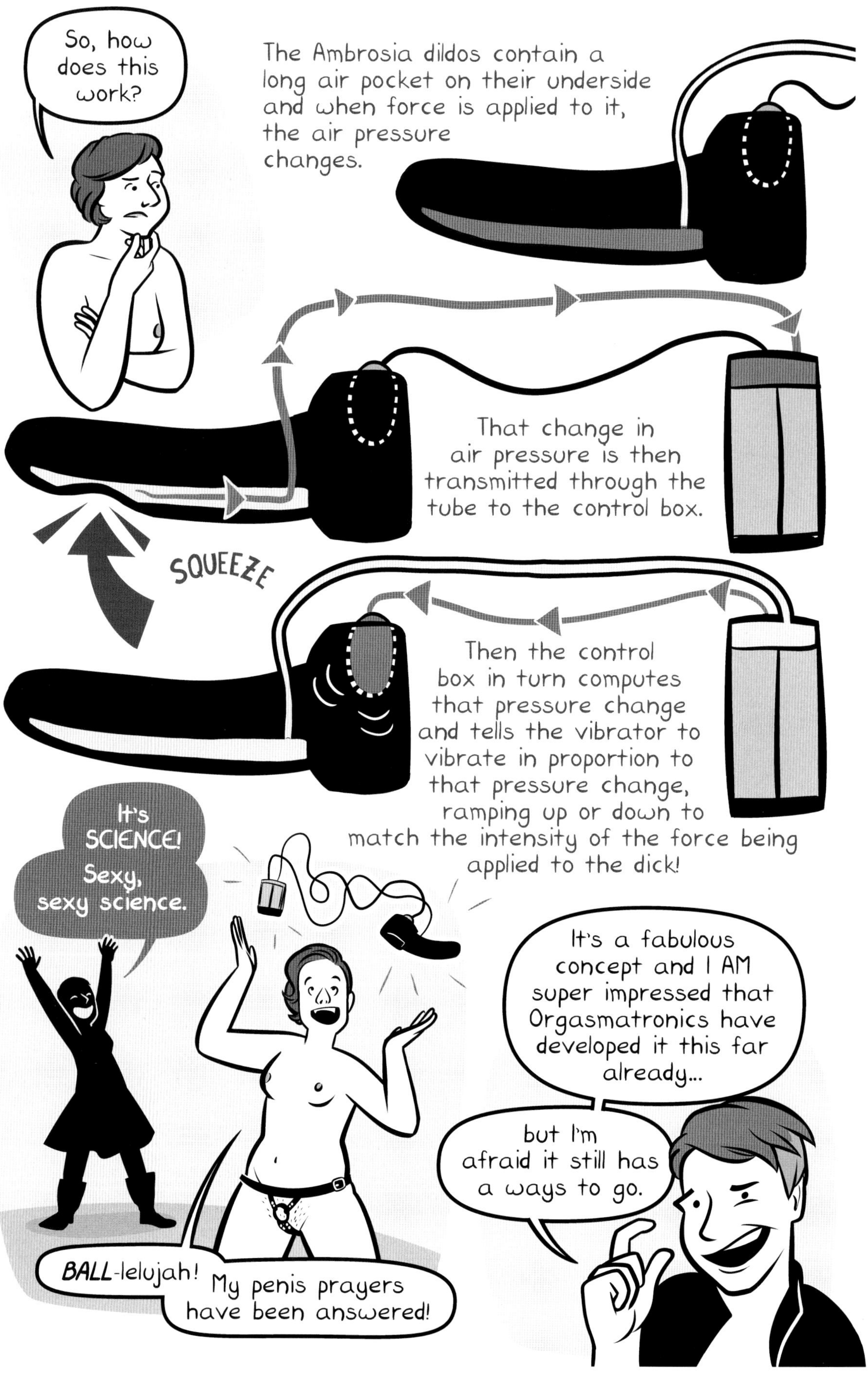

So, how does this work?
The Ambrosia dildos contain a long air pocket on their underside and when force is applied to it, the air pressure changes.
That change in air pressure is then transmitted through the tube to the control box.
SQUEEZE
Then the control box in turn computes that pressure change and tells the vibrator to vibrate in proportion to that pressure change, ramping up or down to match the intensity of the force being applied to the dick!
It's SCIENCE! Sexy, sexy science.
BALL-lelujah!
My penis prayers have been answered!
It's a fabulous concept and I AM super impressed that Orgasmatronics have developed it this far already...
but I'm afraid it still has a ways to go.

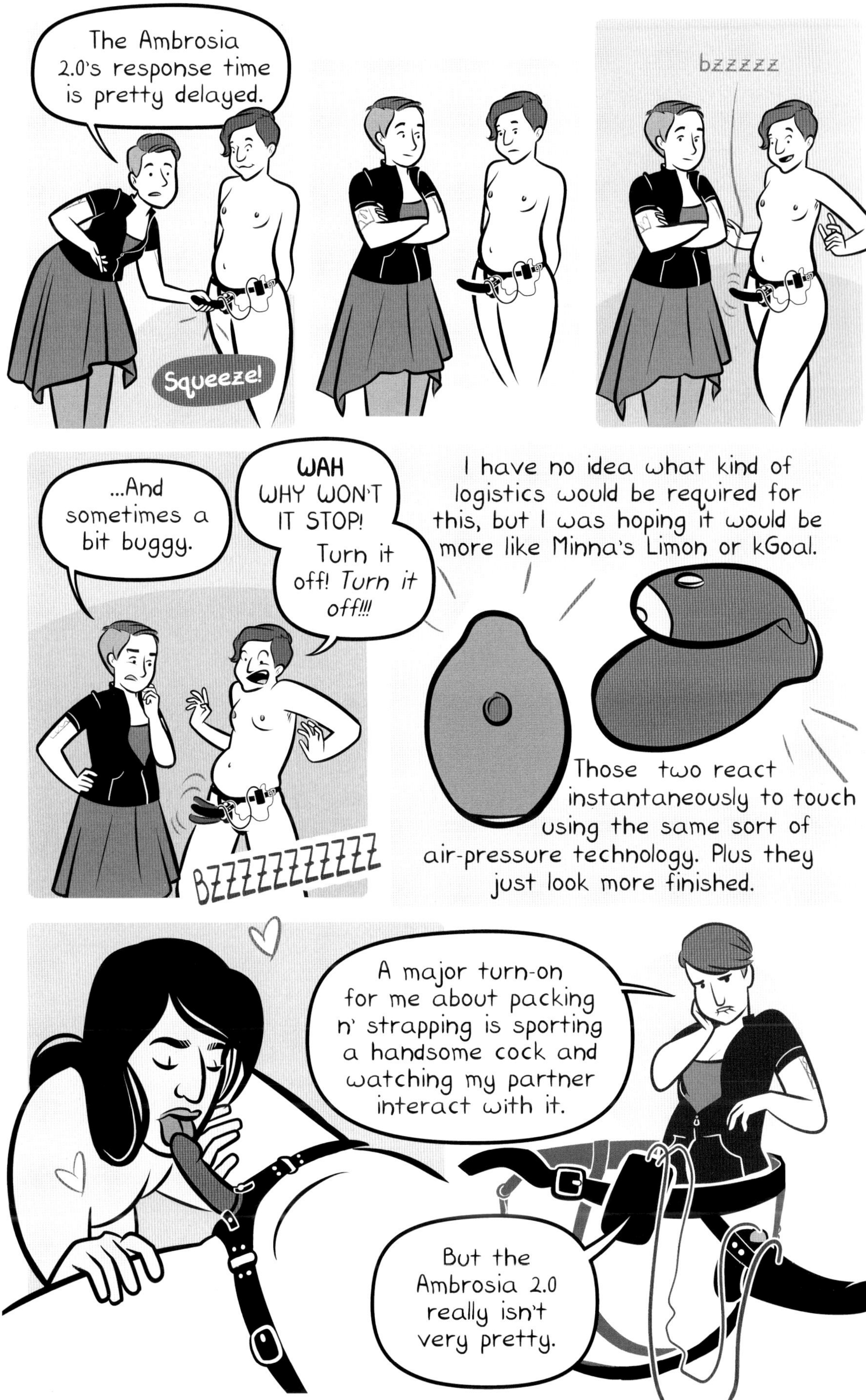
The Ambrosia 2.0's response time is pretty delayed.
Squeeze!
bzzzzz
...And sometimes a bit buggy.
WAH
WHY WON'T IT STOP!
Turn it off! Turn it off!!!
BZZZZZZZZZZZ
I have no idea what kind of logistics would be required for this, but I was hoping it would be more like Minna's Limon or kGoal.
Those two react instantaneously to touch using the same sort of air-pressure technology. Plus they just look more finished.
A major turn-on for me about packing n' strapping is sporting a handsome cock and watching my partner interact with it.
But the Ambrosia 2.0 really isn't very pretty.

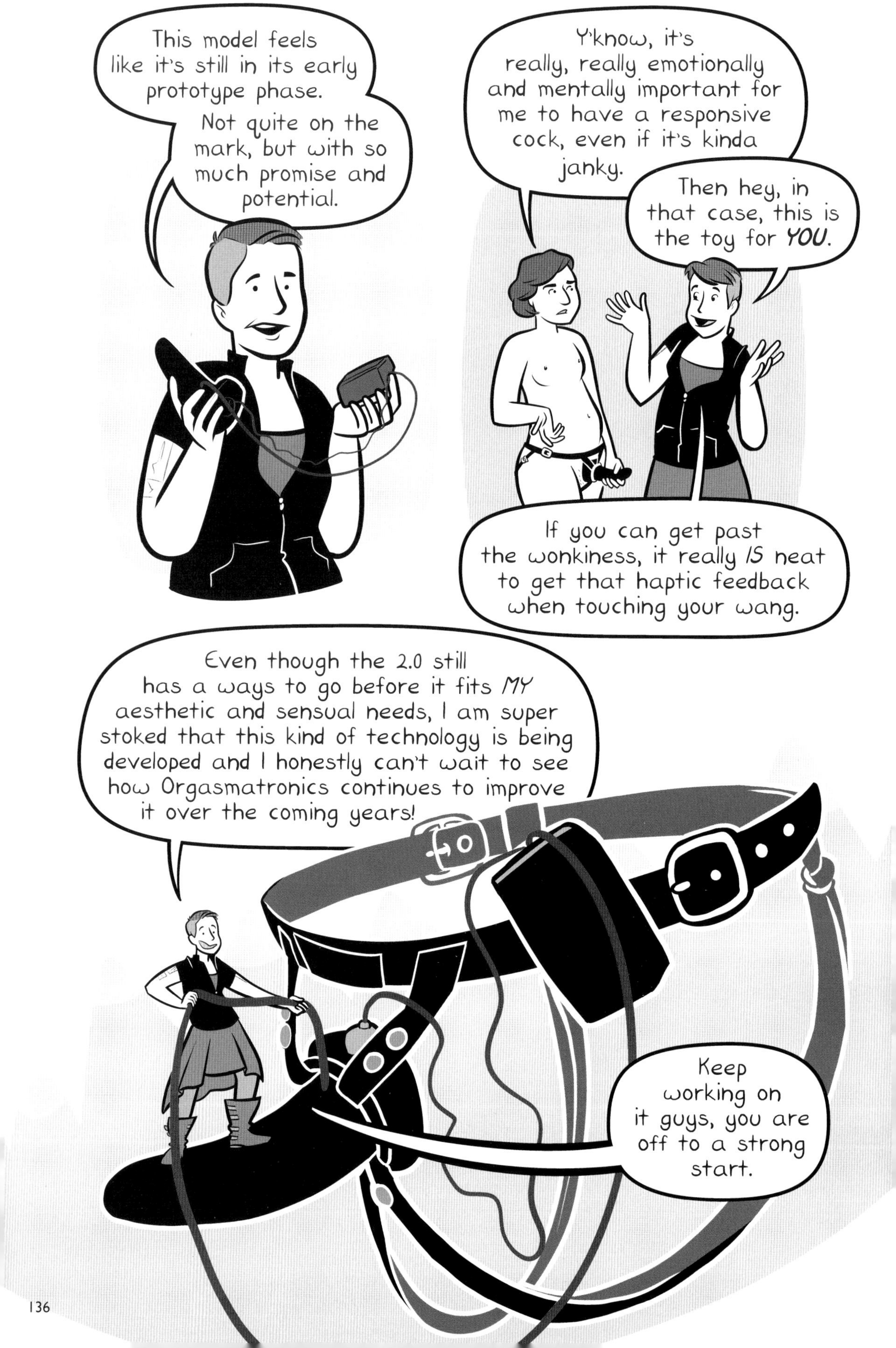
This model feels like it's still in its early prototype phase.
Not quite on the mark, but with so much promise and potential.
Y'know, it's really, really emotionally and mentally important for me to have a responsive cock, even if it's kinda janky.
Then hey, in that case, this is the toy for YOU.
If you can get past the wonkiness, it really IS neat to get that haptic feedback when touching your wang.
Even though the 2.0 still has a ways to go before it fits MY aesthetic and sensual needs, I am super stoked that this kind of technology is being developed and I honestly can't wait to see how Orgasmatronics continues to improve it over the coming years!
Keep working on it guys, you are off to a strong start.

STAG

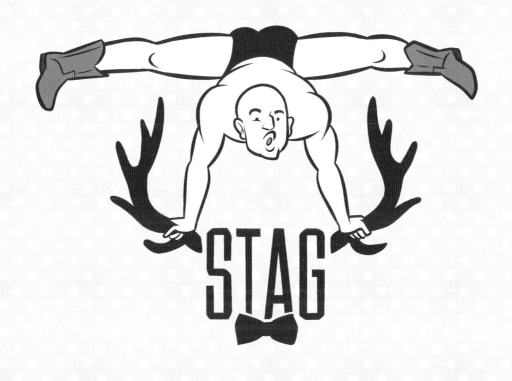

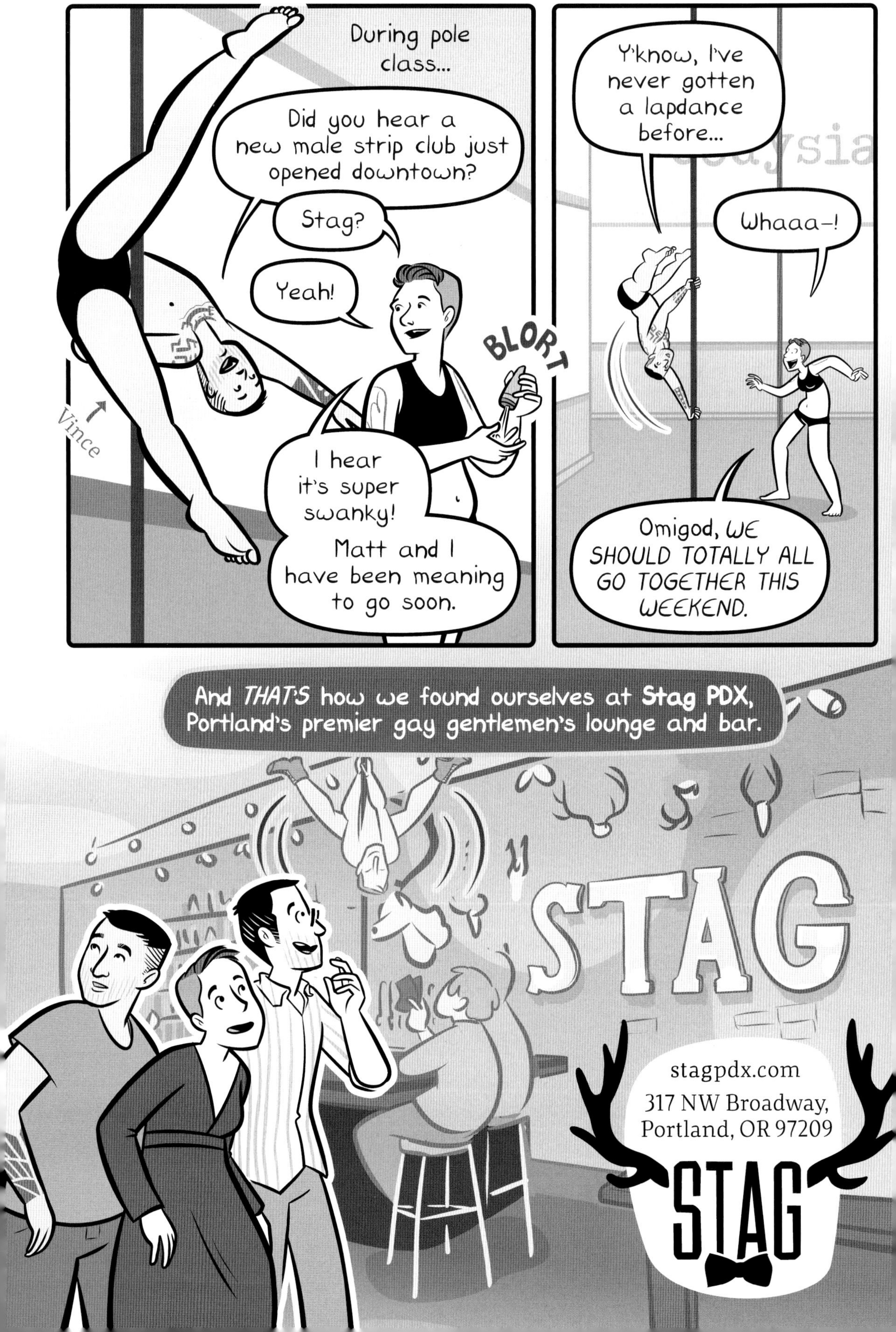
During pole class...
Did you hear a new male strip club just opened downtown?
Stag?
Yeah!
Vince
BLORT
I hear it's super swanky!
Matt and I have been meaning to go soon.
Y'know, I've never gotten a lapdance before...
Whaaa–!
Omigod, WE SHOULD TOTALLY ALL GO TOGETHER THIS WEEKEND.
And THAT'S how we found ourselves at Stag PDX, Portland's premier gay gentlemen's lounge and bar.
STAG
stagpdx.com
317 NW Broadway, Portland, OR 97209
STAG

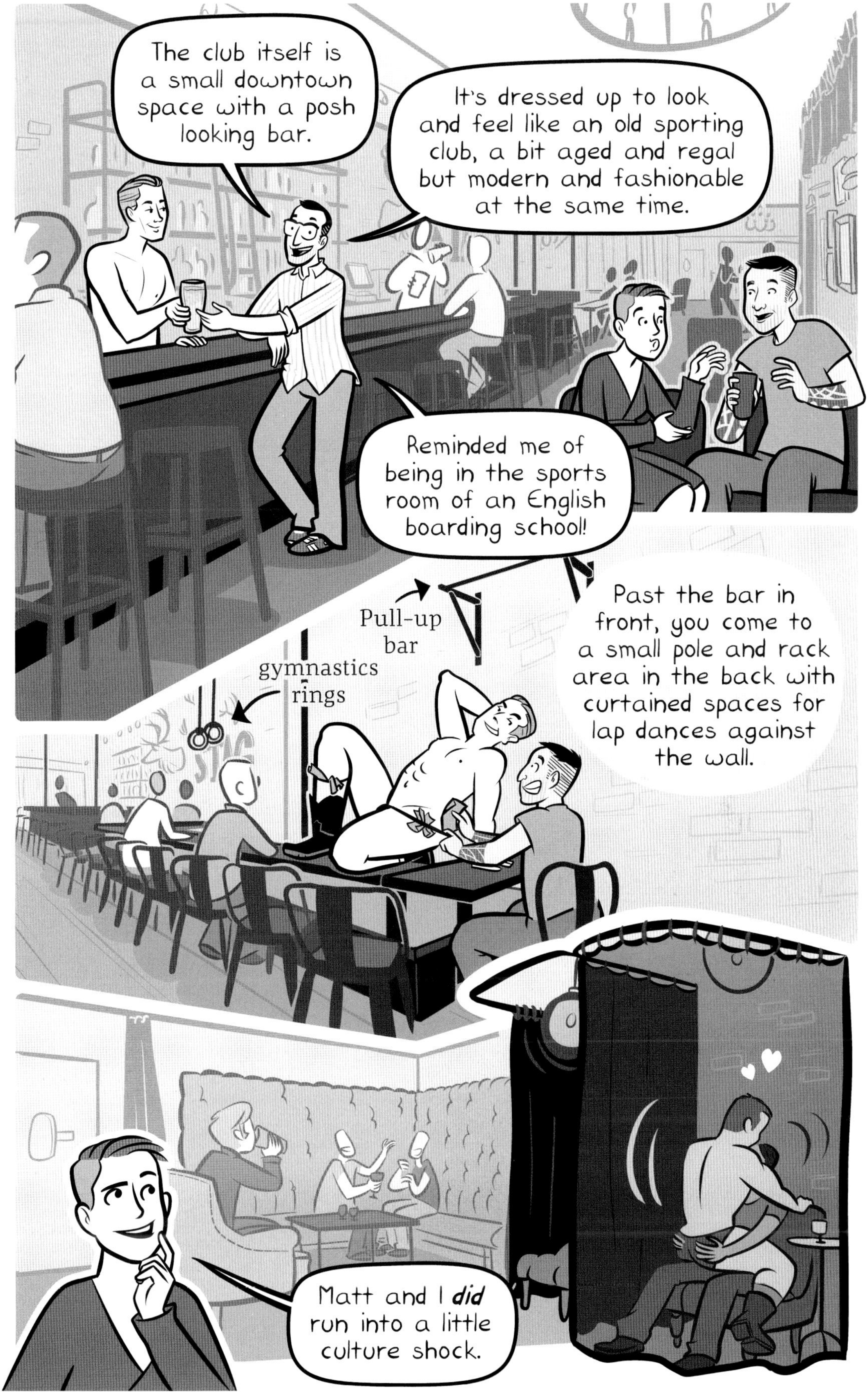
The club itself is a small downtown space with a posh looking bar.
It's dressed up to look and feel like an old sporting club, a bit aged and regal but modern and fashionable at the same time.
Reminded me of being in the sports room of an English boarding school!
Pull-up bar
gymnastics rings
Past the bar in front, you come to a small pole and rack area in the back with curtained spaces for lap dances against the wall.
Matt and I ***did*** run into a little culture shock.

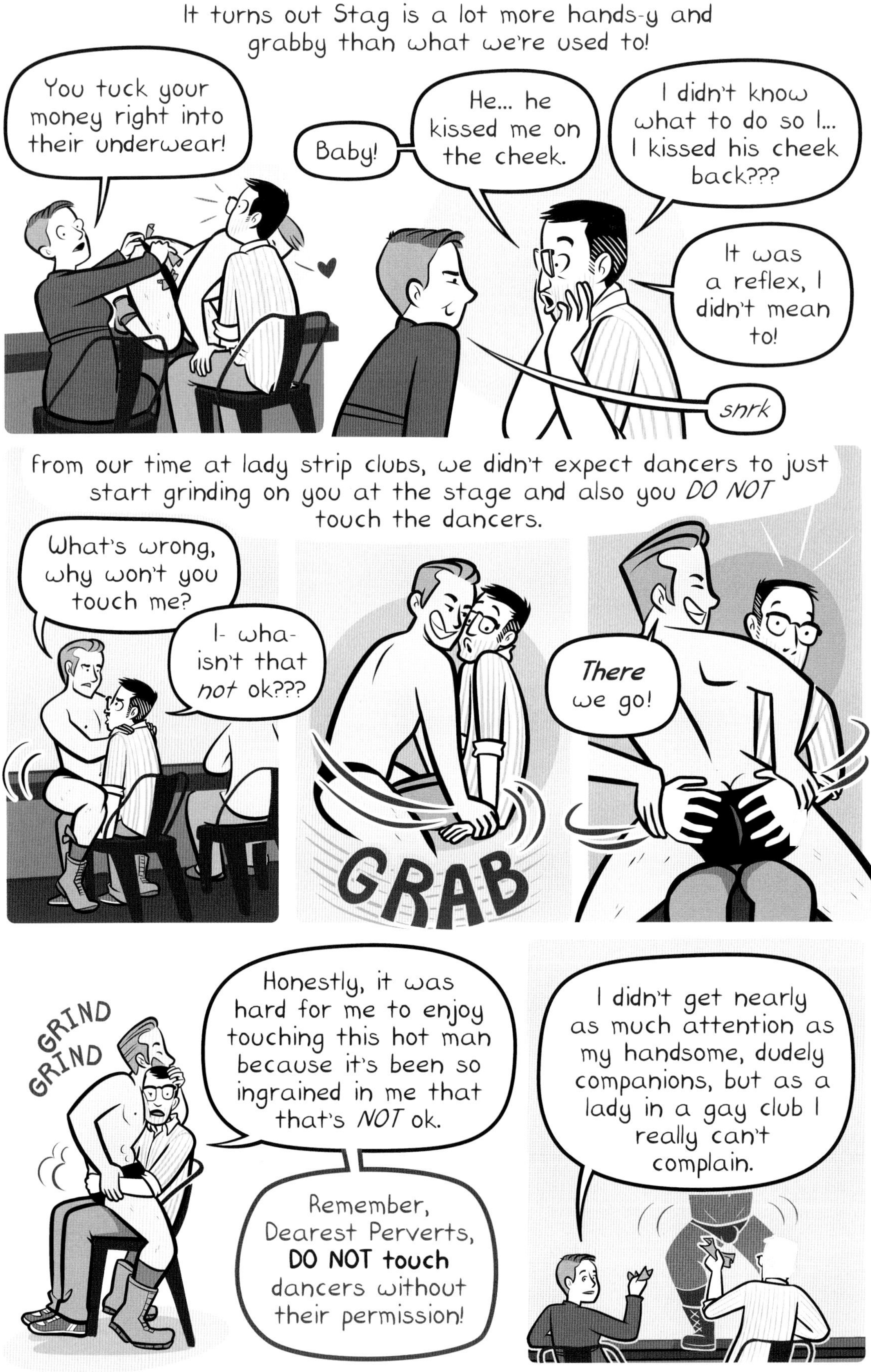
It turns out Stag is a lot more hands-y and grabby than what we're used to!
You tuck your money right into their underwear!
Baby!
He... he kissed me on the cheek.
I didn't know what to do so I... I kissed his cheek back???
It was a reflex, I didn't mean to!
snrk
From our time at lady strip clubs, we didn't expect dancers to just start grinding on you at the stage and also you *DO NOT* touch the dancers.
What's wrong, why won't you touch me?
I- wha- isn't that *not* ok???
GRAB
There we go!
GRIND GRIND
Honestly, it was hard for me to enjoy touching this hot man because it's been so ingrained in me that that's *NOT* ok.
Remember, Dearest Perverts, **DO NOT touch** dancers without their permission!
I didn't get nearly as much attention as my handsome, dudely companions, but as a lady in a gay club I really can't complain.

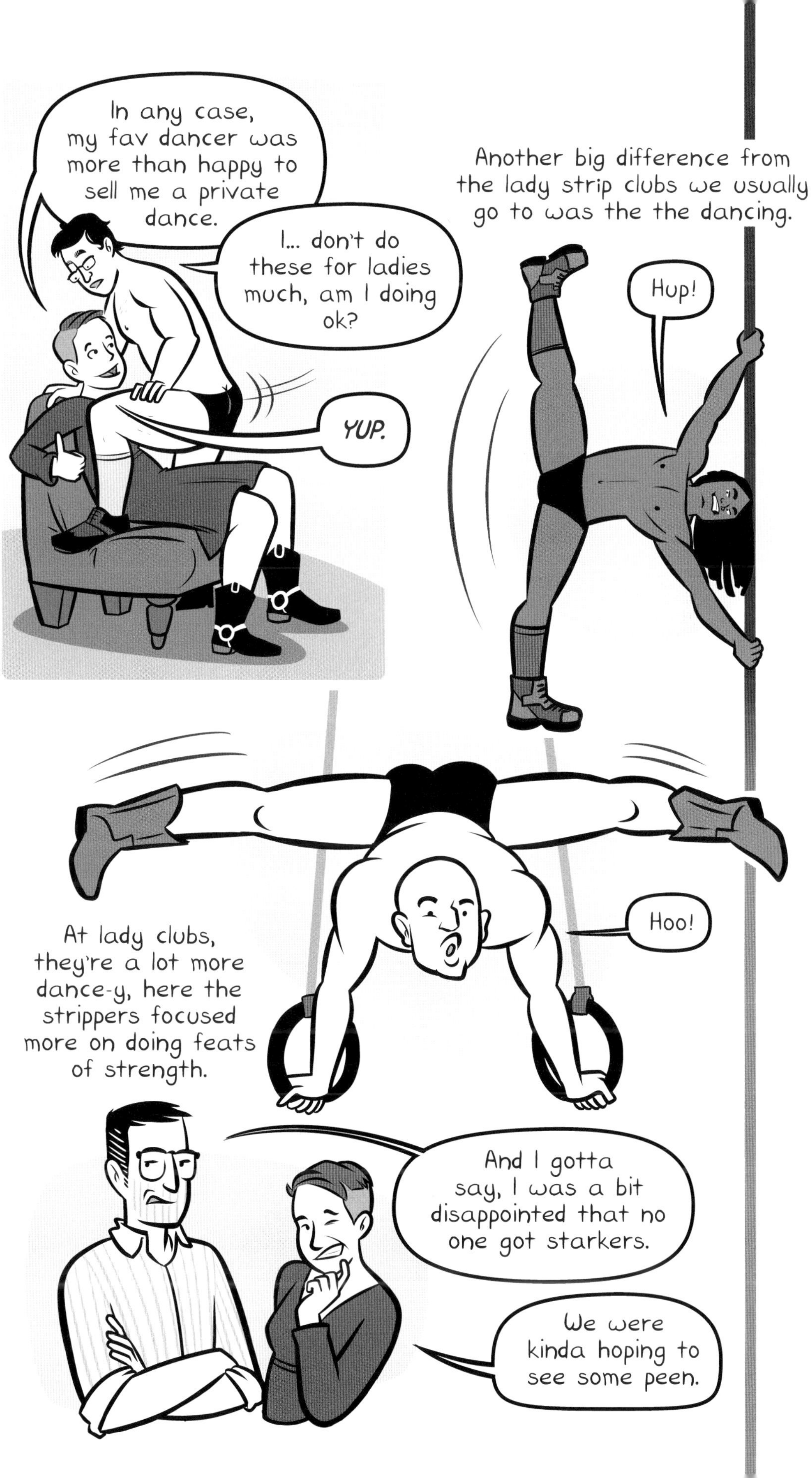
In any case, my fav dancer was more than happy to sell me a private dance.
I... don't do these for ladies much, am I doing ok?
YUP.
Another big difference from the lady strip clubs we usually go to was the the dancing.
Hup!
Hoo!
At lady clubs, they're a lot more dance-y, here the strippers focused more on doing feats of strength.
And I gotta say, I was a bit disappointed that no one got starkers.
We were kinda hoping to see some peen.

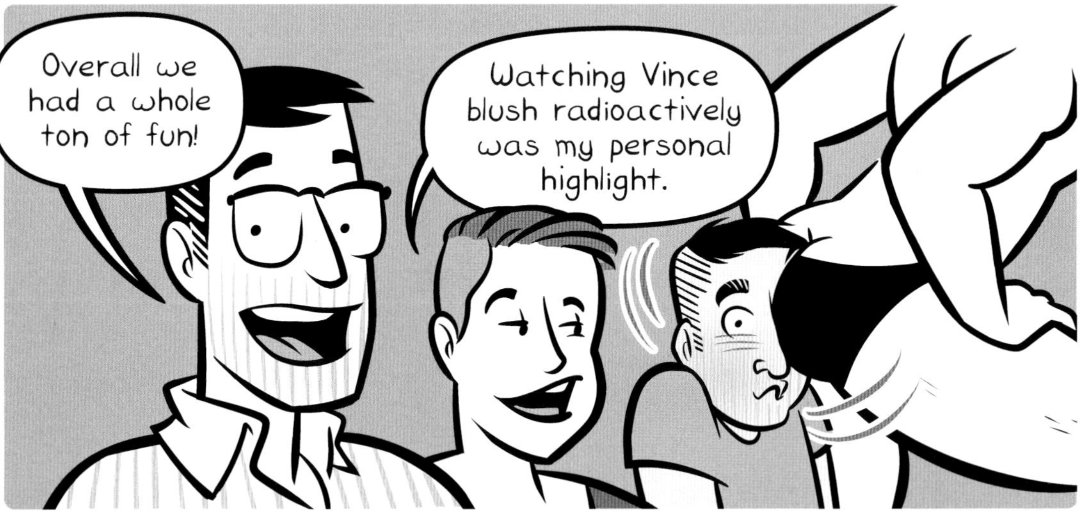
Overall we had a whole ton of fun!
Watching Vince blush radioactively was my personal highlight.

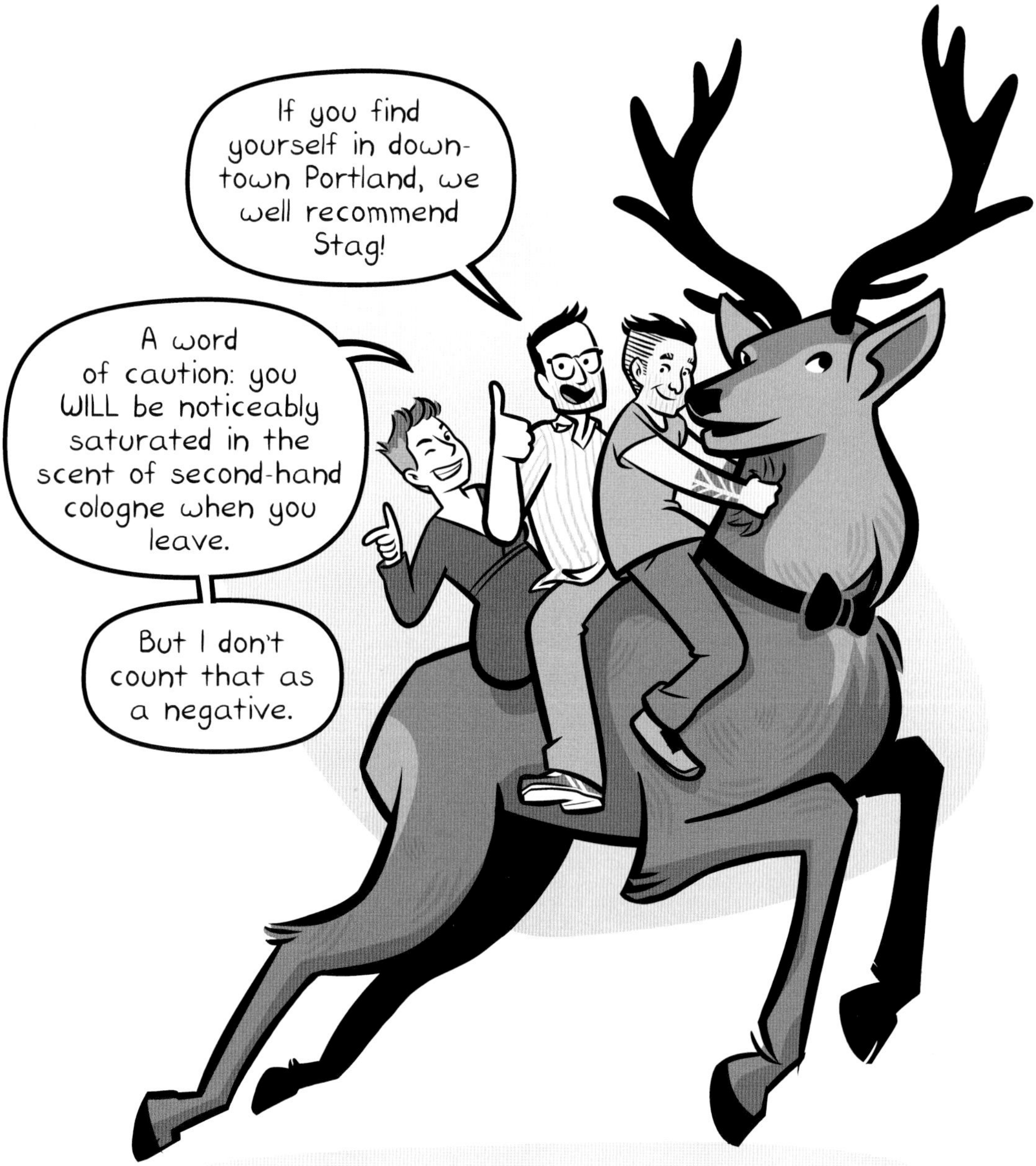
If you find yourself in down-town Portland, we well recommend Stag!
A word of caution: you WILL be noticeably saturated in the scent of second-hand cologne when you leave.
But I don't count that as a negative.

CLAP!

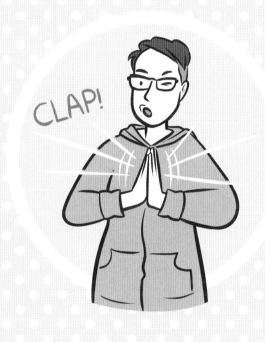

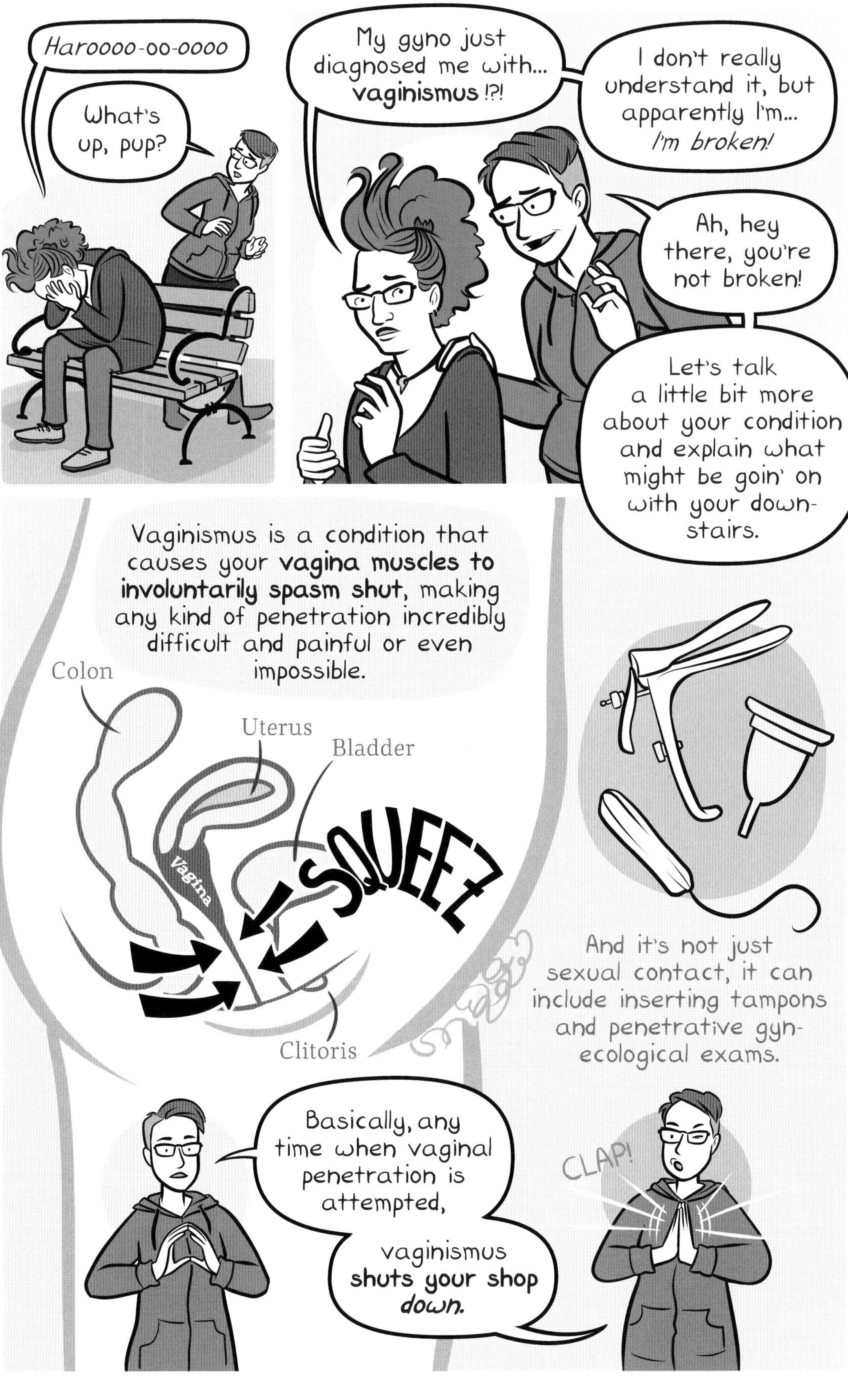

Haroooo-oo-oooo
What's up, pup?
My gyno just diagnosed me with... **vaginismus** !?!
I don't really understand it, but apparently I'm... *I'm broken!*
Ah, hey there, you're not broken!
Let's talk a little bit more about your condition and explain what might be goin' on with your down-stairs.
Vaginismus is a condition that causes your **vagina muscles to involuntarily spasm shut**, making any kind of penetration incredibly difficult and painful or even impossible.
Colon
Uterus
Bladder
Vagina
SQUEEZ
Clitoris
And it's not just sexual contact, it can include inserting tampons and penetrative gyn-ecological exams.
Basically, any time when vaginal penetration is attempted,
vaginismus **shuts your shop** ***down.***
CLAP!

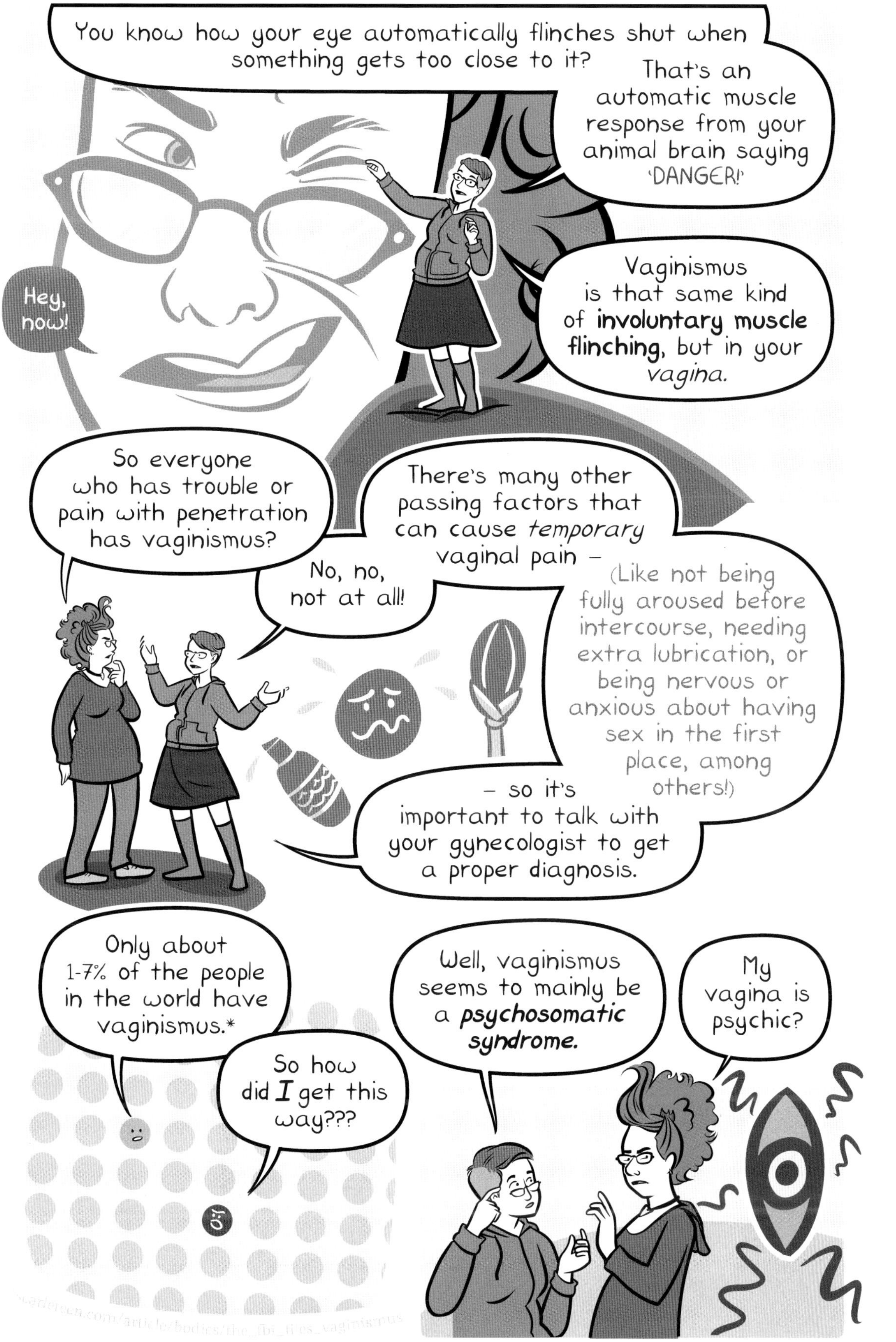
You know how your eye automatically flinches shut when something gets too close to it?
That's an automatic muscle response from your animal brain saying 'DANGER!'
Hey, now!
Vaginismus is that same kind of **involuntary muscle flinching**, but in your *vagina.*
So everyone who has trouble or pain with penetration has vaginismus?
No, no, not at all!
There's many other passing factors that can cause *temporary* vaginal pain –
(Like not being fully aroused before intercourse, needing extra lubrication, or being nervous or anxious about having sex in the first place, among others!)
– so it's important to talk with your gynecologist to get a proper diagnosis.
Only about 1-7% of the people in the world have vaginismus.*
So how did *I* get this way???
Well, vaginismus seems to mainly be a ***psychosomatic syndrome.***
My vagina is psychic?

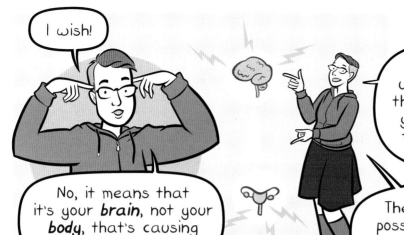

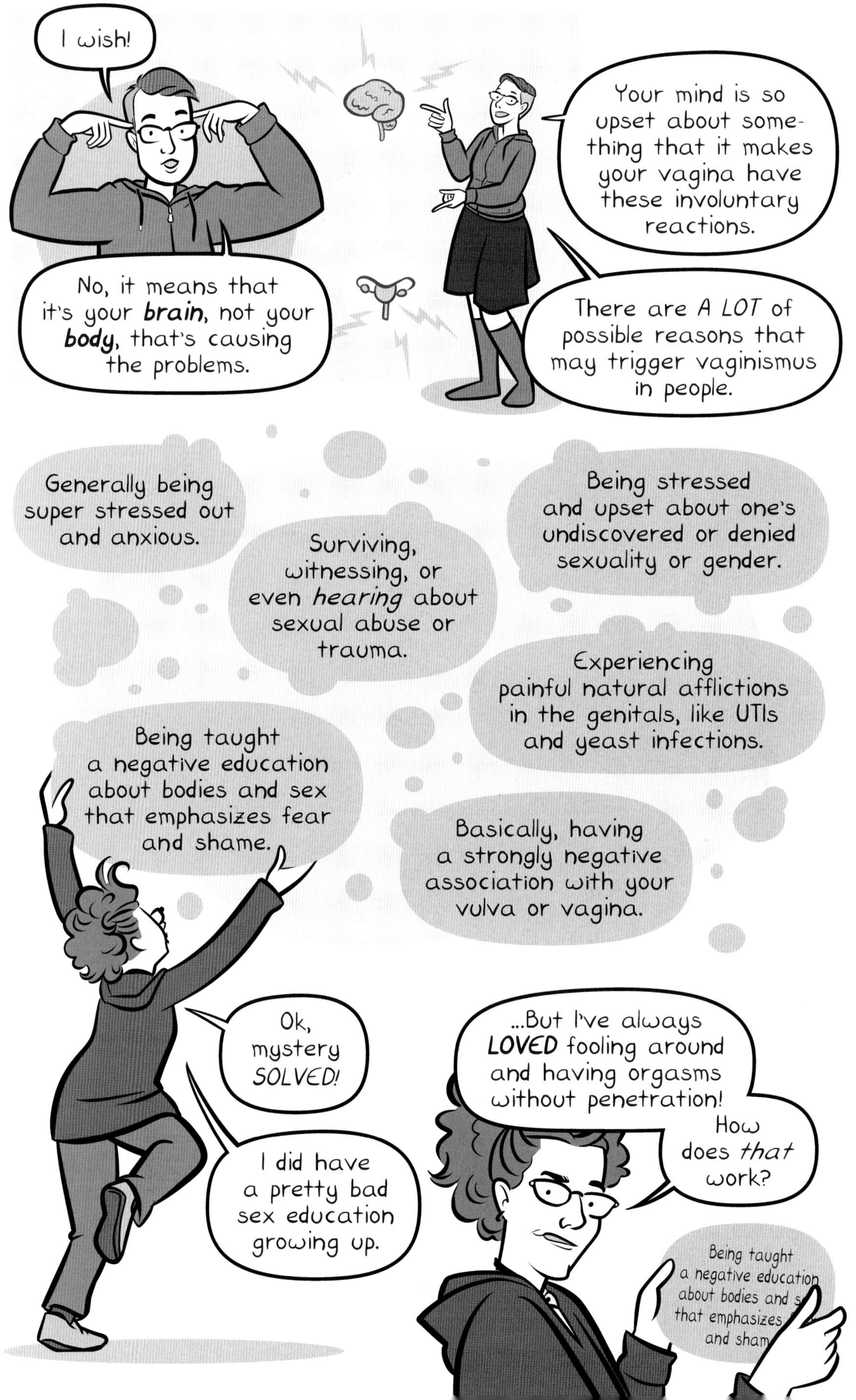

I wish!

Your mind is so upset about something that it makes your vagina have these involuntary reactions.

No, it means that it's your **brain**, not your **body**, that's causing the problems.

There are A LOT of possible reasons that may trigger vaginismus in people.

Generally being super stressed out and anxious.

Surviving, witnessing, or even *hearing* about sexual abuse or trauma.

Being stressed and upset about one's undiscovered or denied sexuality or gender.

Experiencing painful natural afflictions in the genitals, like UTIs and yeast infections.

Being taught a negative education about bodies and sex that emphasizes fear and shame.

Basically, having a strongly negative association with your vulva or vagina.

Ok, mystery SOLVED!

I did have a pretty bad sex education growing up.

...But I've always **LOVED** fooling around and having orgasms without penetration! How does *that* work?

Being taught a negative education about bodies and s that emphasizes and sham

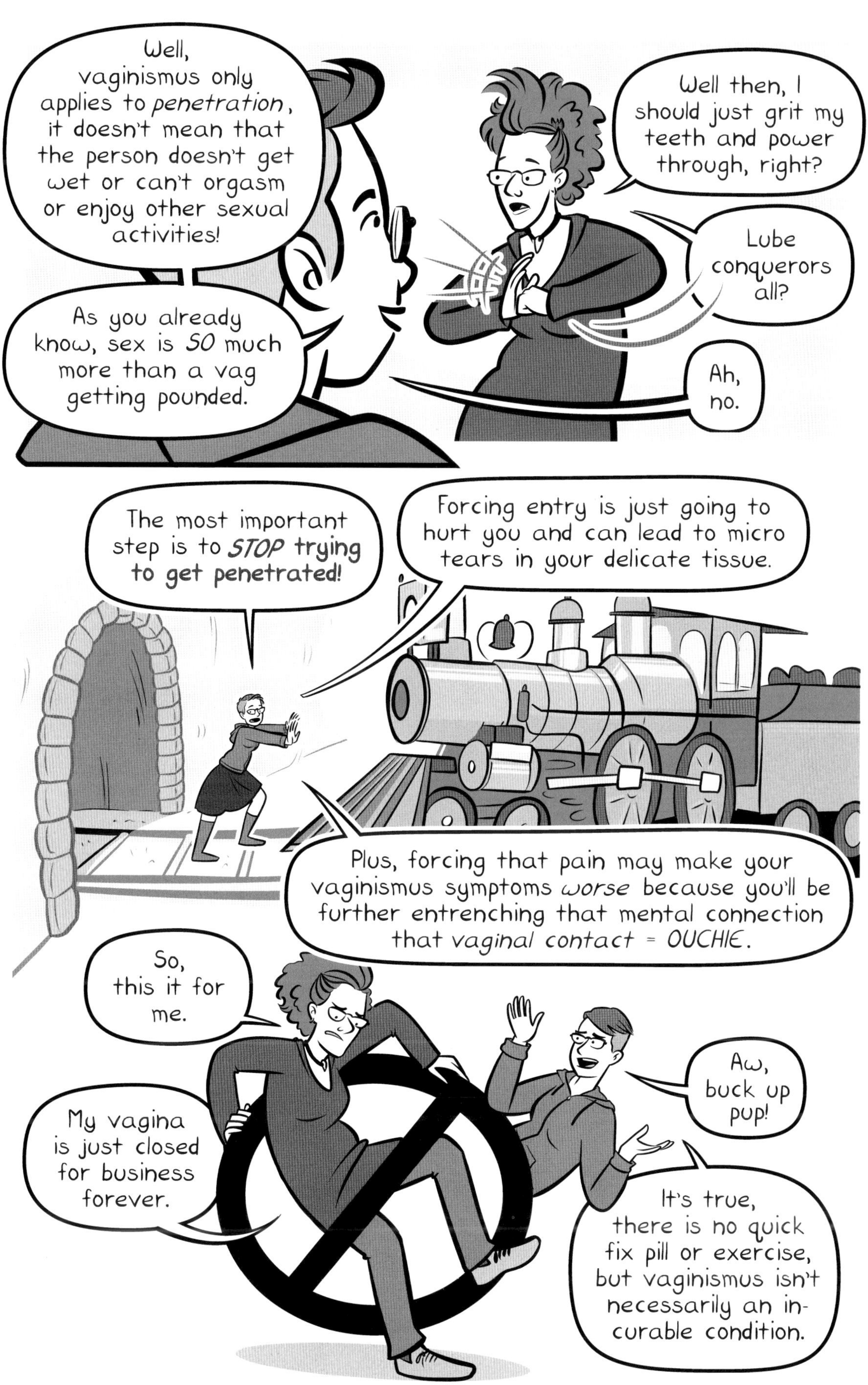
Well, vaginismus only applies to *penetration*, it doesn't mean that the person doesn't get wet or can't orgasm or enjoy other sexual activities!
As you already know, sex is *SO* much more than a vag getting pounded.
Well then, I should just grit my teeth and power through, right?
Lube conquerors all?
Ah, no.
The most important step is to *STOP* trying to get penetrated!
Forcing entry is just going to hurt you and can lead to micro tears in your delicate tissue.
Plus, forcing that pain may make your vaginismus symptoms *worse* because you'll be further entrenching that mental connection that *vaginal contact* = *OUCHIE*.
So, this it for me.
My vagina is just closed for business forever.
Aw, buck up pup!
It's true, there is no quick fix pill or exercise, but vaginismus isn't necessarily an in-curable condition.

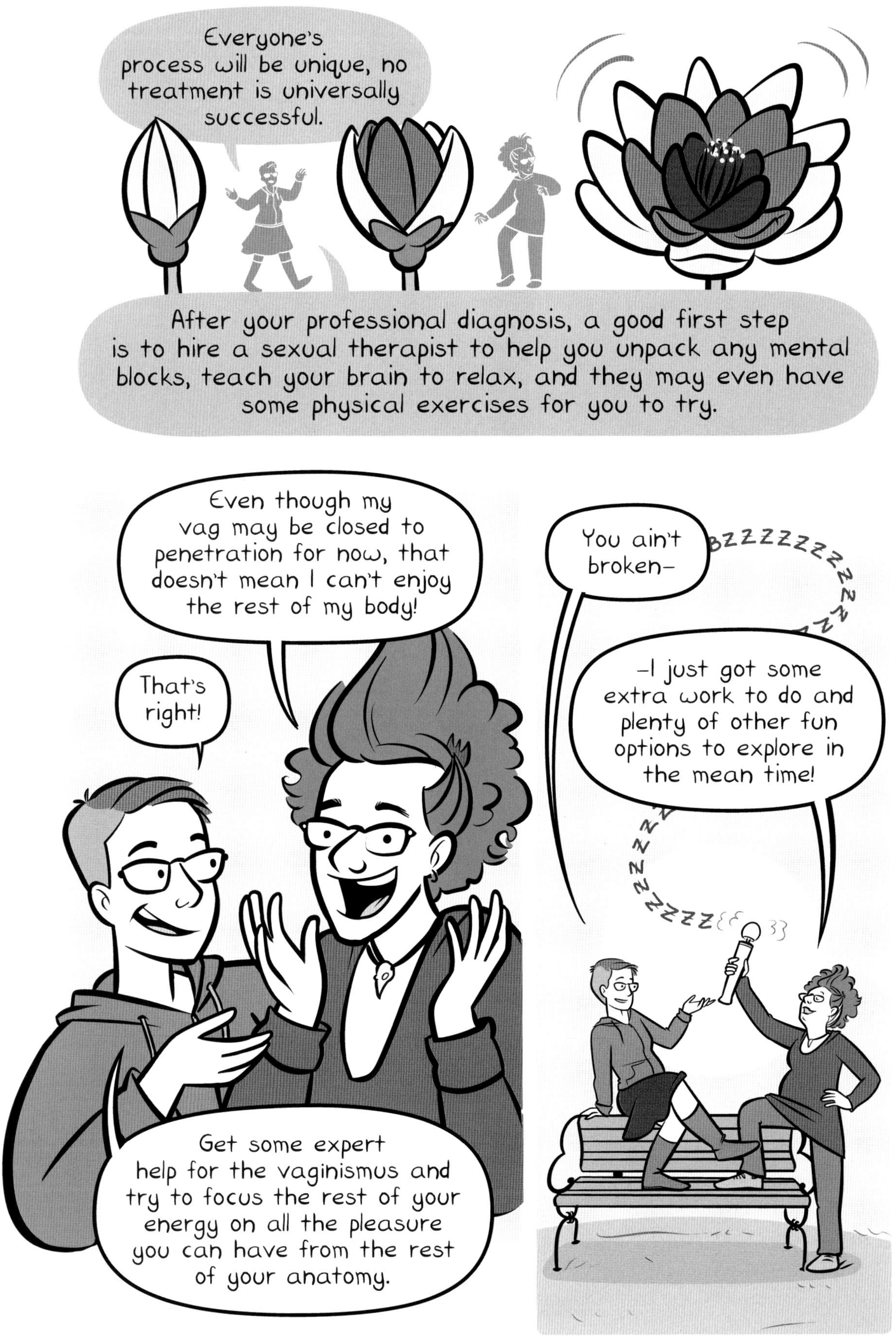
Everyone's process will be unique, no treatment is universally successful.
After your professional diagnosis, a good first step is to hire a sexual therapist to help you unpack any mental blocks, teach your brain to relax, and they may even have some physical exercises for you to try.
Even though my vag may be closed to penetration for now, that doesn't mean I can't enjoy the rest of my body!
That's right!
Get some expert help for the vaginismus and try to focus the rest of your energy on all the pleasure you can have from the rest of your anatomy.
You ain't broken–
–I just got some extra work to do and plenty of other fun options to explore in the mean time!

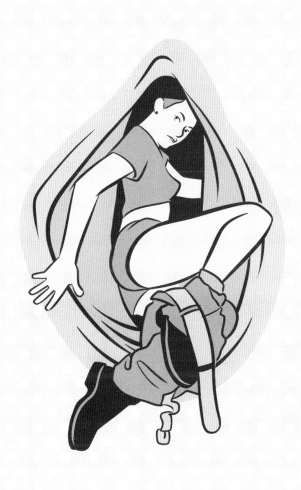

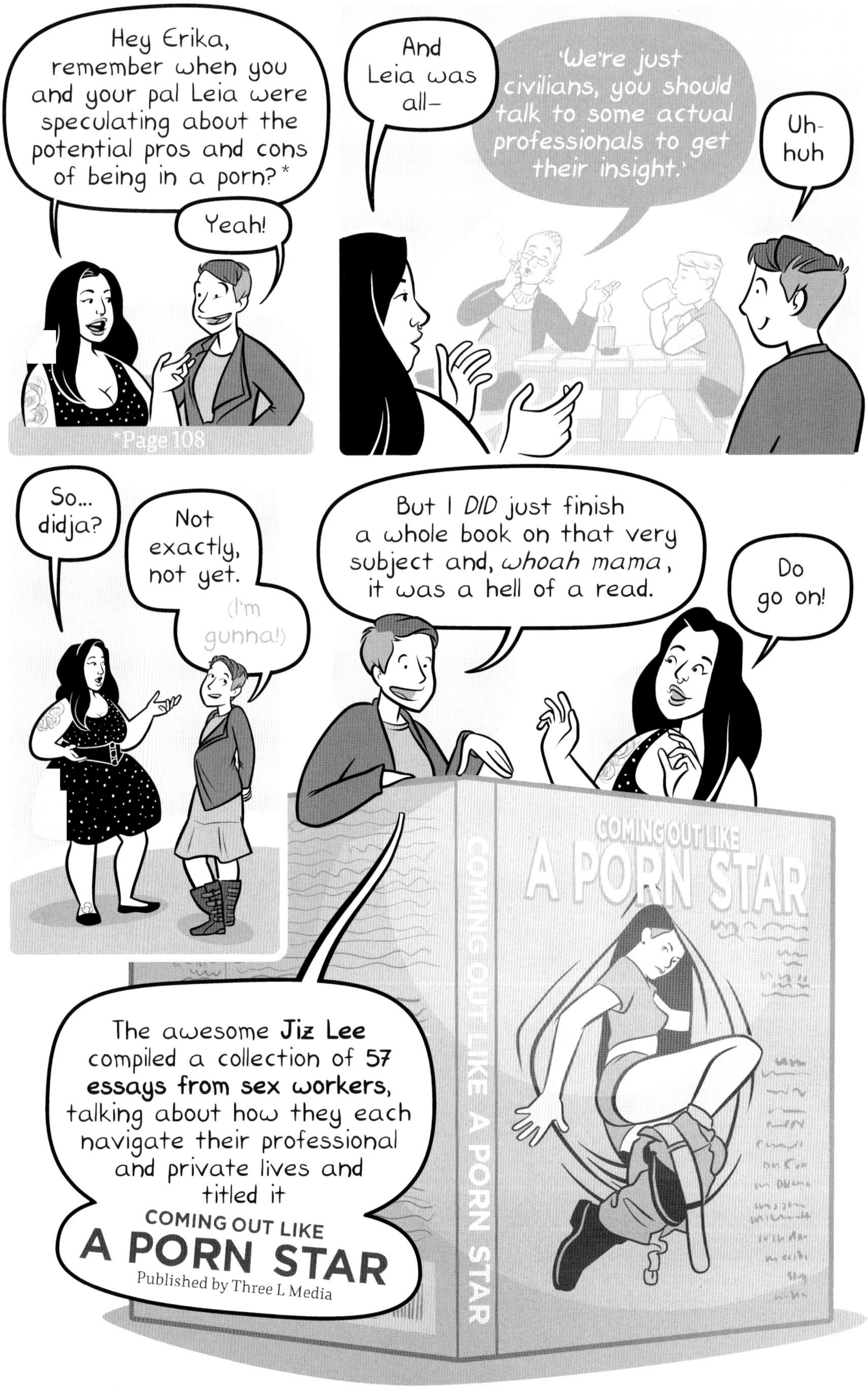

Hey Erika, remember when you and your pal Leia were speculating about the potential pros and cons of being in a porn?*
Yeah!
*Page 108
And Leia was all–
'We're just civilians, you should talk to some actual professionals to get their insight.'
Uh-huh
So... didja?
Not exactly, not yet.
(I'm gunna!)
But I *DID* just finish a whole book on that very subject and, *whoah mama*, it was a hell of a read.
Do go on!
COMING OUT LIKE A PORN STAR
COMING OUT LIKE A PORN STAR
The awesome **Jiz Lee** compiled a collection of **57 essays from sex workers,** talking about how they each navigate their professional and private lives and titled it
COMING OUT LIKE A PORN STAR
Published by Three L Media

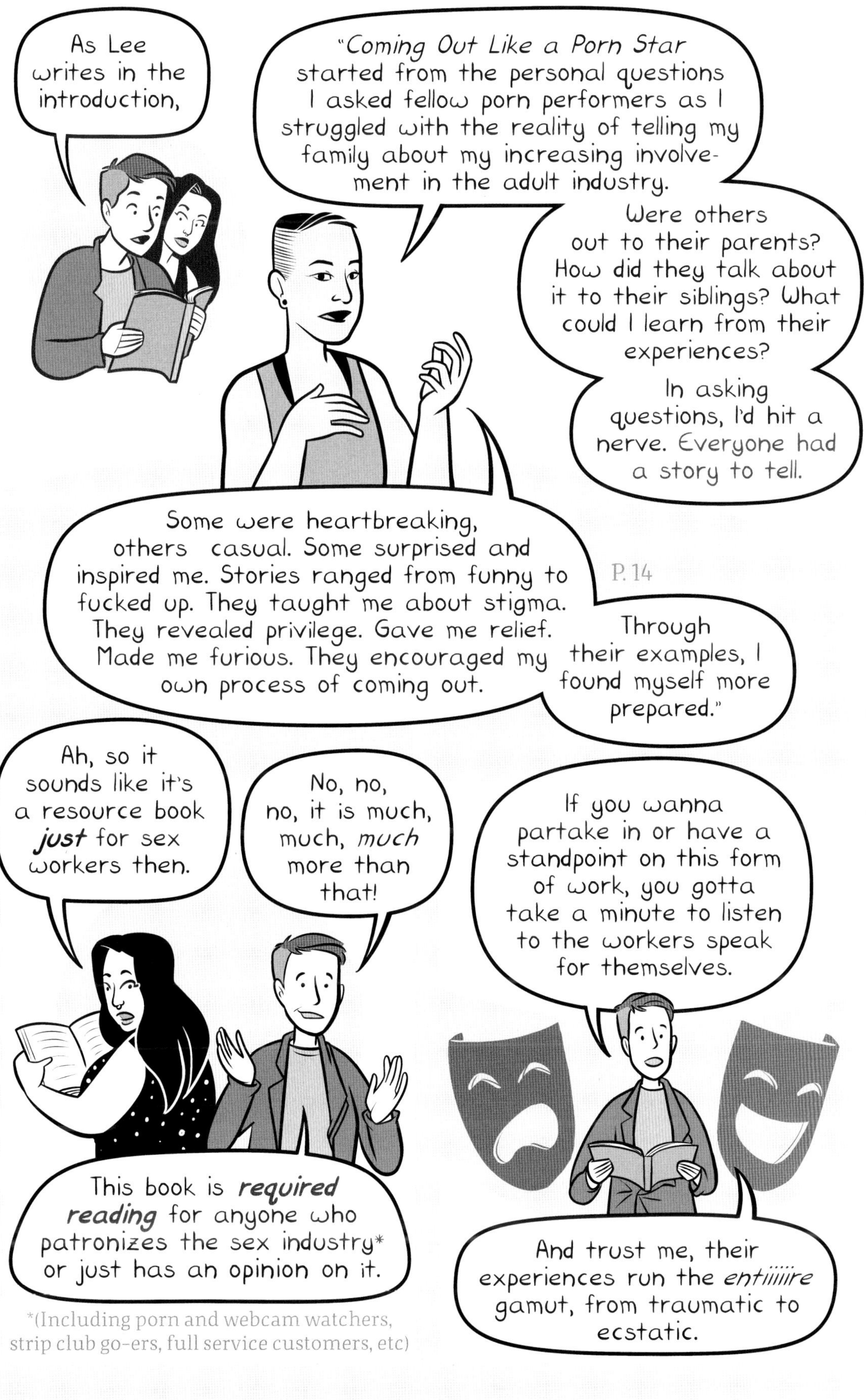

As Lee writes in the introduction,
"*Coming Out Like a Porn Star* started from the personal questions I asked fellow porn performers as I struggled with the reality of telling my family about my increasing involvement in the adult industry.
Were others out to their parents? How did they talk about it to their siblings? What could I learn from their experiences?
In asking questions, I'd hit a nerve. Everyone had a story to tell.
Some were heartbreaking, others casual. Some surprised and inspired me. Stories ranged from funny to fucked up. They taught me about stigma. They revealed privilege. Gave me relief. Made me furious. They encouraged my own process of coming out.
P. 14
Through their examples, I found myself more prepared."
Ah, so it sounds like it's a resource book ***just*** for sex workers then.
No, no, no, it is much, much, *much* more than that!
This book is ***required reading*** for anyone who patronizes the sex industry* or just has an opinion on it.
*(Including porn and webcam watchers, strip club go-ers, full service customers, etc)
If you wanna partake in or have a standpoint on this form of work, you gotta take a minute to listen to the workers speak for themselves.
And trust me, their experiences run the *entiiiiire* gamut, from traumatic to ecstatic.

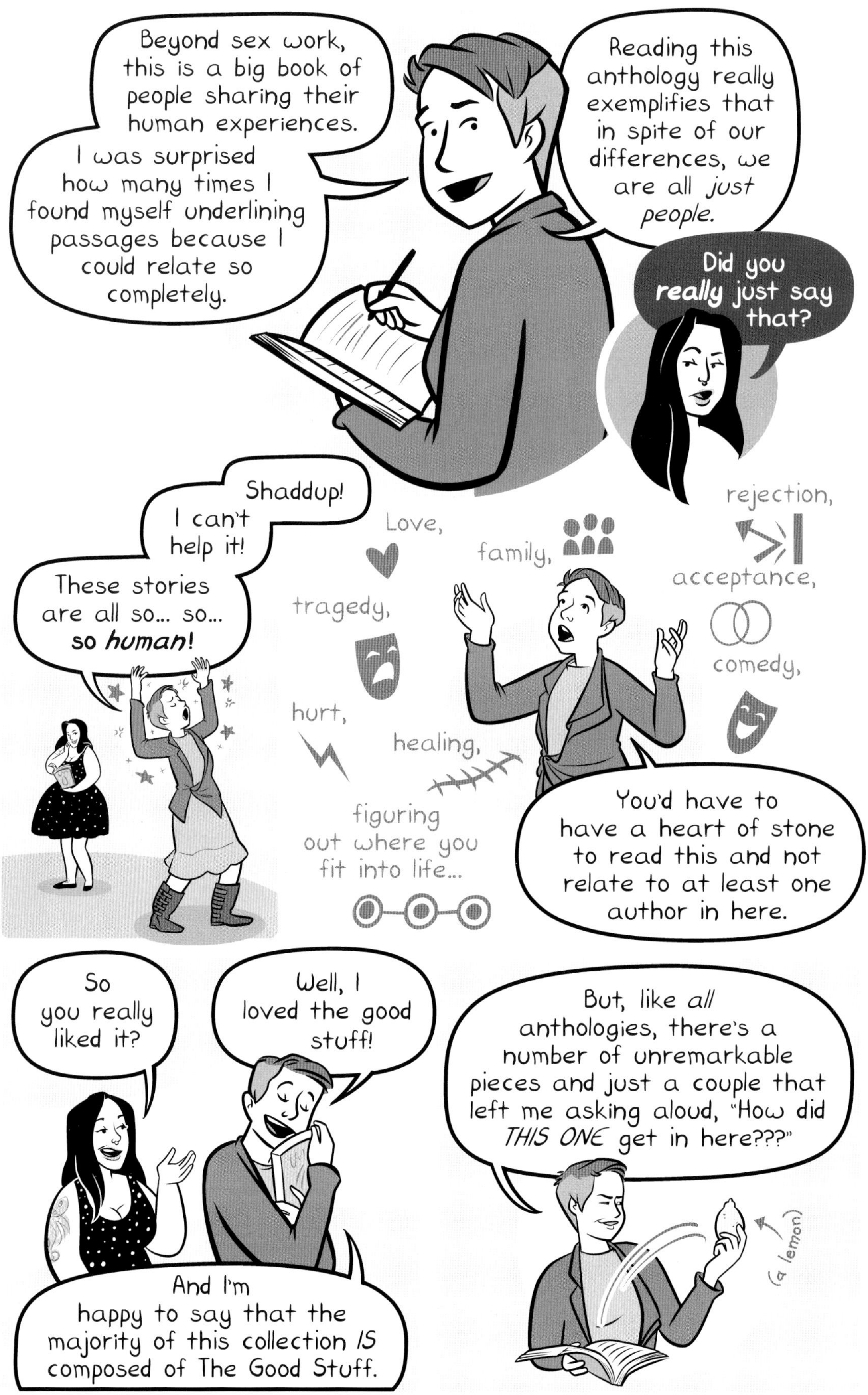
Beyond sex work, this is a big book of people sharing their human experiences.
I was surprised how many times I found myself underlining passages because I could relate so completely.
Reading this anthology really exemplifies that in spite of our differences, we are all *just people.*
Did you ***really*** just say that?
Shaddup!
I can't help it!
These stories are all so... so... **so *human*!**
Love,
family,
rejection,
acceptance,
tragedy,
comedy,
hurt,
healing,
figuring out where you fit into life...
You'd have to have a heart of stone to read this and not relate to at least one author in here.
So you really liked it?
Well, I loved the good stuff!
And I'm happy to say that the majority of this collection *IS* composed of The Good Stuff.
But, like *all* anthologies, there's a number of unremarkable pieces and just a couple that left me asking aloud, "How did *THIS ONE* get in here???"
(a lemon)

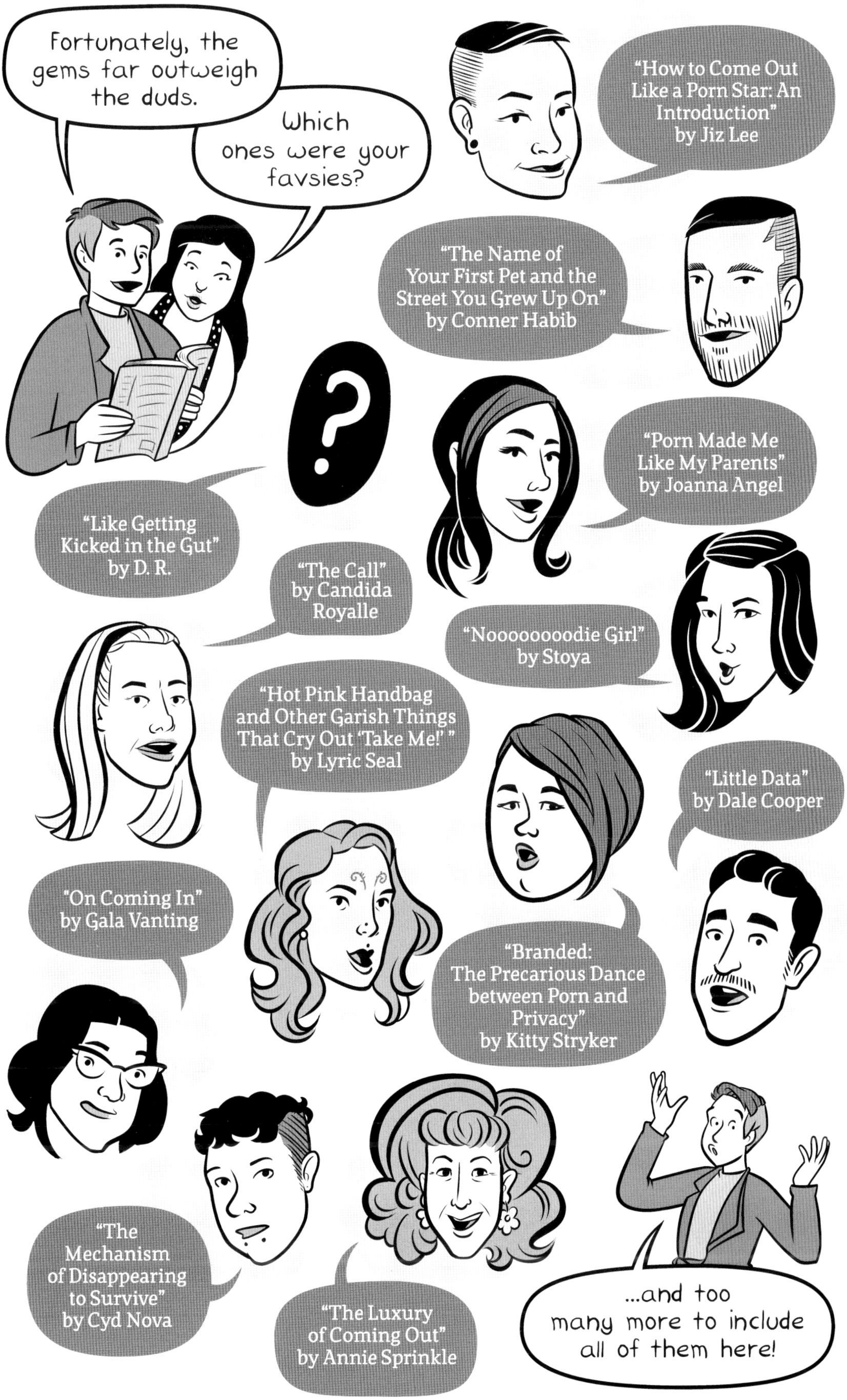
Fortunately, the gems far outweigh the duds.
Which ones were your favsies?
"How to Come Out Like a Porn Star: An Introduction" by Jiz Lee
"The Name of Your First Pet and the Street You Grew Up On" by Conner Habib
?
"Porn Made Me Like My Parents" by Joanna Angel
"Like Getting Kicked in the Gut" by D. R.
"The Call" by Candida Royalle
"Nooooooooodie Girl" by Stoya
"Hot Pink Handbag and Other Garish Things That Cry Out 'Take Me!'" by Lyric Seal
"Little Data" by Dale Cooper
"On Coming In" by Gala Vanting
"Branded: The Precarious Dance between Porn and Privacy" by Kitty Stryker
"The Mechanism of Disappearing to Survive" by Cyd Nova
"The Luxury of Coming Out" by Annie Sprinkle
...and too many more to include all of them here!

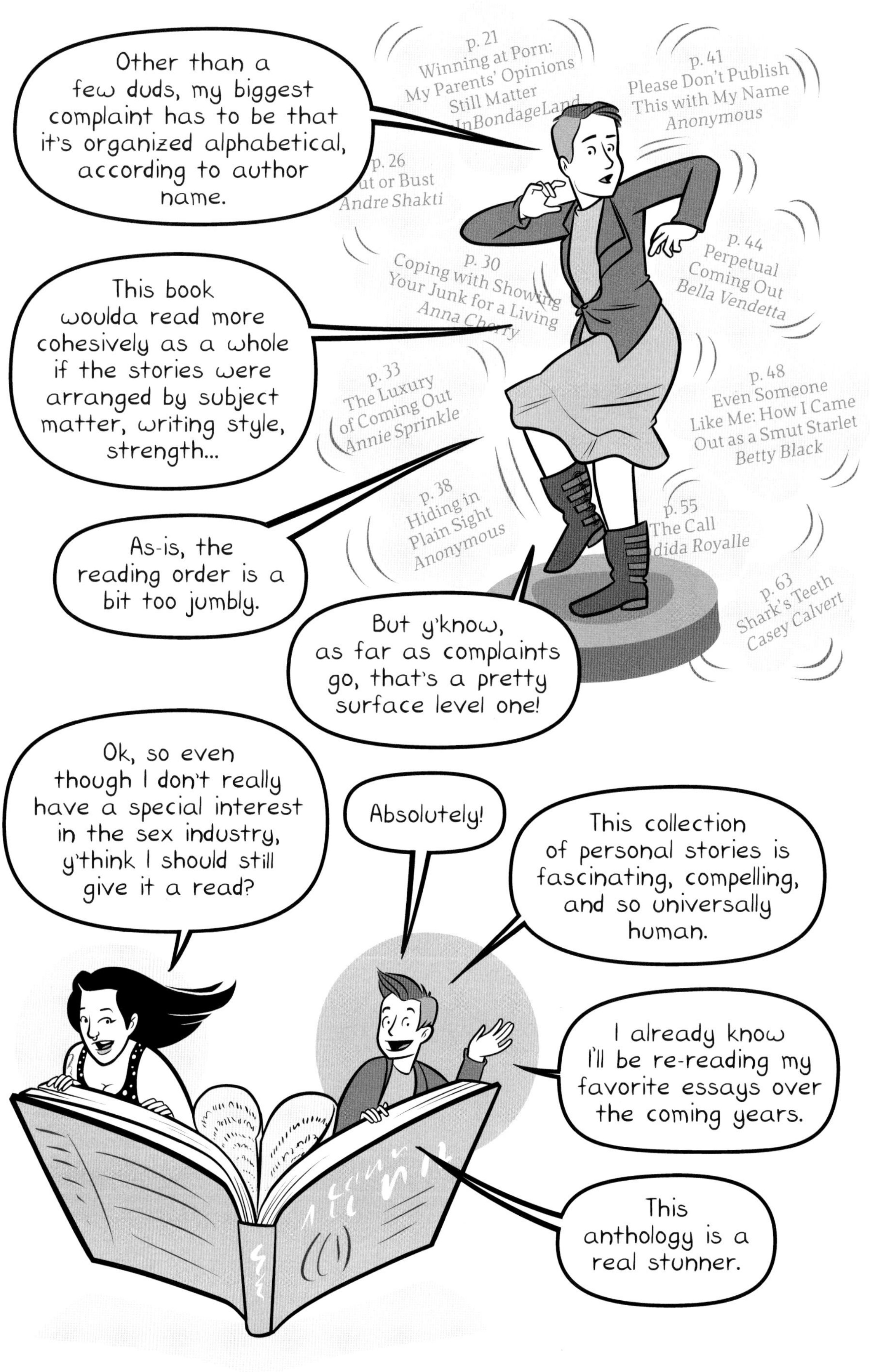
Other than a few duds, my biggest complaint has to be that it's organized alphabetical, according to author name.
p. 21 Winning at Porn: My Parents' Opinions Still Matter InBondageLand
p. 41 Please Don't Publish This with My Name Anonymous
p. 26 ut or Bust Andre Shakti
p. 30 Coping with Showing Your Junk for a Living Anna Cherry
p. 44 Perpetual Coming Out Bella Vendetta
This book woulda read more cohesively as a whole if the stories were arranged by subject matter, writing style, strength...
p. 33 The Luxury of Coming Out Annie Sprinkle
p. 48 Even Someone Like Me: How I Came Out as a Smut Starlet Betty Black
p. 38 Hiding in Plain Sight Anonymous
p. 55 The Call ndida Royalle
p. 63 Shark's Teeth Casey Calvert
As-is, the reading order is a bit too jumbly.
But y'know, as far as complaints go, that's a pretty surface level one!
Ok, so even though I don't really have a special interest in the sex industry, y'think I should still give it a read?
Absolutely!
This collection of personal stories is fascinating, compelling, and so universally human.
I already know I'll be re-reading my favorite essays over the coming years.
This anthology is a real stunner.

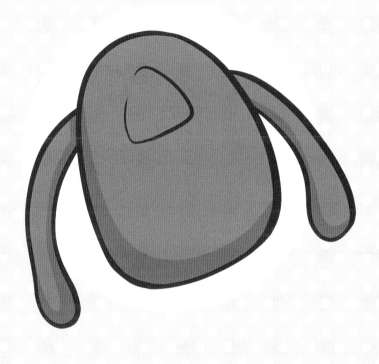

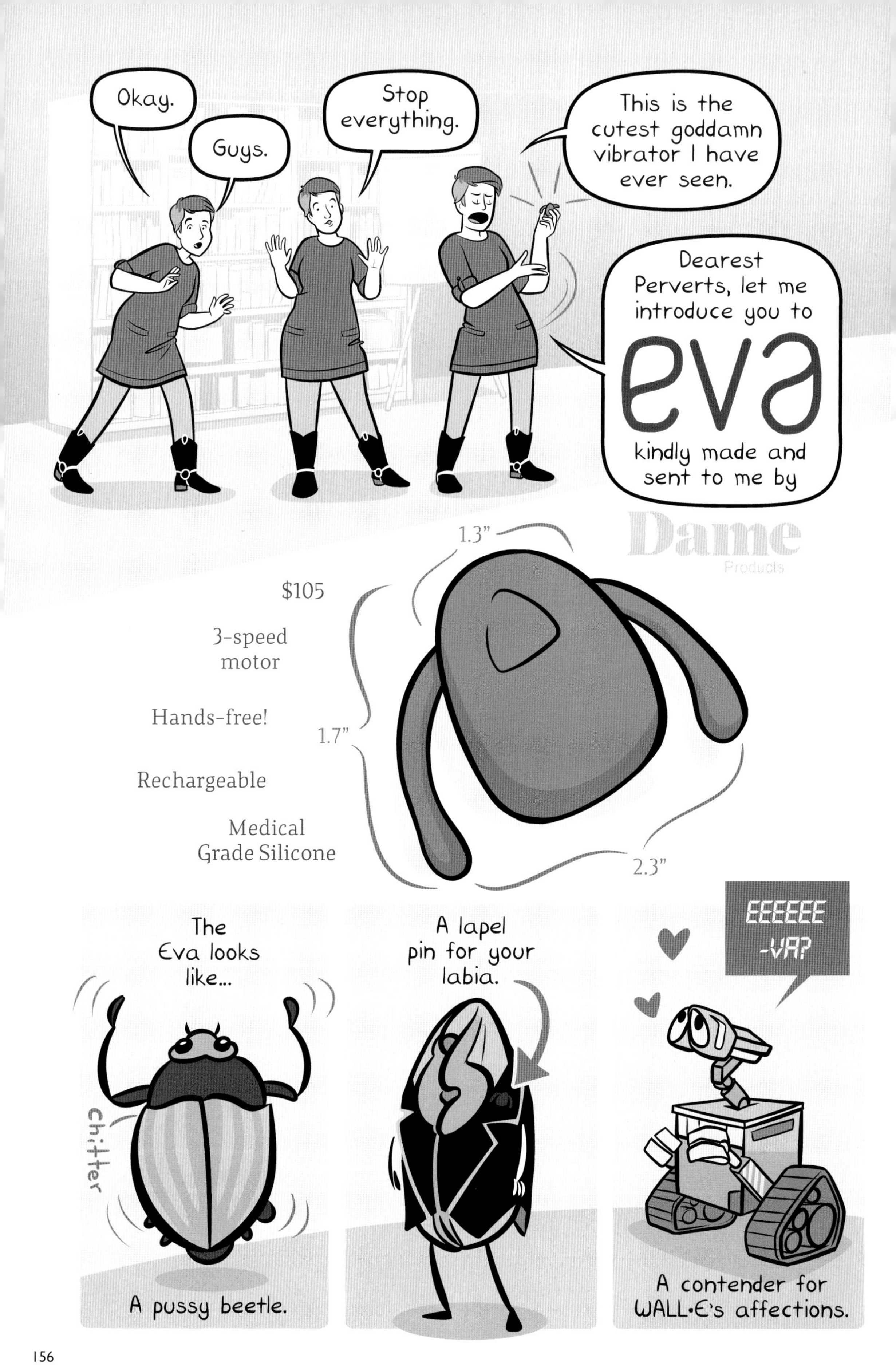
Okay.
Guys.
Stop everything.
This is the cutest goddamn vibrator I have ever seen.
Dearest Perverts, let me introduce you to
eva
kindly made and sent to me by
Dame
Products
1.3"
$105
3-speed motor
Hands-free!
1.7"
Rechargeable
Medical Grade Silicone
2.3"
The Eva looks like...
chitter
A pussy beetle.
A lapel pin for your labia.
EEEEEE -VA?
A contender for WALL•E's affections.

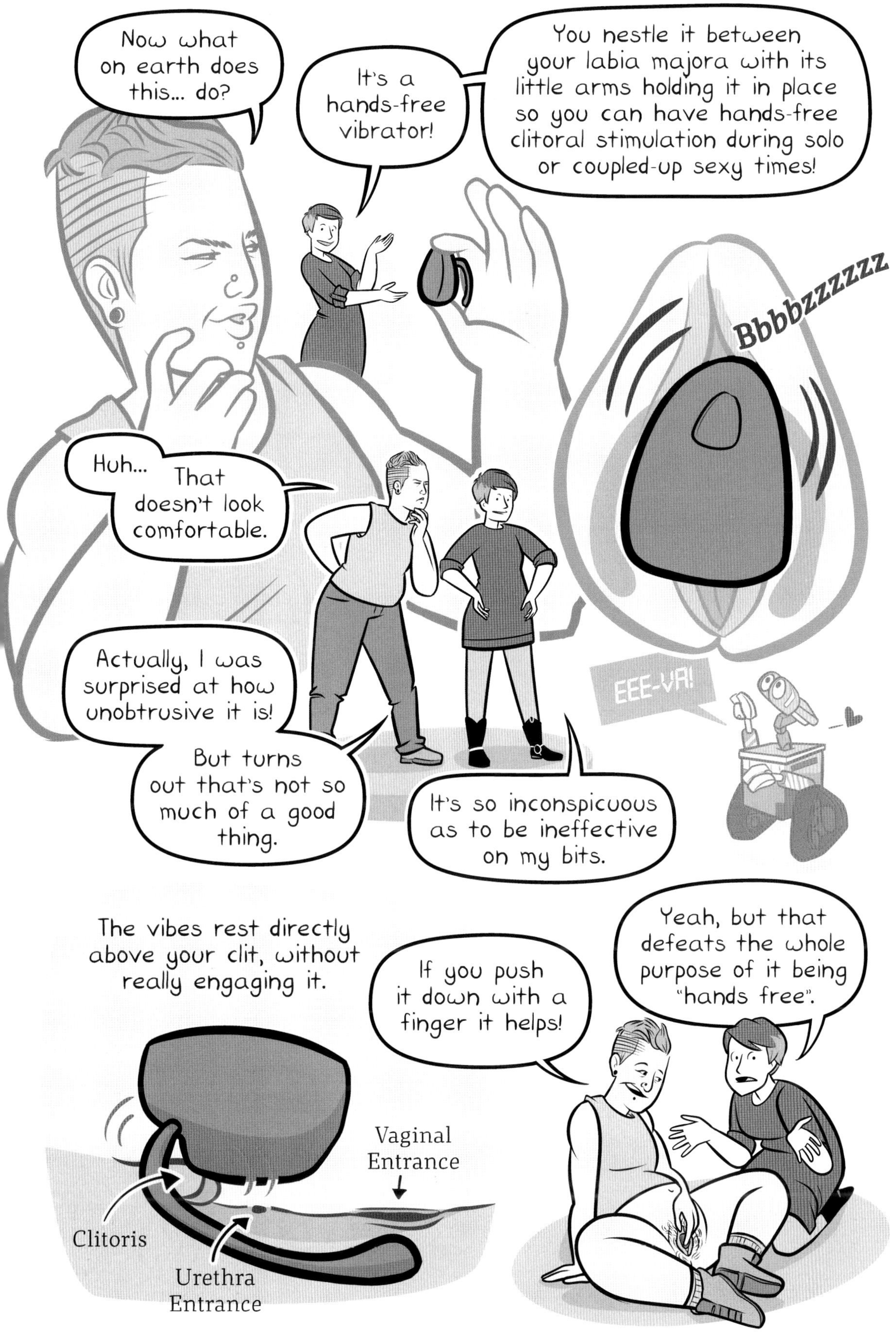
Now what on earth does this... do?
It's a hands-free vibrator!
You nestle it between your labia majora with its little arms holding it in place so you can have hands-free clitoral stimulation during solo or coupled-up sexy times!
Bbbbzzzzzz
Huh... That doesn't look comfortable.
Actually, I was surprised at how unobtrusive it is!
But turns out that's not so much of a good thing.
It's so inconspicuous as to be ineffective on my bits.
EEE-VA!
The vibes rest directly above your clit, without really engaging it.
Vaginal Entrance
Clitoris
Urethra Entrance
If you push it down with a finger it helps!
Yeah, but that defeats the whole purpose of it being "hands free".

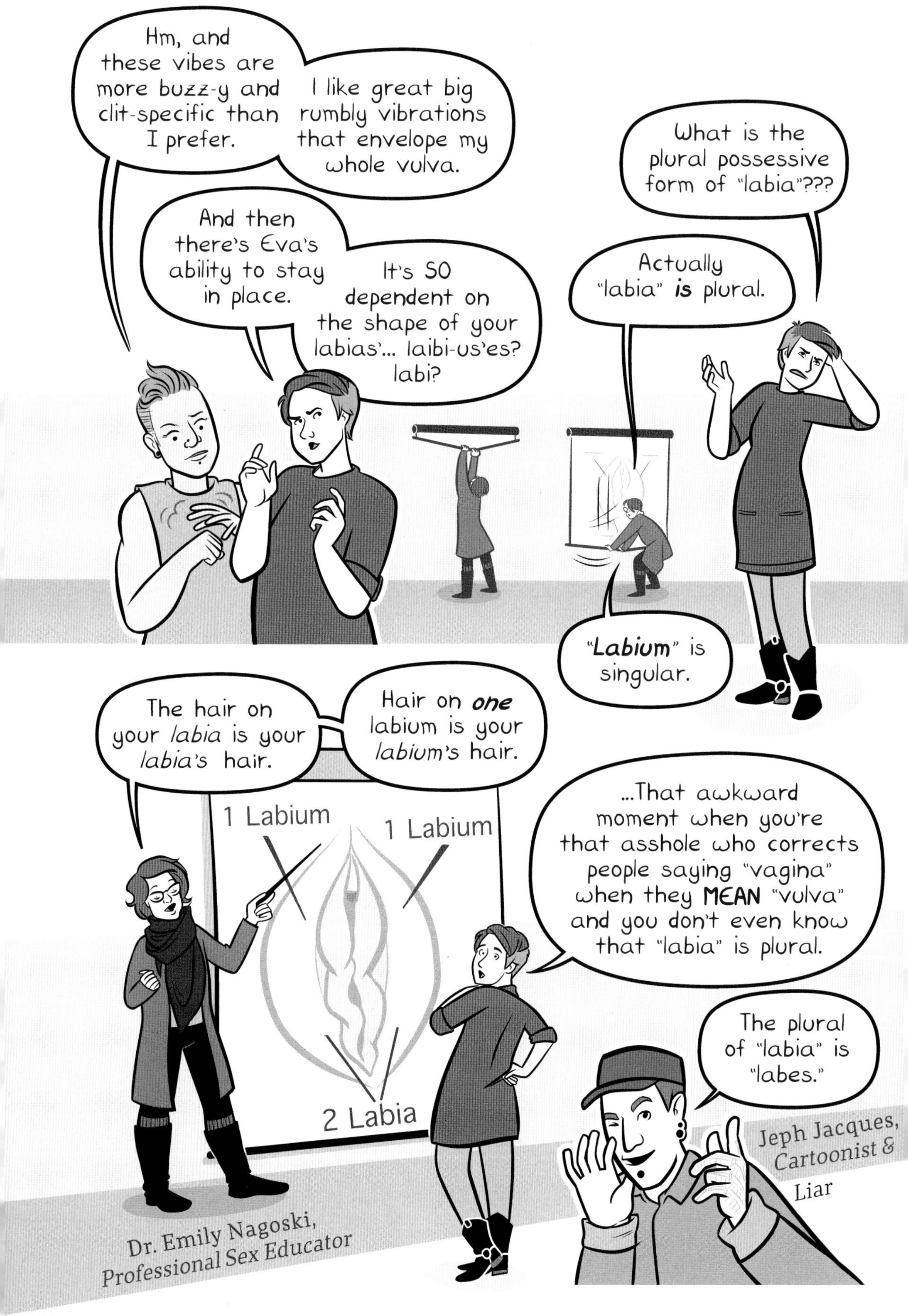
Hm, and these vibes are more buzz-y and clit-specific than I prefer.
I like great big rumbly vibrations that envelope my whole vulva.
And then there's Eva's ability to stay in place.
It's SO **dependent** on the shape of your labias'... laibi-us'es? labi?
What is the plural possessive form of "labia"???
Actually "labia" **is** plural.
"**Labium**" is singular.
The hair on your *labia* is your *labia*'s hair.
Hair on ***one*** labium is your *labium*'s hair.
1 Labium
1 Labium
2 Labia
...That awkward moment when you're that asshole who corrects people saying "vagina" when they **MEAN** "vulva" and you don't even know that "labia" is plural.
The plural of "labia" is "labes."
Dr. Emily Nagoski, Professional Sex Educator
Jeph Jacques, Cartoonist & Liar

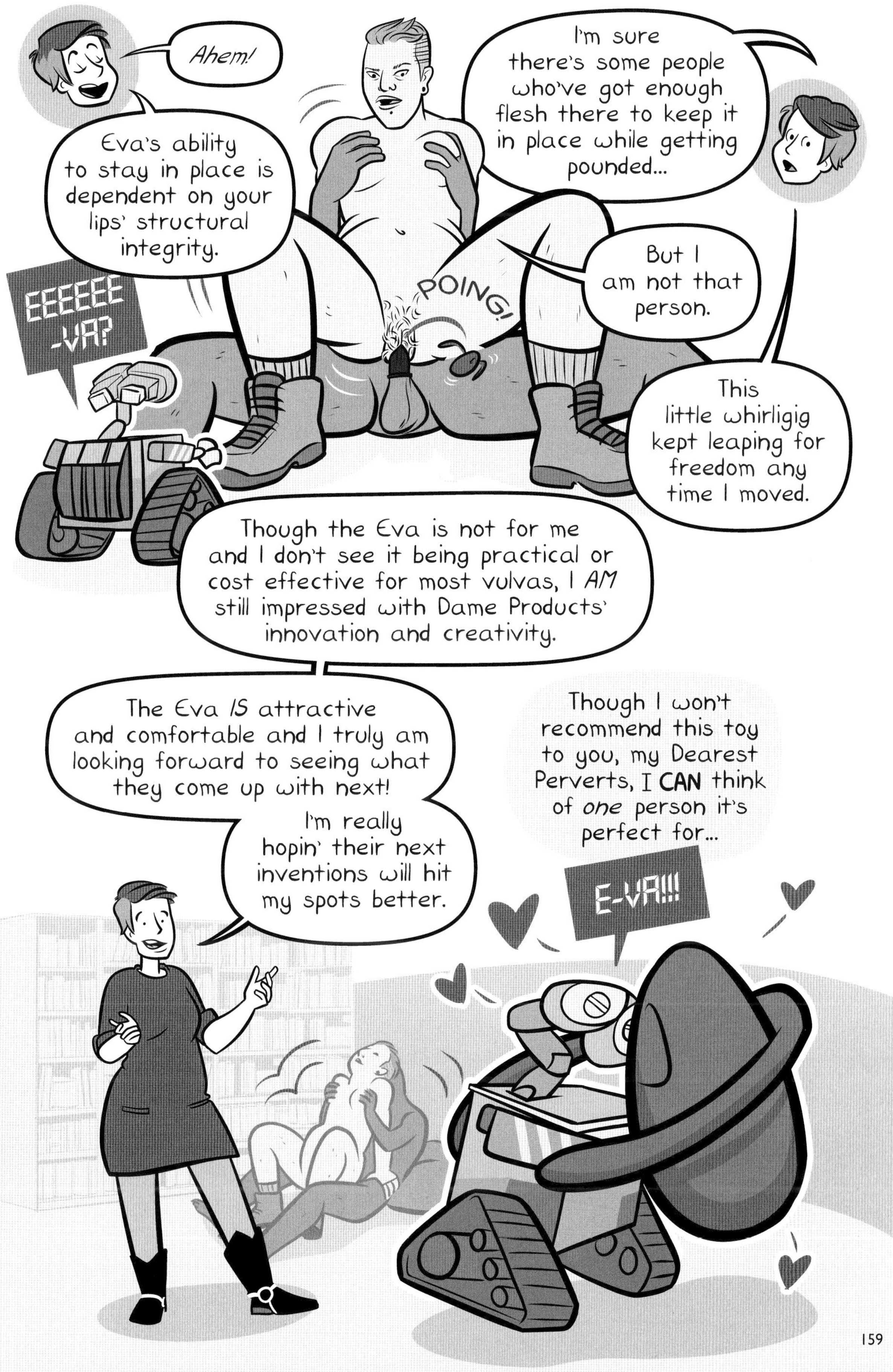

Ahem!
Eva's ability to stay in place is dependent on your lips' structural integrity.
I'm sure there's some people who've got enough flesh there to keep it in place while getting pounded...
EEEEEE -VA?
POING!
But I am not that person.
This little whirligig kept leaping for freedom any time I moved.
Though the Eva is not for me and I don't see it being practical or cost effective for most vulvas, I *AM* still impressed with Dame Products' innovation and creativity.
The Eva *IS* attractive and comfortable and I truly am looking forward to seeing what they come up with next!
I'm really hopin' their next inventions will hit my spots better.
Though I won't recommend this toy to you, my Dearest Perverts, I **CAN** think of *one* person it's perfect for...
E-VA!!!

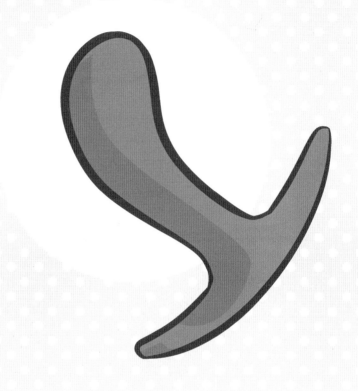

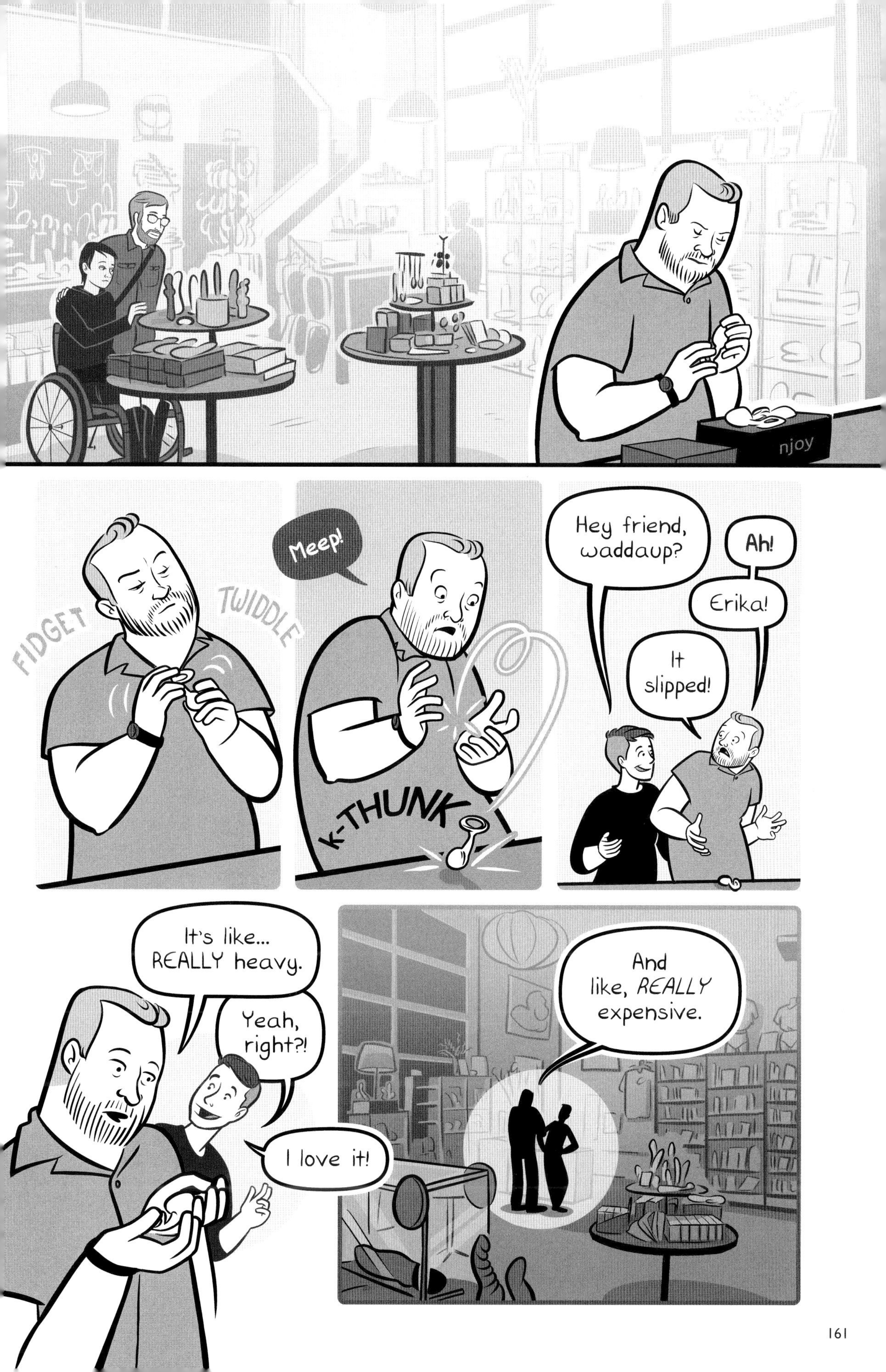
njoy
FIDGET
TWIDDLE
Meep!
K-THUNK
Hey friend, waddaup?
Ah!
Erika!
It slipped!
It's like... REALLY heavy.
Yeah, right?!
I love it!
And like, *REALLY* expensive.

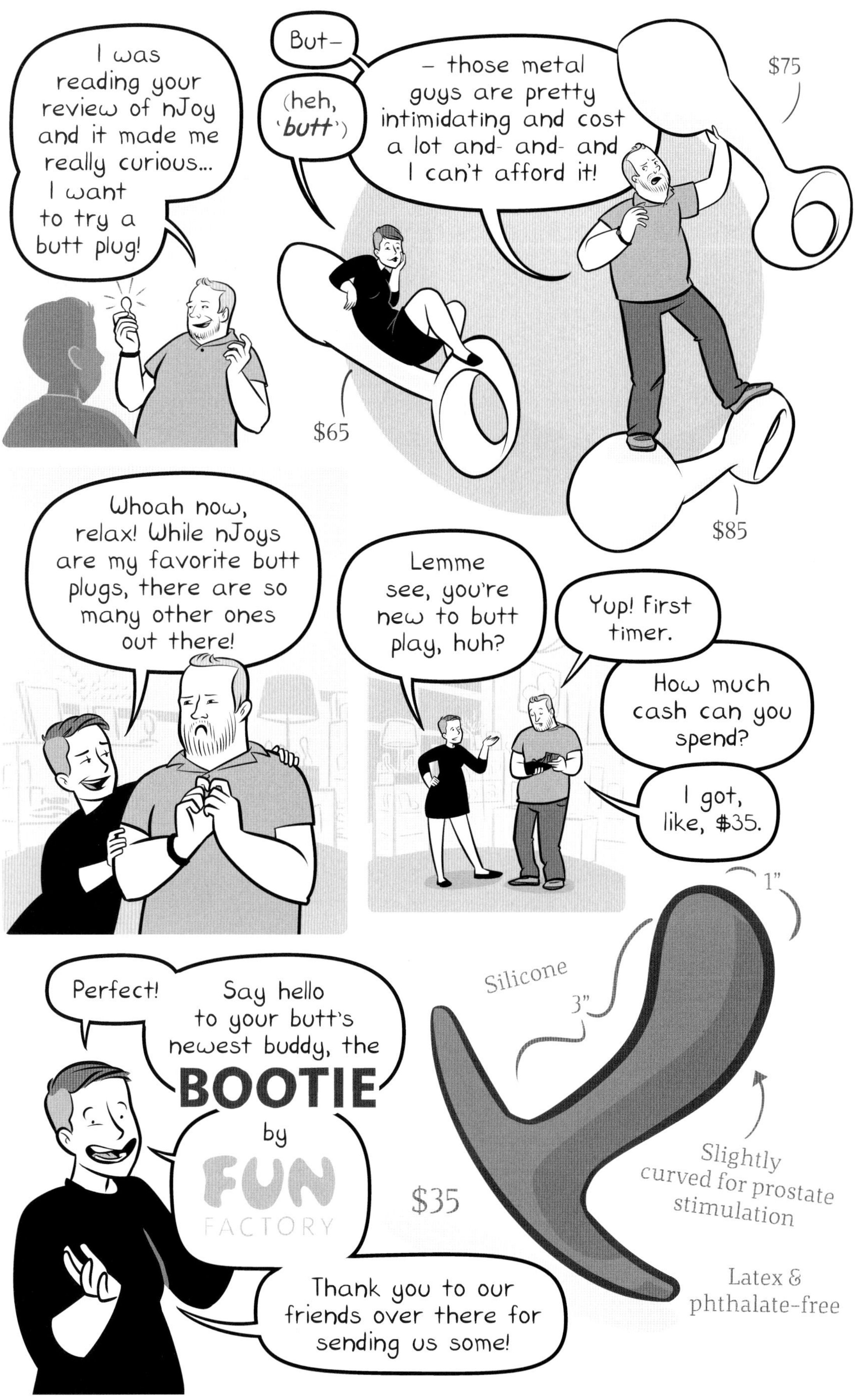
I was reading your review of nJoy and it made me really curious... I want to try a butt plug!
But–
(heh, '*butt*')
– those metal guys are pretty intimidating and cost a lot and- and- and I can't afford it!
$75
$65
$85
Whoah now, relax! While nJoys are my favorite butt plugs, there are so many other ones out there!
Lemme see, you're new to butt play, huh?
Yup! First timer.
How much cash can you spend?
I got, like, $35.
Perfect!
Say hello to your butt's newest buddy, the
BOOTIE
by
FUN FACTORY
$35
1"
Silicone
3"
Slightly curved for prostate stimulation
Latex & phthalate-free
Thank you to our friends over there for sending us some!

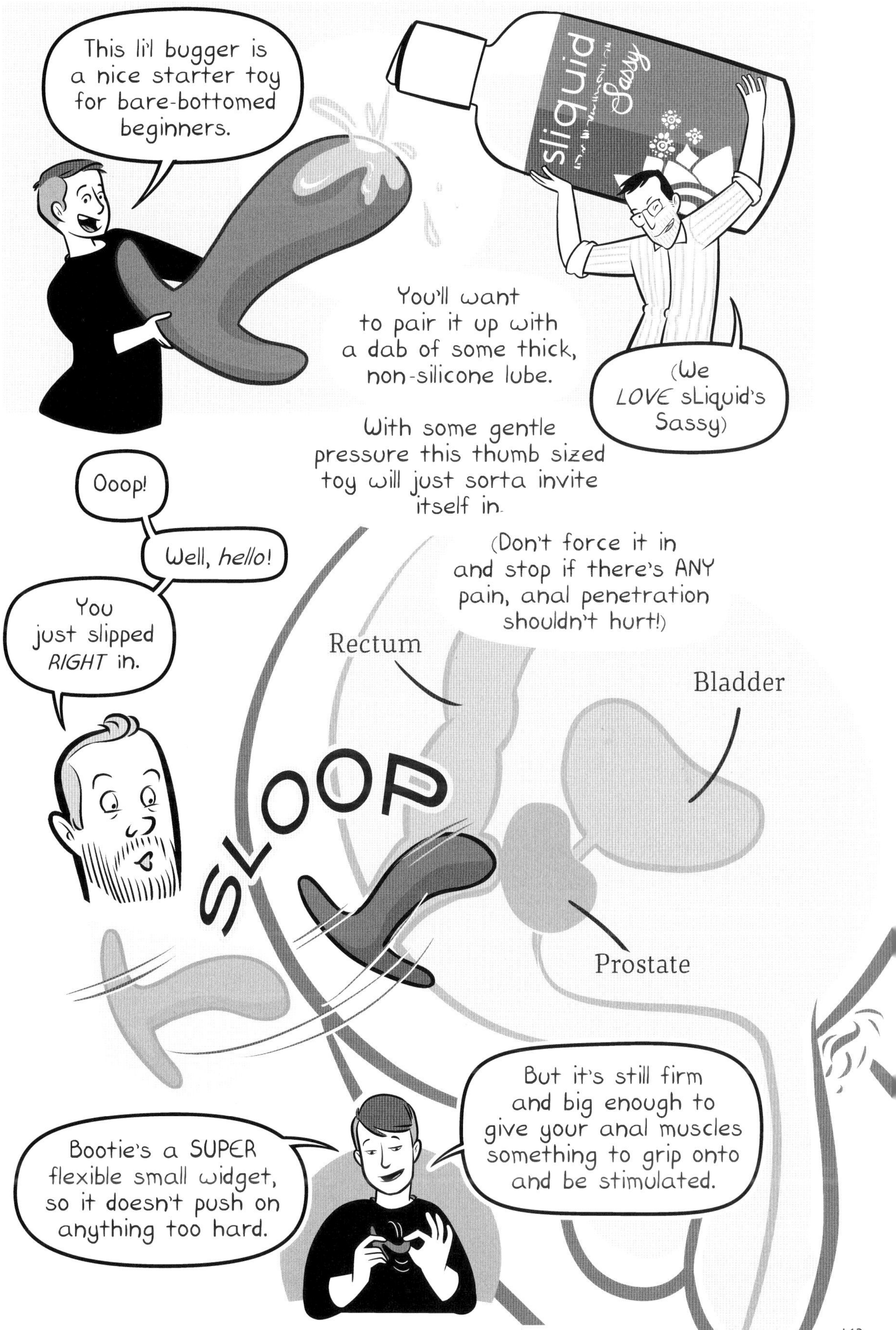

This li'l bugger is a nice starter toy for bare-bottomed beginners.
sliquid
Sassy
You'll want to pair it up with a dab of some thick, non-silicone lube.
(We LOVE sLiquid's Sassy)
With some gentle pressure this thumb sized toy will just sorta invite itself in.
Ooop!
Well, *hello*!
You just slipped *RIGHT* in.
(Don't force it in and stop if there's ANY pain, anal penetration shouldn't hurt!)
Rectum
Bladder
SLOOP
Prostate
Bootie's a SUPER flexible small widget, so it doesn't push on anything too hard.
But it's still firm and big enough to give your anal muscles something to grip onto and be stimulated.

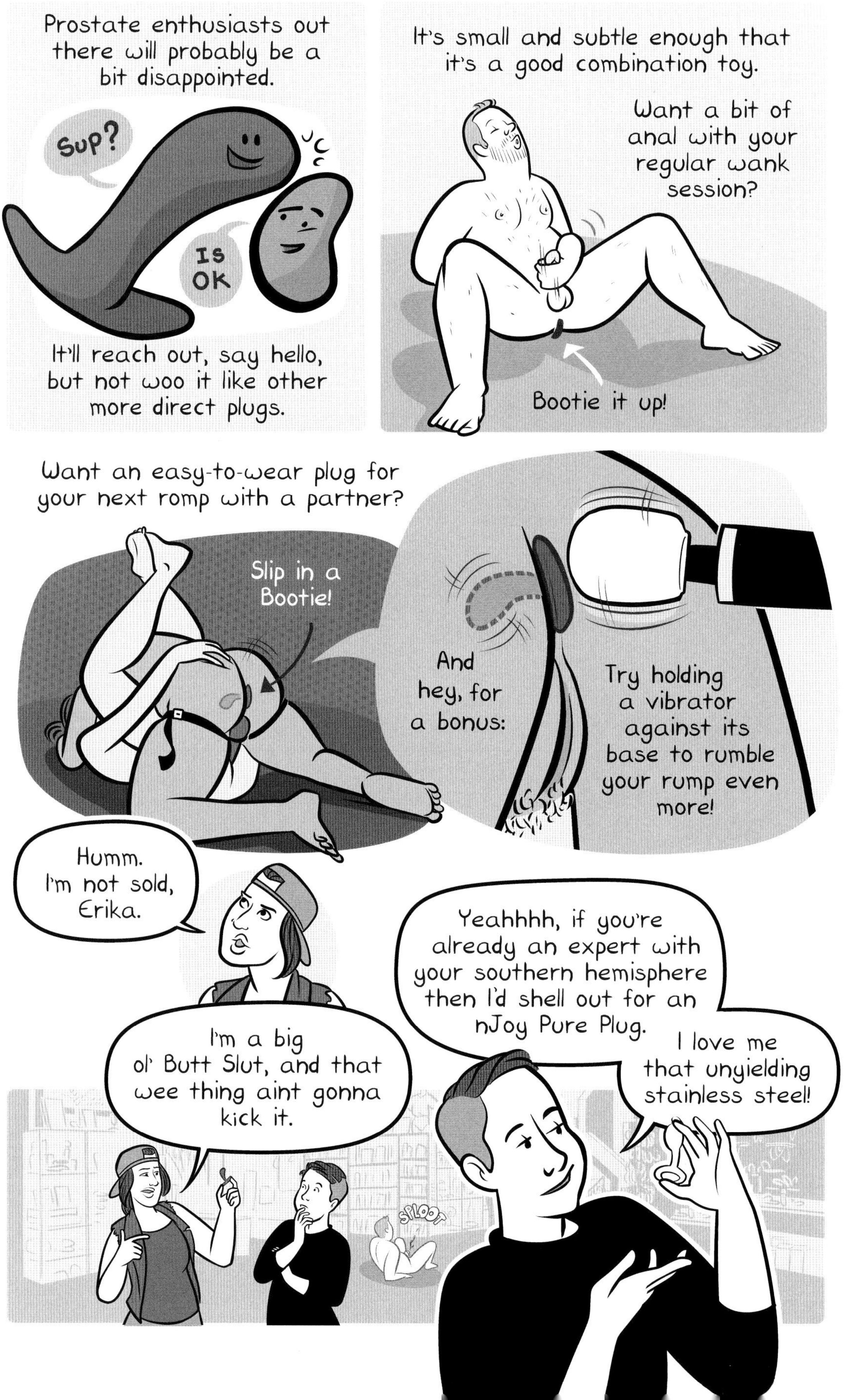
Prostate enthusiasts out there will probably be a bit disappointed.
Sup?
Is OK
It'll reach out, say hello, but not woo it like other more direct plugs.
It's small and subtle enough that it's a good combination toy.
Want a bit of anal with your regular wank session?
Bootie it up!
Want an easy-to-wear plug for your next romp with a partner?
Slip in a Bootie!
And hey, for a bonus:
Try holding a vibrator against its base to rumble your rump even more!
Humm. I'm not sold, Erika.
I'm a big ol' Butt Slut, and that wee thing aint gonna kick it.
SPLOOT
Yeahhhh, if you're already an expert with your southern hemisphere then I'd shell out for an nJoy Pure Plug.
I love me that unyielding stainless steel!

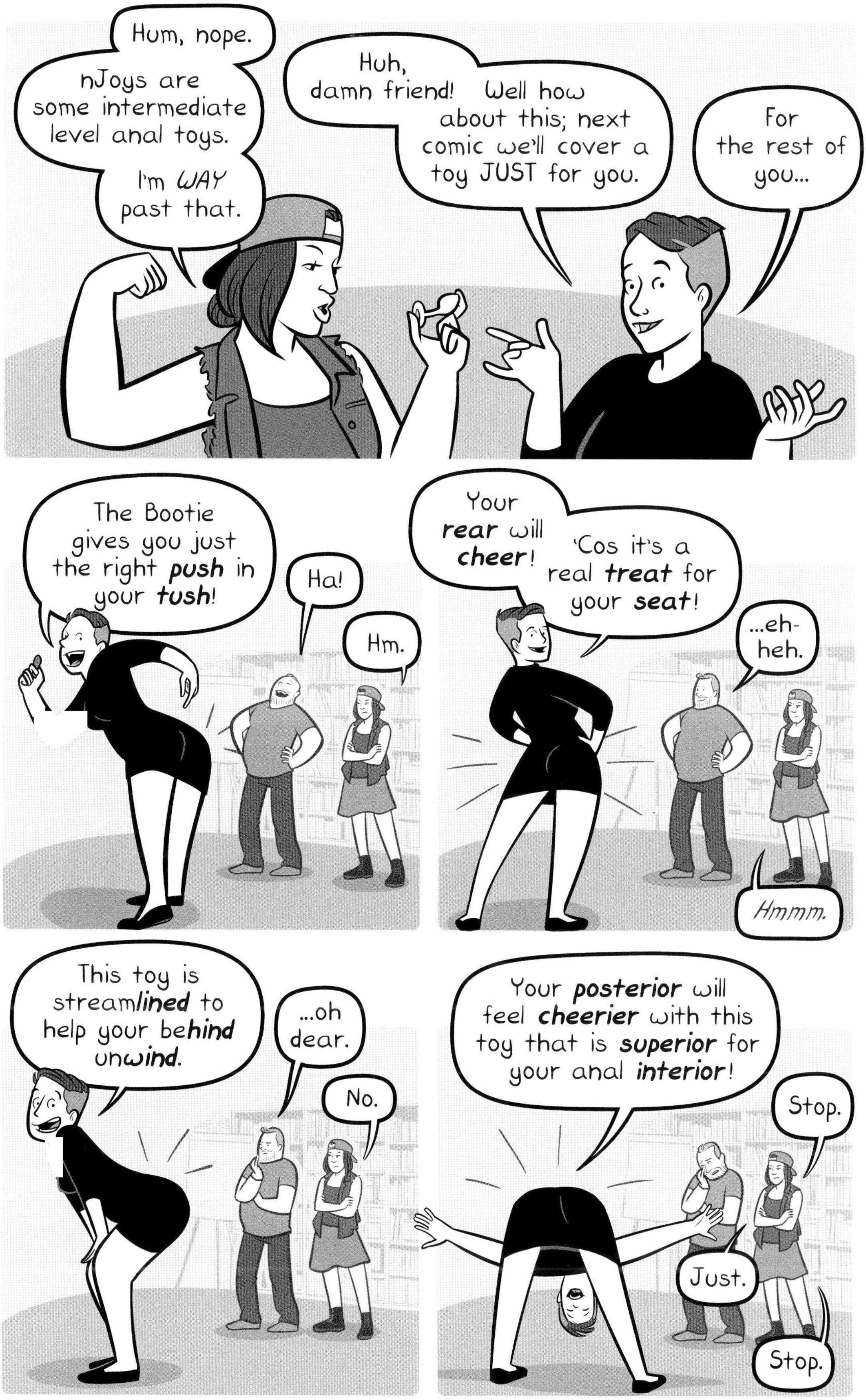
Hum, nope.
nJoys are some intermediate level anal toys.
I'm *WAY* past that.
Huh, damn friend!
Well how about this; next comic we'll cover a toy JUST for you.
For the rest of you...
The Bootie gives you just the right **push** in your **tush**!
Ha!
Hm.
Your **rear** will **cheer**!
'Cos it's a real **treat** for your **seat**!
...eh-heh.
Hmmm.
This toy is stream**lined** to help your be**hind** un**wind**.
...oh dear.
No.
Your **posterior** will feel **cheerier** with this toy that is **superior** for your anal **interior**!
Stop.
Just.
Stop.

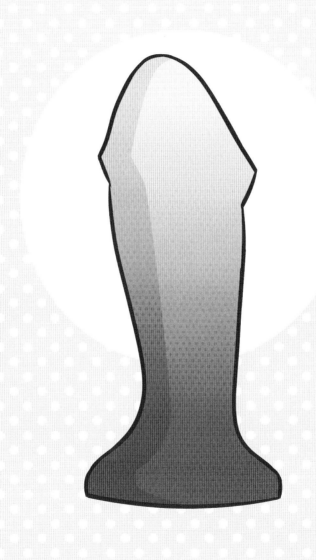

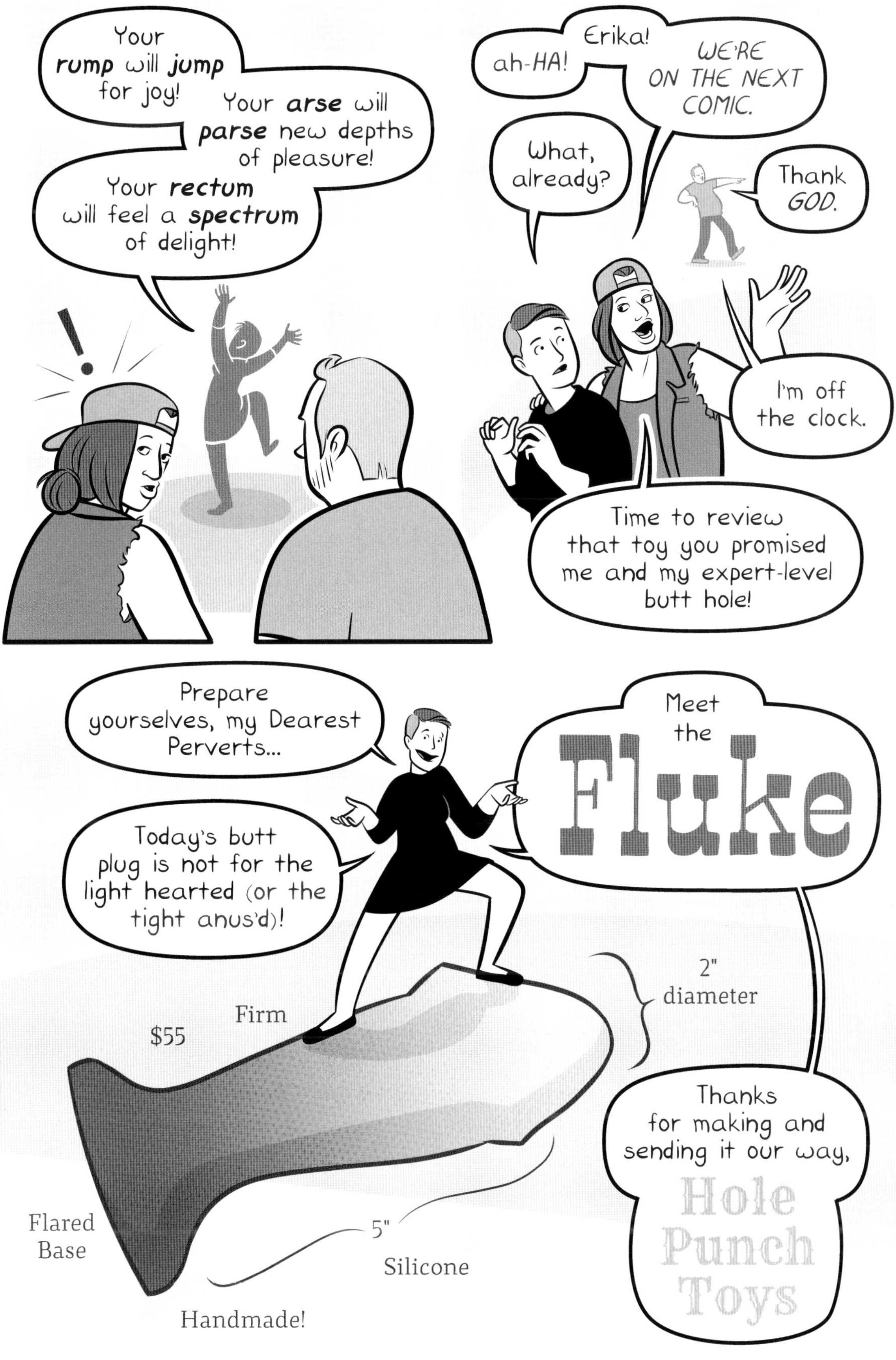
Your **rump** will **jump** for joy!
Your **arse** will **parse** new depths of pleasure!
Your **rectum** will feel a **spectrum** of delight!
!
Erika!
ah-HA!
WE'RE ON THE NEXT COMIC.
What, already?
Thank GOD.
I'm off the clock.
Time to review that toy you promised me and my expert-level butt hole!
Prepare yourselves, my Dearest Perverts...
Today's butt plug is not for the light hearted (or the tight anus'd)!
Meet the Fluke
Thanks for making and sending it our way, Hole Punch Toys
2" diameter
Firm
$55
Flared Base
5"
Silicone
Handmade!

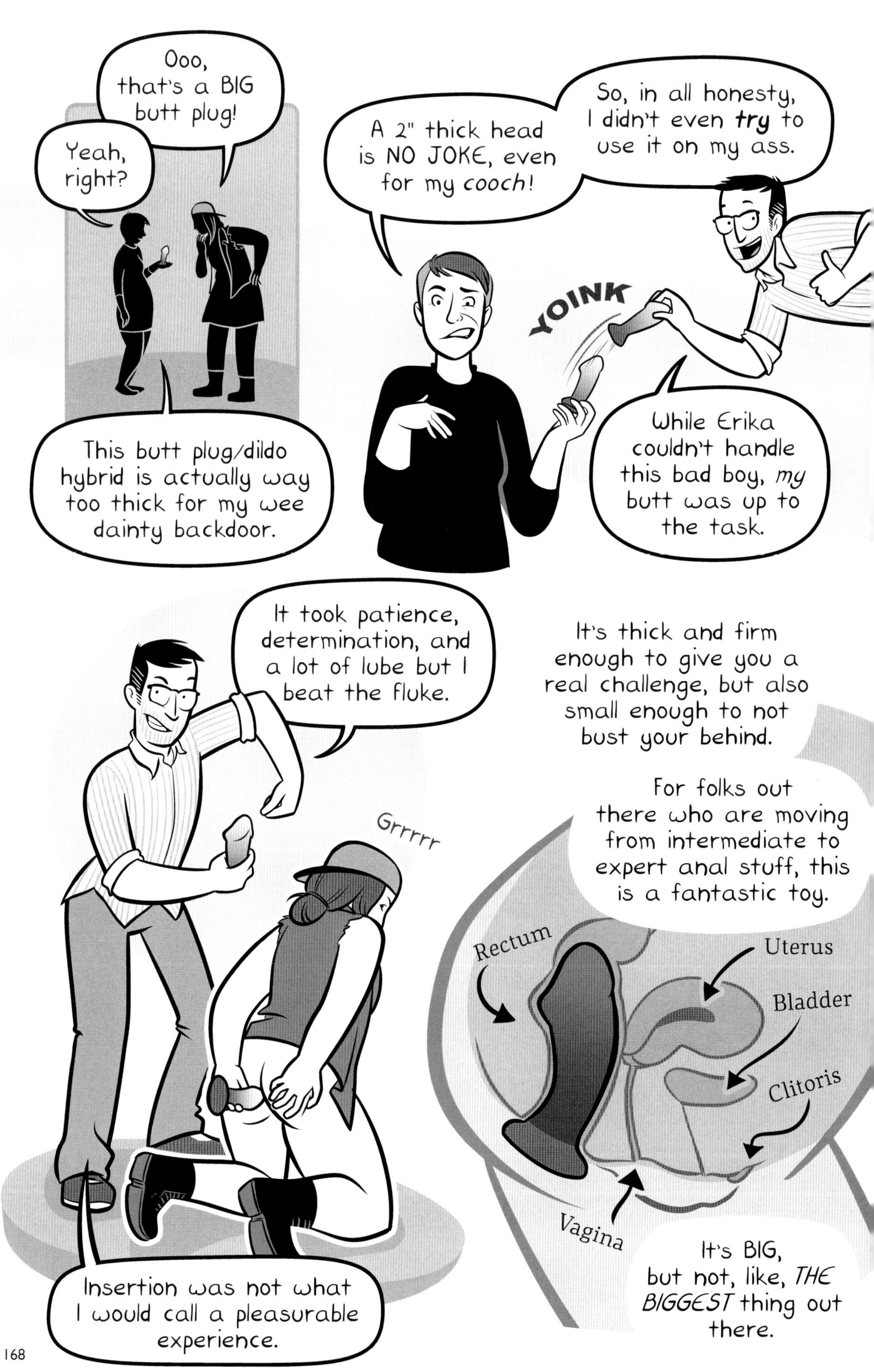
Ooo, that's a BIG butt plug!
Yeah, right?
This butt plug/dildo hybrid is actually way too thick for my wee dainty backdoor.
A 2" thick head is NO JOKE, even for my *cooch*!
So, in all honesty, I didn't even **try** to use it on my ass.
YOINK
While Erika couldn't handle this bad boy, *my* butt was up to the task.
It took patience, determination, and a lot of lube but I beat the fluke.
Grrrrr
Insertion was not what I would call a pleasurable experience.
It's thick and firm enough to give you a real challenge, but also small enough to not bust your behind.
For folks out there who are moving from intermediate to expert anal stuff, this is a fantastic toy.
Rectum
Uterus
Bladder
Clitoris
Vagina
It's BIG, but not, like, *THE BIGGEST* thing out there.

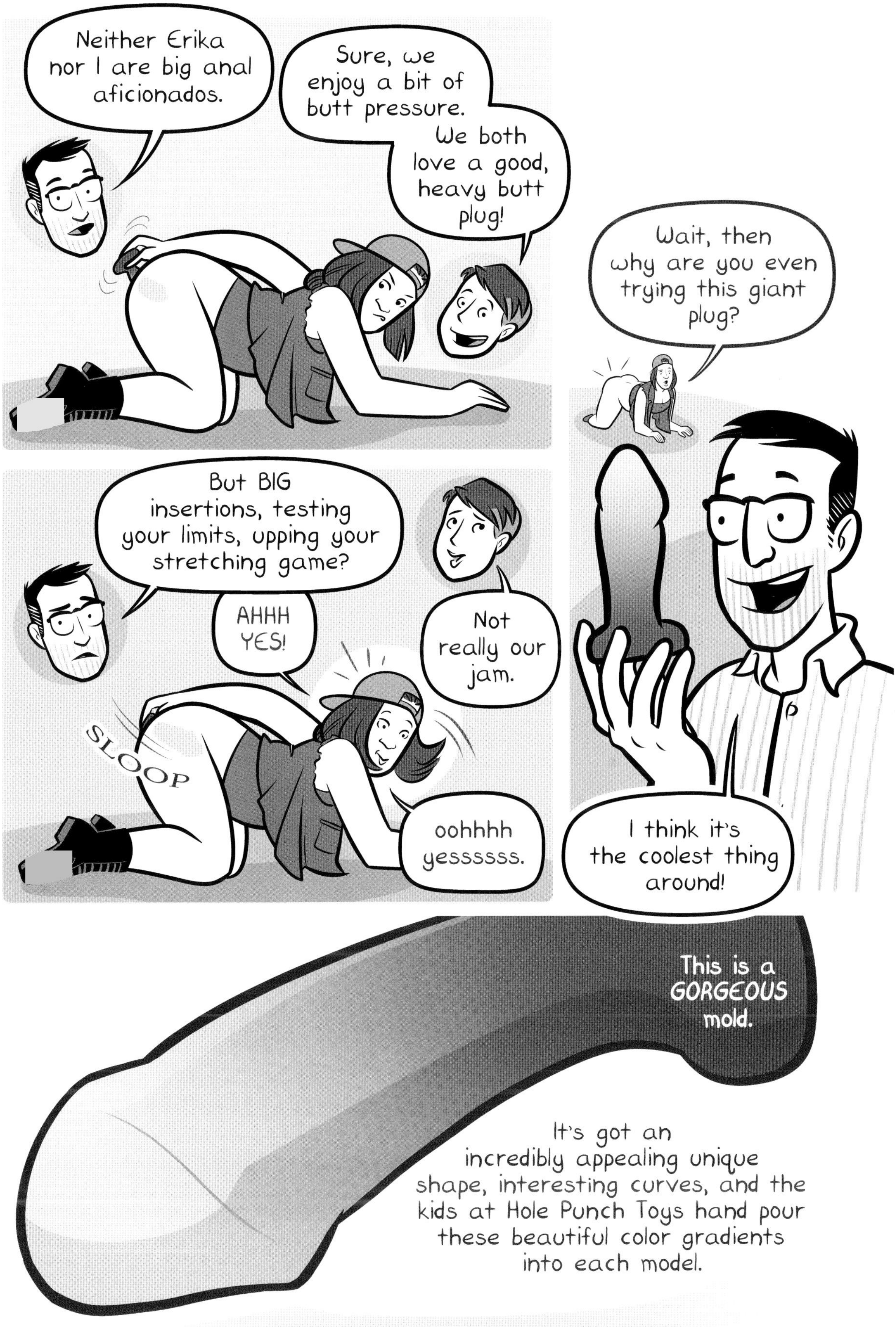

Neither Erika nor I are big anal aficionados.
Sure, we enjoy a bit of butt pressure.
We both love a good, heavy butt plug!
But BIG insertions, testing your limits, upping your stretching game?
AHHH YES!
Not really our jam.
SLOOP
oohhhh yessssss.
Wait, then why are you even trying this giant plug?
I think it's the coolest thing around!
This is a GORGEOUS mold.
It's got an incredibly appealing unique shape, interesting curves, and the kids at Hole Punch Toys hand pour these beautiful color gradients into each model.

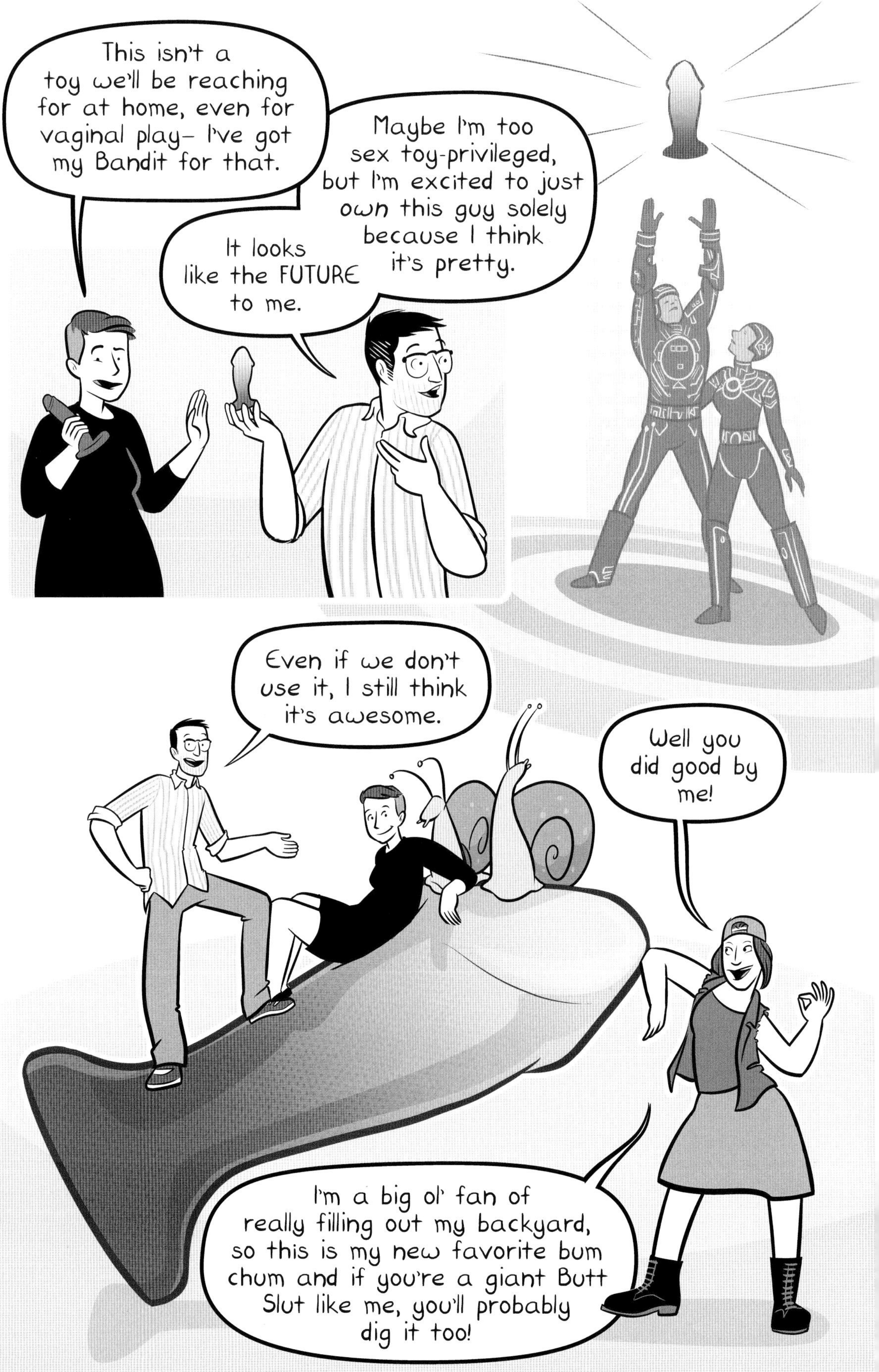
This isn't a toy we'll be reaching for at home, even for vaginal play– I've got my Bandit for that.
It looks like the FUTURE to me.
Maybe I'm too sex toy-privileged, but I'm excited to just own this guy solely because I think it's pretty.
Even if we don't use it, I still think it's awesome.
Well you did good by me!
I'm a big ol' fan of really filling out my backyard, so this is my new favorite bum chum and if you're a giant Butt Slut like me, you'll probably dig it too!

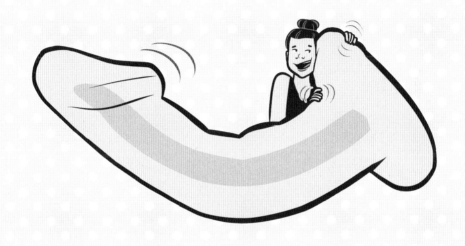

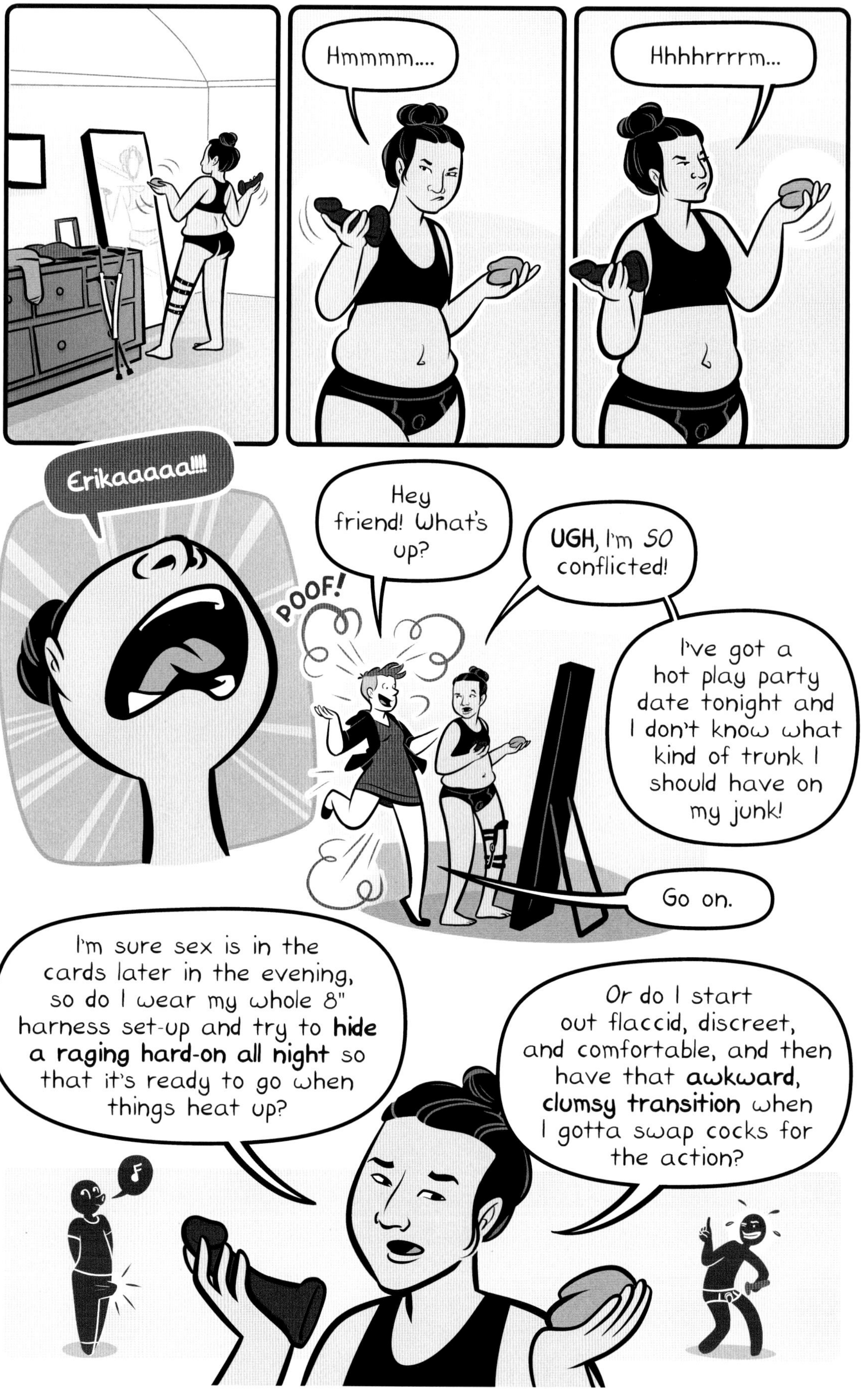
Hmmmm....
Hhhhrrrrm...
Erikaaaaa!!!
POOF!
Hey friend! What's up?
UGH, I'm *SO* conflicted!
I've got a hot play party date tonight and I don't know what kind of trunk I should have on my junk!
Go on.
I'm sure sex is in the cards later in the evening, so do I wear my whole 8" harness set-up and try to **hide a raging hard-on all night** so that it's ready to go when things heat up?
Or do I start out flaccid, discreet, and comfortable, and then have that **awkward, clumsy transition** when I gotta swap cocks for the action?

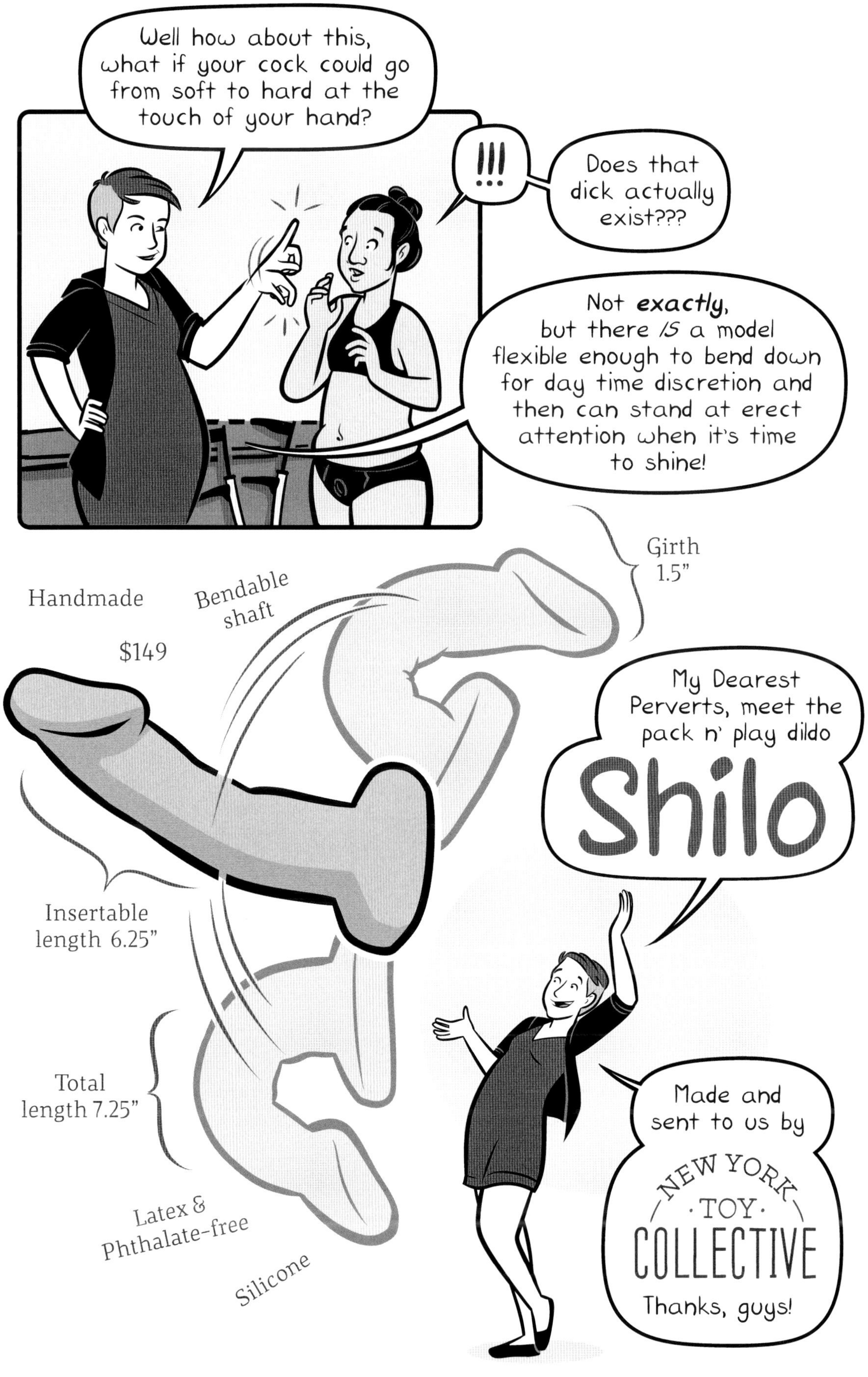

Well how about this, what if your cock could go from soft to hard at the touch of your hand?
!!!
Does that dick actually exist???
Not **exactly**, but there IS a model flexible enough to bend down for day time discretion and then can stand at erect attention when it's time to shine!
Handmade
Bendable shaft
$149
Girth 1.5"
Insertable length 6.25"
Total length 7.25"
Latex & Phthalate-free
Silicone
My Dearest Perverts, meet the pack n' play dildo
Shilo
Made and sent to us by
NEW YORK TOY COLLECTIVE
Thanks, guys!

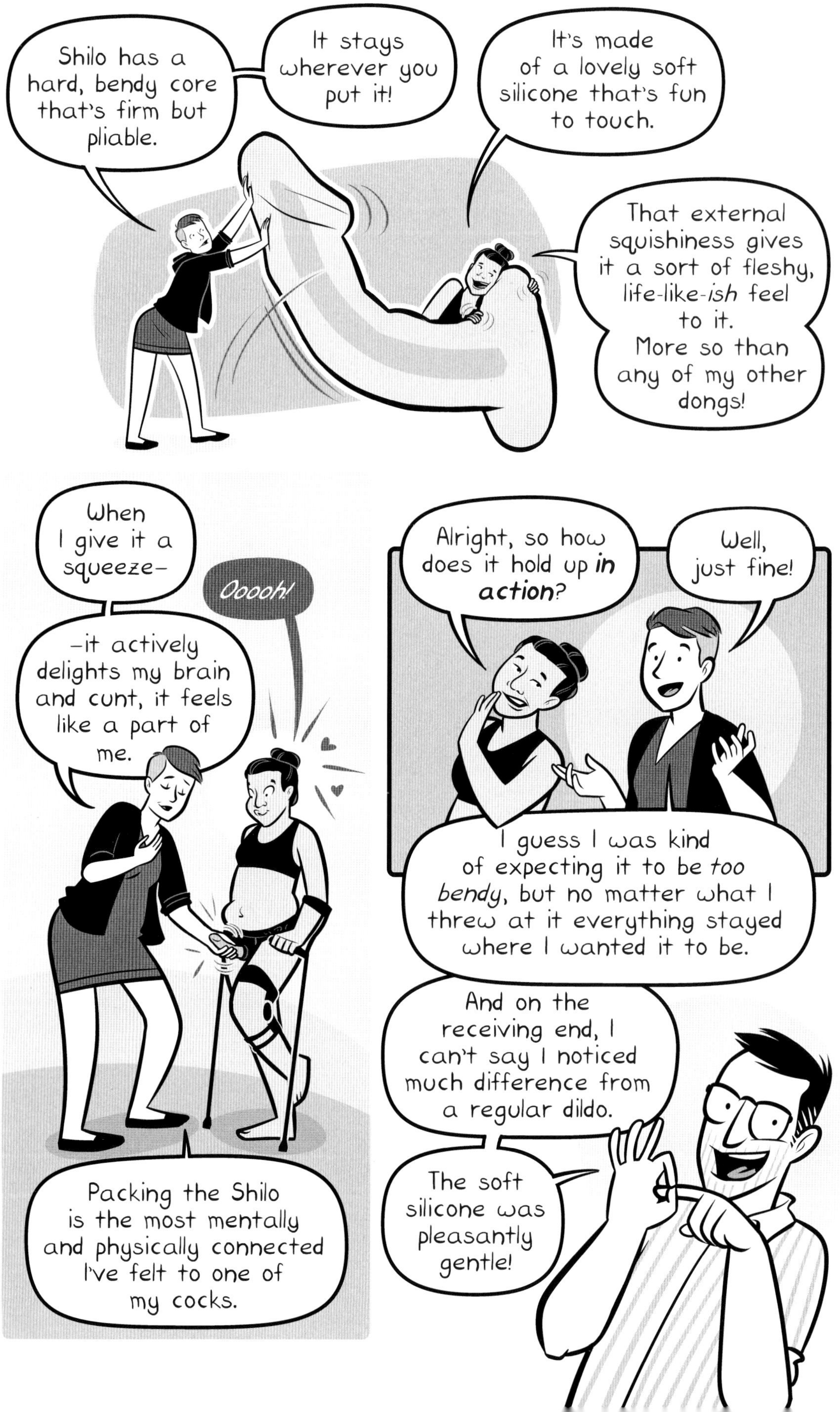
Shilo has a hard, bendy core that's firm but pliable.
It stays wherever you put it!
It's made of a lovely soft silicone that's fun to touch.
That external squishiness gives it a sort of fleshy, life-like-*ish* feel to it. More so than any of my other dongs!
When I give it a squeeze–
Ooooh!
–it actively delights my brain and cunt, it feels like a part of me.
Packing the Shilo is the most mentally and physically connected I've felt to one of my cocks.
Alright, so how does it hold up **in action**?
Well, just fine!
I guess I was kind of expecting it to be *too bendy*, but no matter what I threw at it everything stayed where I wanted it to be.
And on the receiving end, I can't say I noticed much difference from a regular dildo.
The soft silicone was pleasantly gentle!

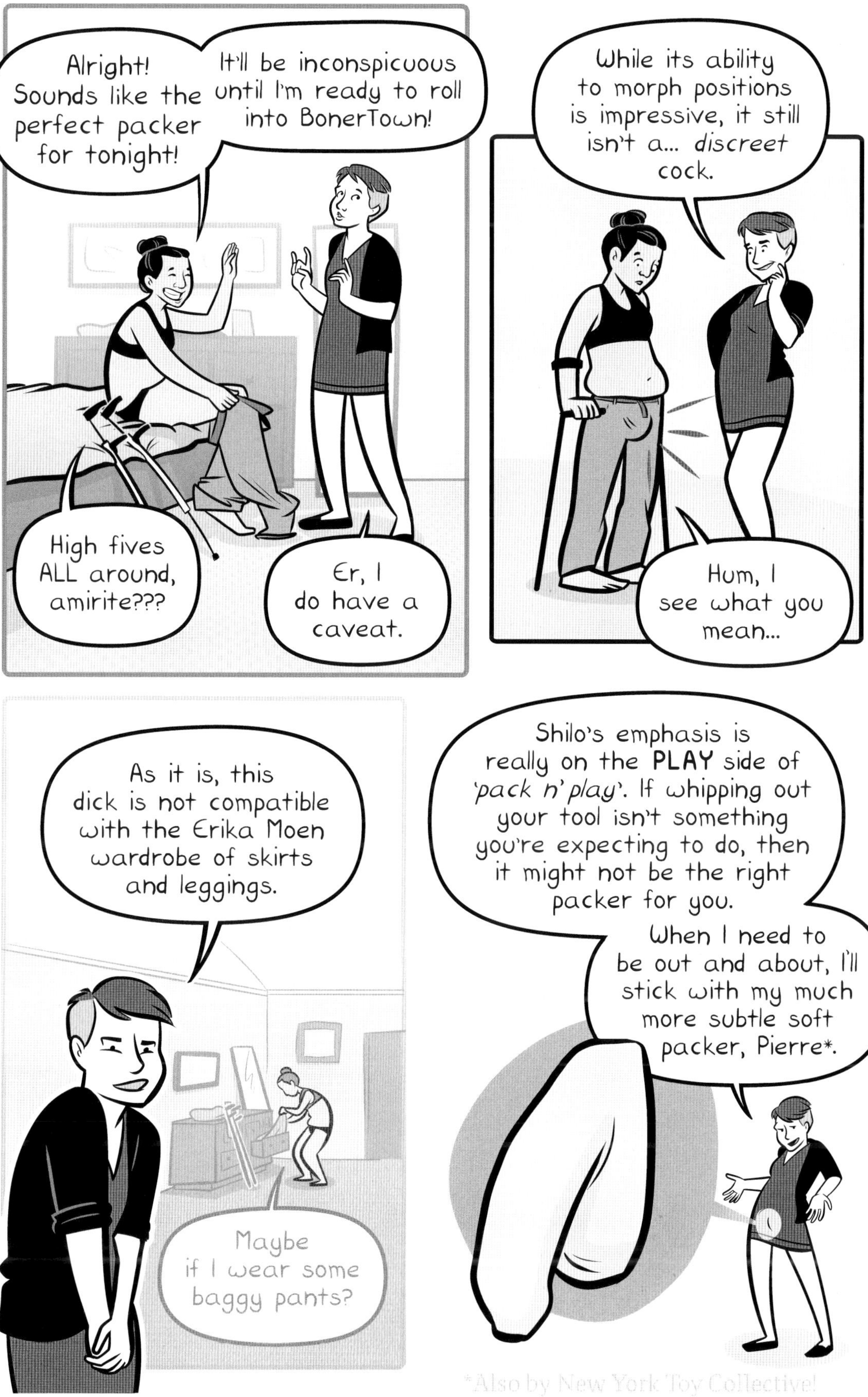
Alright! Sounds like the perfect packer for tonight!
It'll be inconspicuous until I'm ready to roll into BonerTown!
High fives ALL around, amirite???
Er, I do have a caveat.
While its ability to morph positions is impressive, it still isn't a... *discreet* cock.
Hum, I see what you mean...
As it is, this dick is not compatible with the Erika Moen wardrobe of skirts and leggings.
Maybe if I wear some baggy pants?
Shilo's emphasis is really on the **PLAY** side of *'pack n' play'*. If whipping out your tool isn't something you're expecting to do, then it might not be the right packer for you.
When I need to be out and about, I'll stick with my much more subtle soft packer, Pierre*.
*Also by New York Toy Collective!

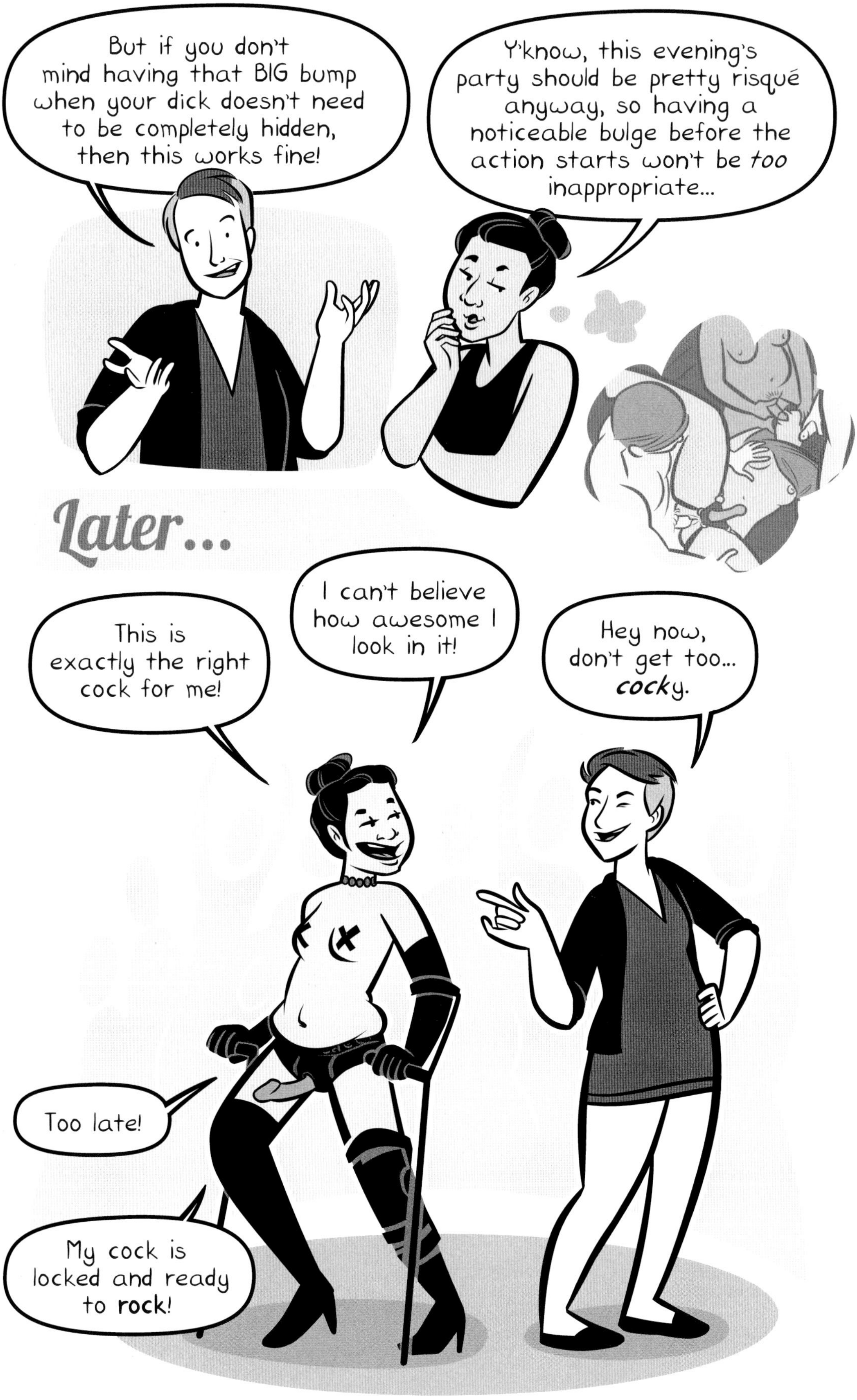

But if you don't mind having that BIG bump when your dick doesn't need to be completely hidden, then this works fine!
Y'know, this evening's party should be pretty risqué anyway, so having a noticeable bulge before the action starts won't be *too* inappropriate...
Later...
This is exactly the right cock for me!
I can't believe how awesome I look in it!
Hey now, don't get too... ***cock***y.
Too late!
My cock is locked and ready to **rock**!

Respect

Consent Joy

Exploration

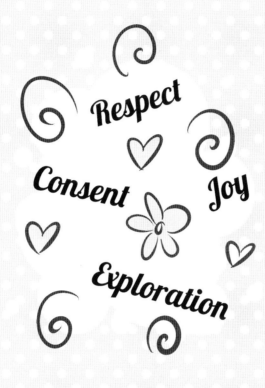

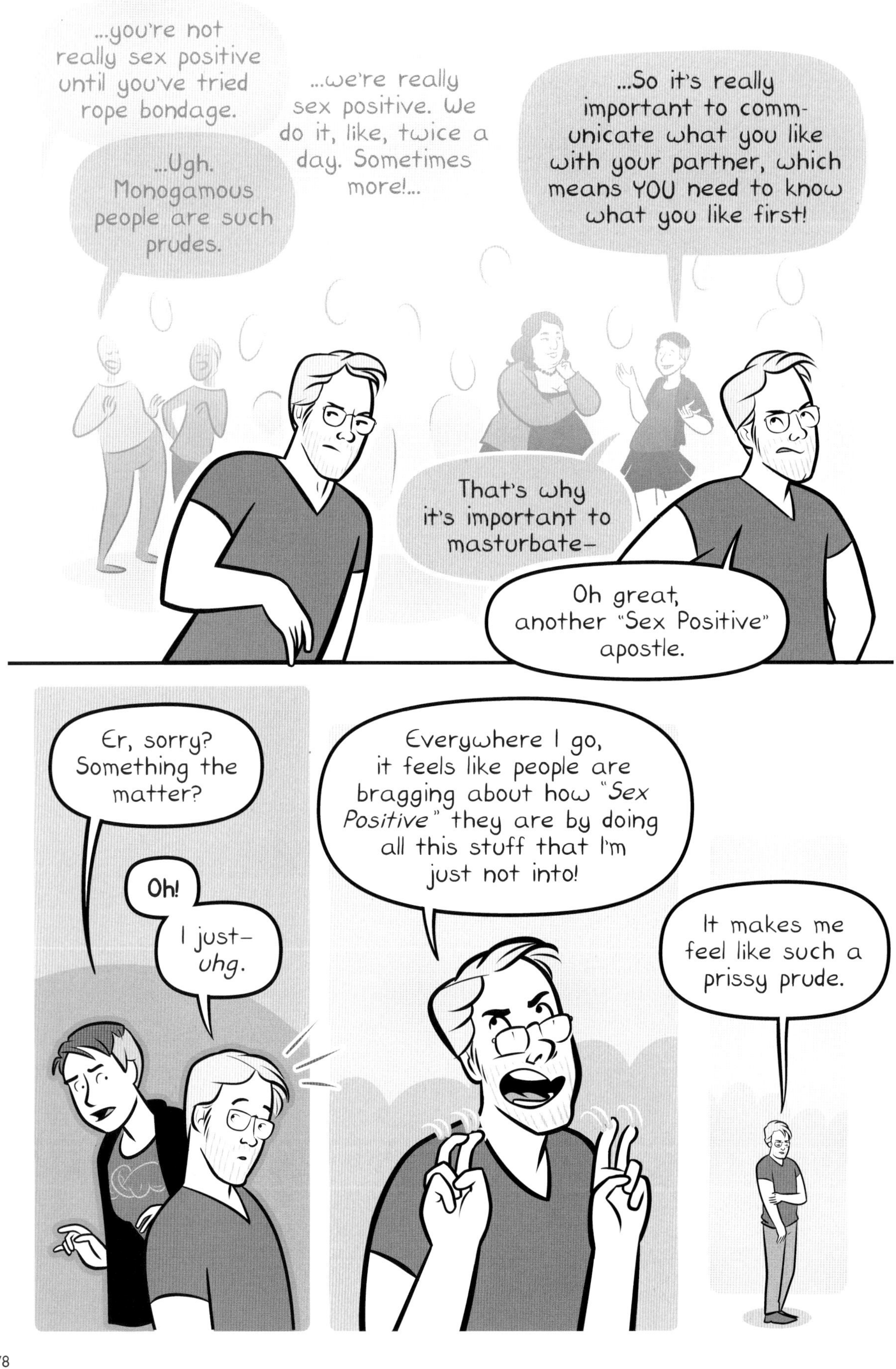

...you're not really sex positive until you've tried rope bondage.
...Ugh. Monogamous people are such prudes.
...we're really sex positive. We do it, like, twice a day. Sometimes more!...
...So it's really important to communicate what you like with your partner, which means YOU need to know what you like first!
That's why it's important to masturbate–
Oh great, another "Sex Positive" apostle.
Er, sorry? Something the matter?
Oh!
I just–uhg.
Everywhere I go, it feels like people are bragging about how "Sex Positive" they are by doing all this stuff that I'm just not into!
It makes me feel like such a prissy prude.

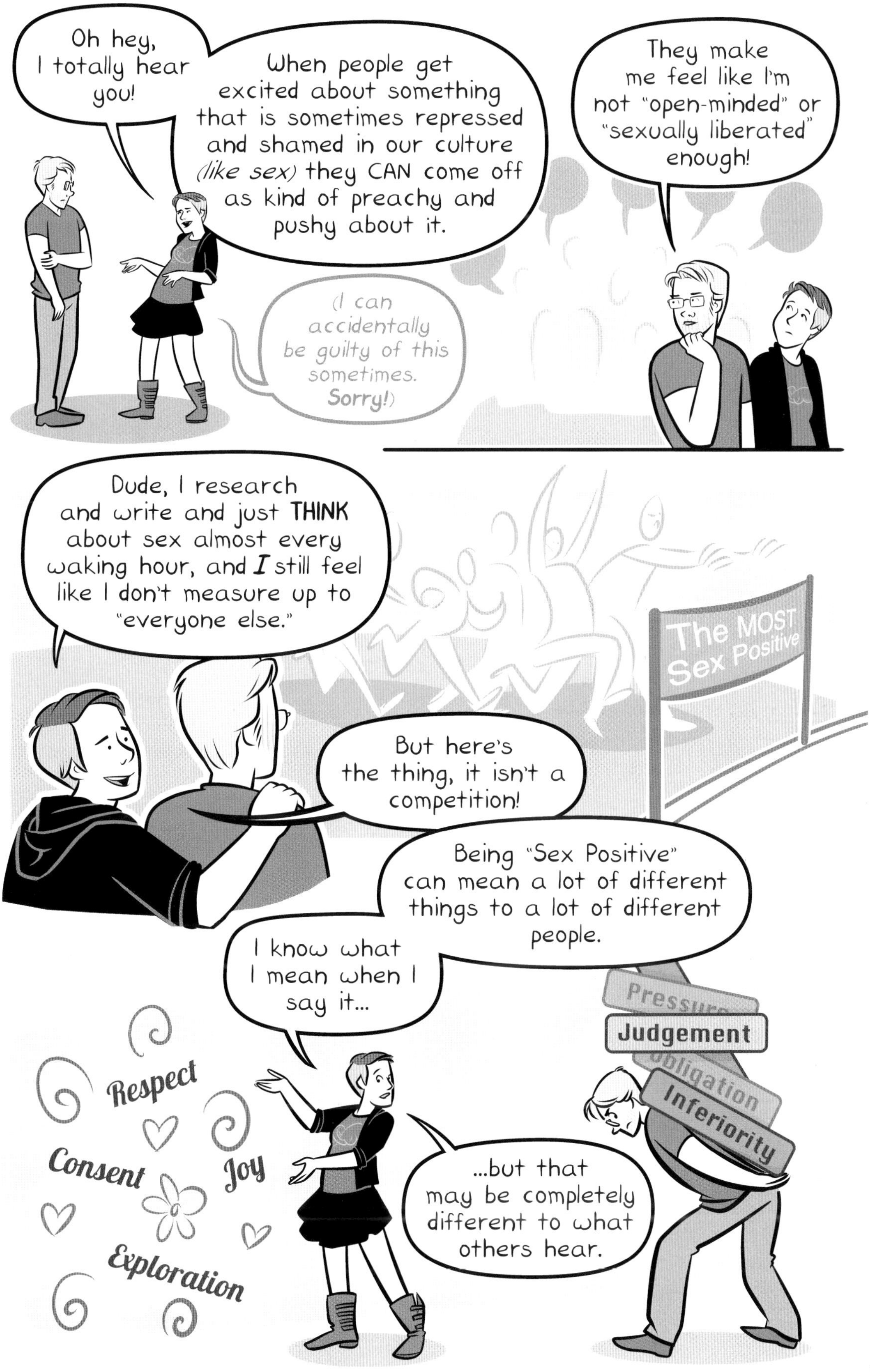
Oh hey, I totally hear you!
When people get excited about something that is sometimes repressed and shamed in our culture (like sex) they CAN come off as kind of preachy and pushy about it.
(I can accidentally be guilty of this sometimes. Sorry!)
They make me feel like I'm not "open-minded" or "sexually liberated" enough!
Dude, I research and write and just THINK about sex almost every waking hour, and I still feel like I don't measure up to "everyone else."
The MOST Sex Positive
But here's the thing, it isn't a competition!
Being "Sex Positive" can mean a lot of different things to a lot of different people.
I know what I mean when I say it...
Respect
Consent
Joy
Exploration
...but that may be completely different to what others hear.
Judgement
Obligation
Inferiority

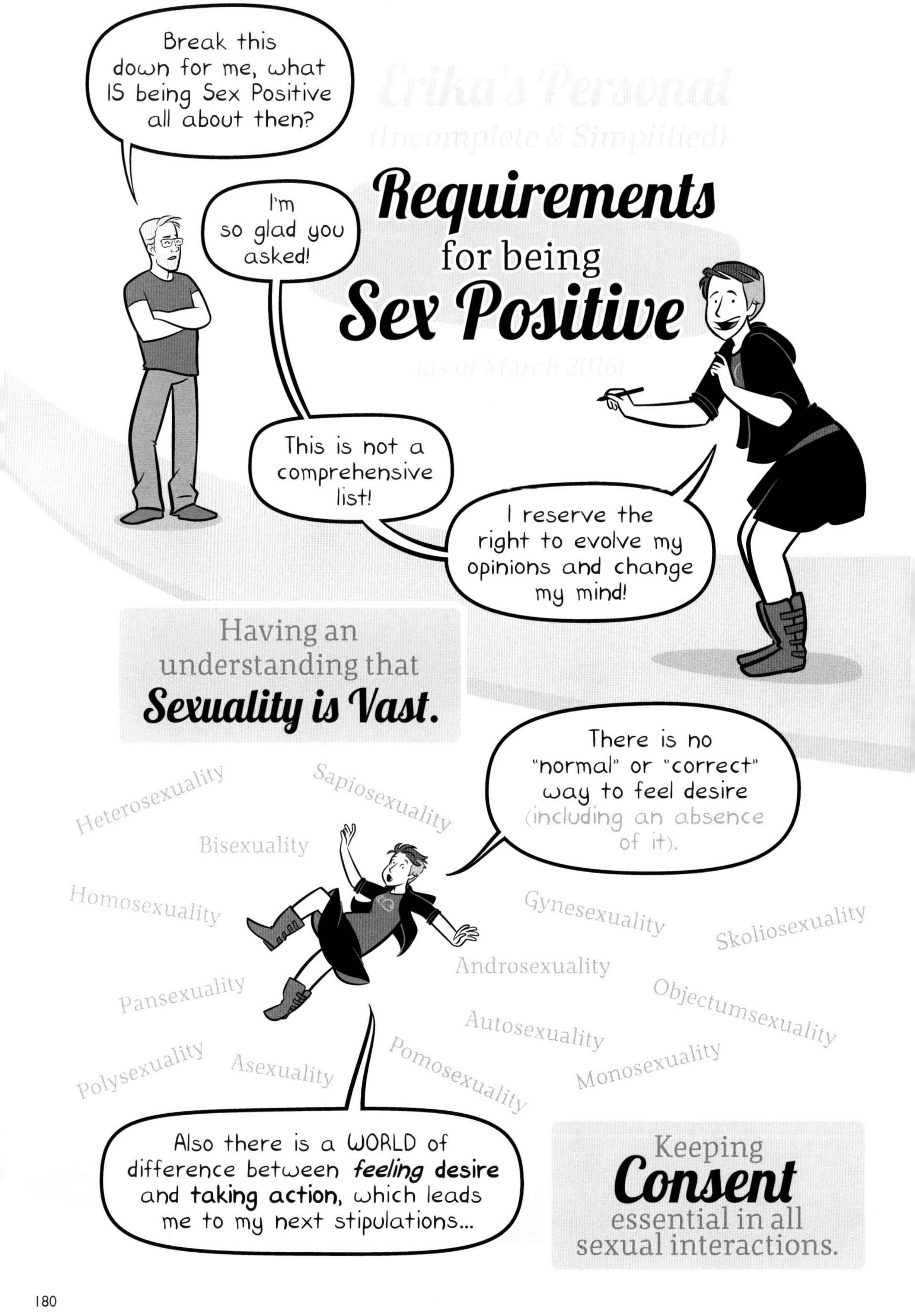

Break this down for me, what IS being Sex Positive all about then?
I'm so glad you asked!
Erika's Personal
(Incomplete & Simplified)
Requirements
for being
Sex Positive
(as of March 2016)
This is not a comprehensive list!
I reserve the right to evolve my opinions and change my mind!
Having an understanding that Sexuality is Vast.
There is no "normal" or "correct" way to feel desire (including an absence of it).
Heterosexuality
Sapiosexuality
Bisexuality
Homosexuality
Gynesexuality
Skoliosexuality
Androsexuality
Pansexuality
Objectumsexuality
Autosexuality
Polysexuality
Asexuality
Pomosexuality
Monosexuality
Also there is a WORLD of difference between feeling desire and taking action, which leads me to my next stipulations...
Keeping Consent essential in all sexual interactions.

Fostering
Tolerance
for identities, orientations and consensual practices that differ from your own.

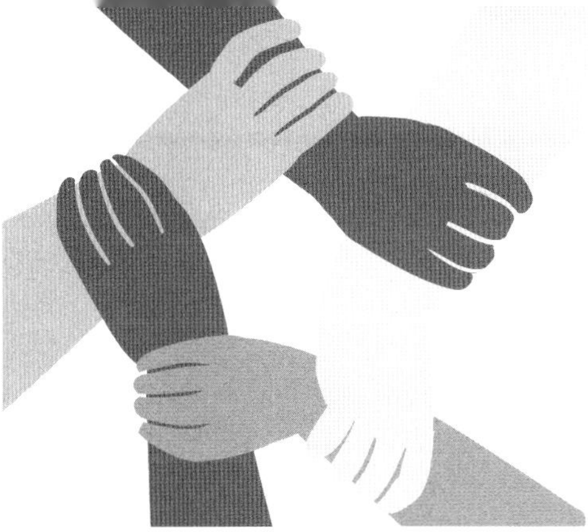

Knowing that everyone is entitled to
Comprehensive Sex Education
that teaches function, safety, choice, and pleasure without moral judgement, shaming, or pressure.

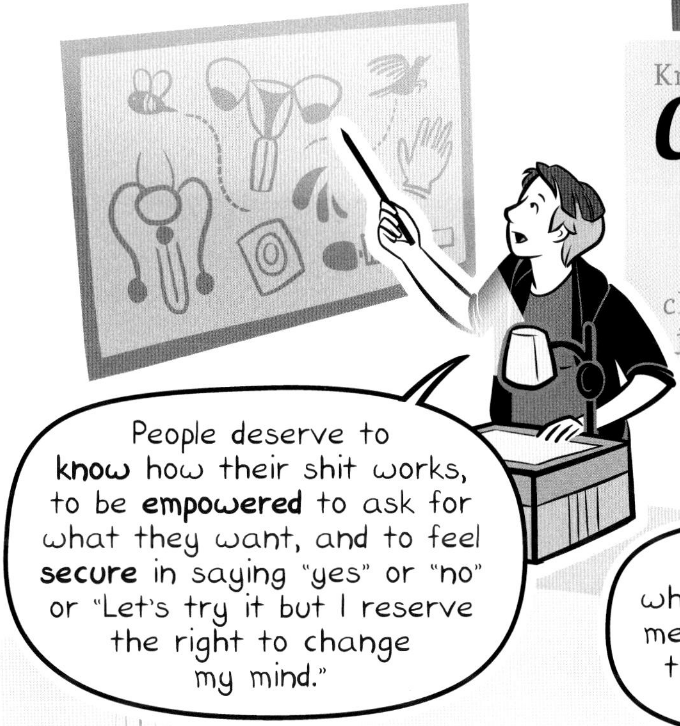
People deserve to **know** how their shit works, to be **empowered** to ask for what they want, and to feel **secure** in saying "yes" or "no" or "Let's try it but I reserve the right to change my mind."

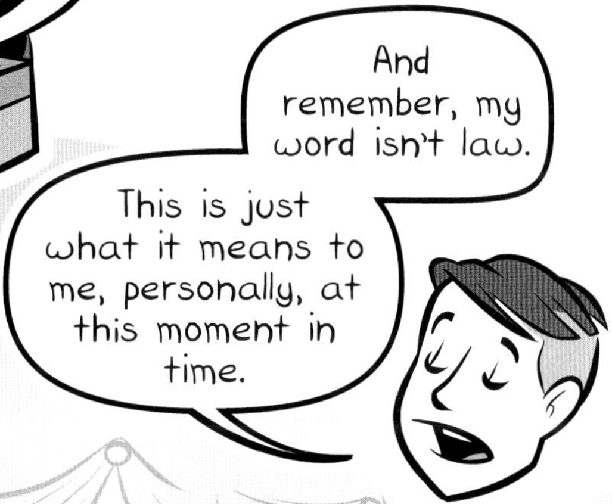
And remember, my word isn't law.
This is just what it means to me, personally, at this moment in time.

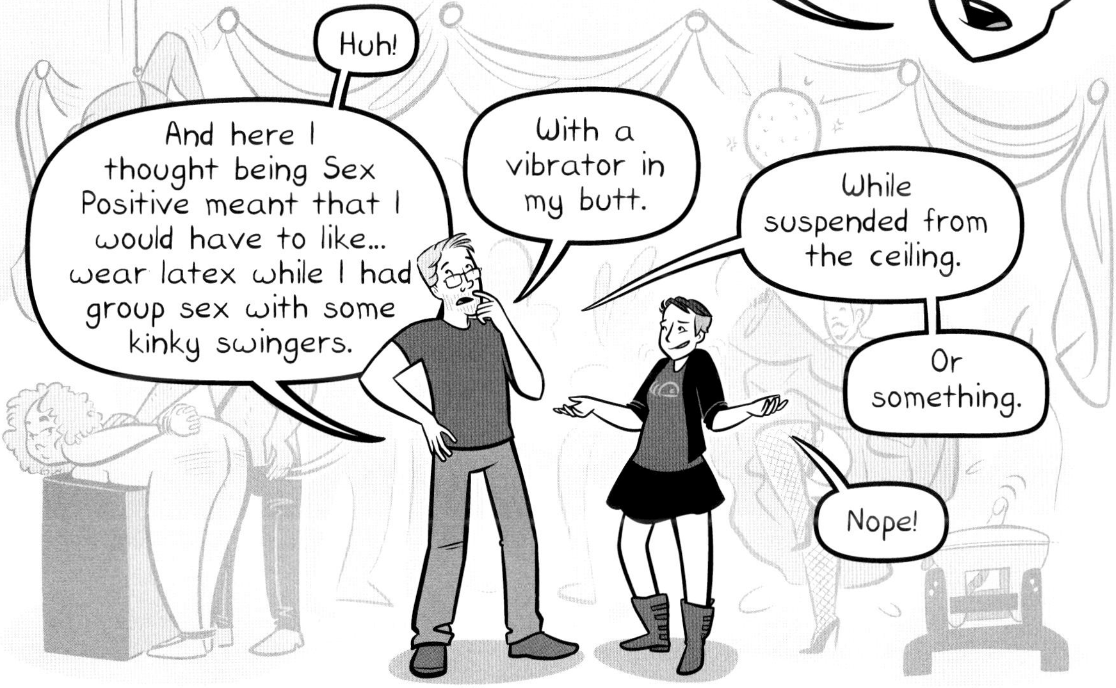
Huh!
And here I thought being Sex Positive meant that I would have to like... wear latex while I had group sex with some kinky swingers.
With a vibrator in my butt.
While suspended from the ceiling.
Or something.
Nope!

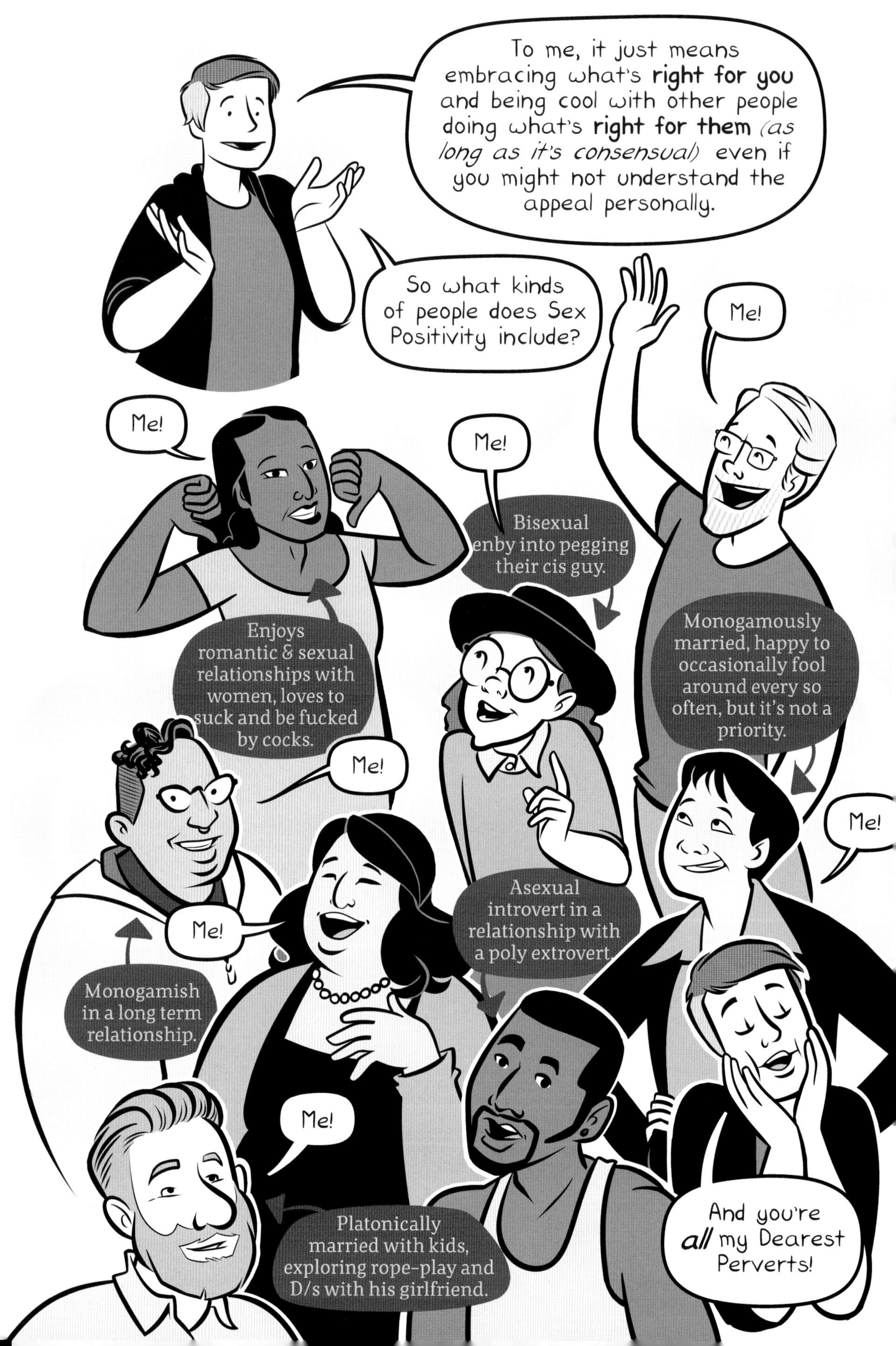
To me, it just means embracing what's **right for you** and being cool with other people doing what's **right for them** *(as long as it's consensual)* even if you might not understand the appeal personally.
So what kinds of people does Sex Positivity include?
Me!
Me!
Me!
Bisexual enby into pegging their cis guy.
Enjoys romantic & sexual relationships with women, loves to suck and be fucked by cocks.
Monogamously married, happy to occasionally fool around every so often, but it's not a priority.
Me!
Me!
Me!
Asexual introvert in a relationship with a poly extrovert.
Monogamish in a long term relationship.
Me!
Platonically married with kids, exploring rope-play and D/s with his girlfriend.
And you're *all* my Dearest Perverts!

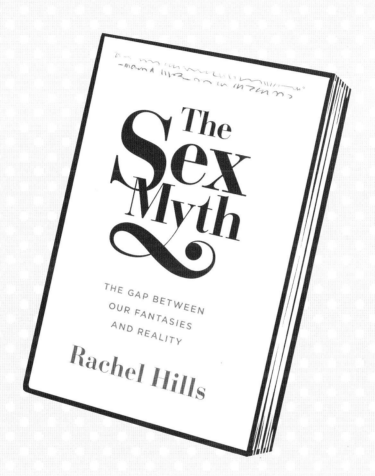

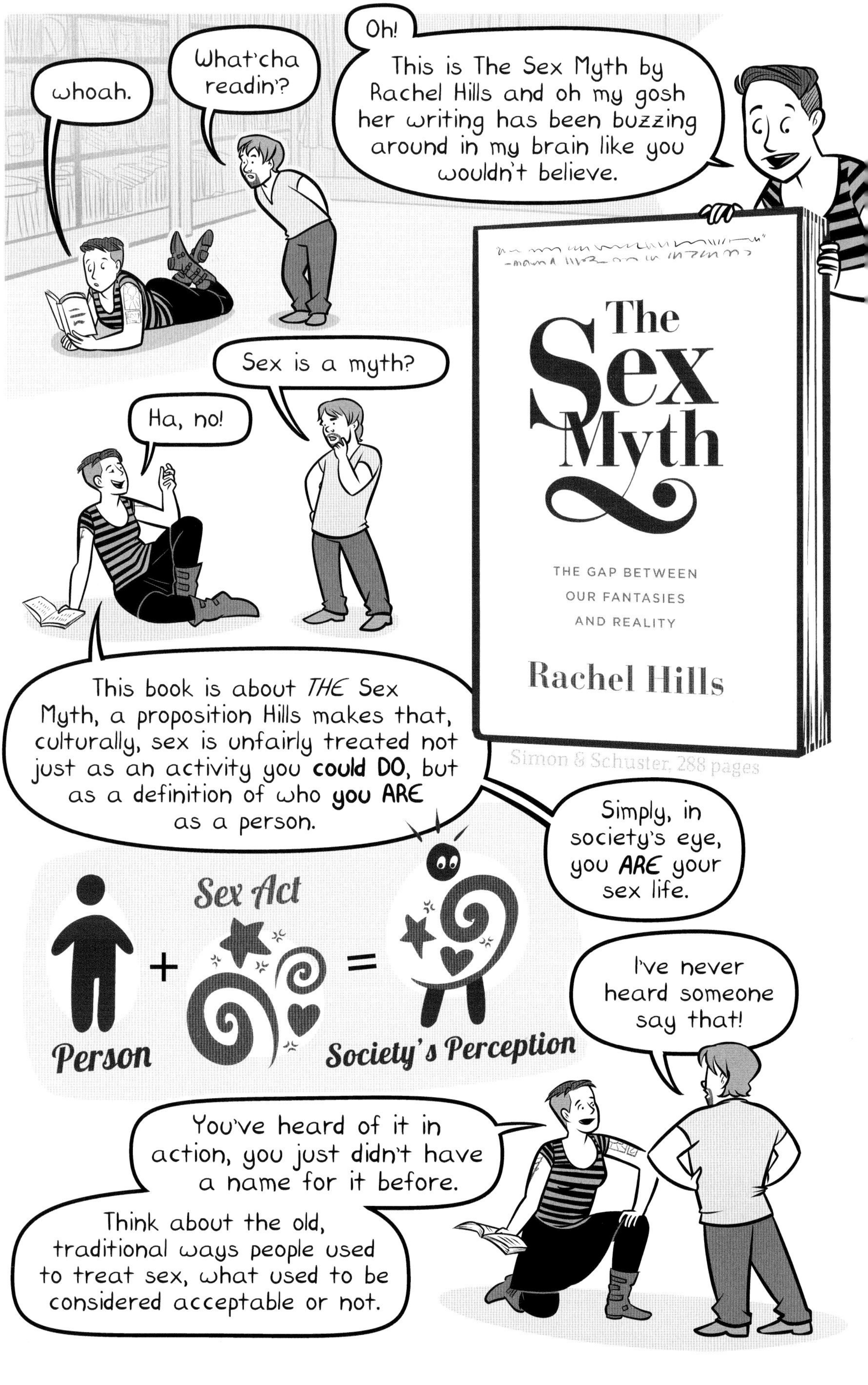
whoah.
What'cha readin'?
Oh!
This is The Sex Myth by Rachel Hills and oh my gosh her writing has been buzzing around in my brain like you wouldn't believe.
The Sex Myth
THE GAP BETWEEN OUR FANTASIES AND REALITY
Rachel Hills
Simon & Schuster, 288 pages
Sex is a myth?
Ha, no!
This book is about *THE* Sex Myth, a proposition Hills makes that, culturally, sex is unfairly treated not just as an activity you **could DO**, but as a definition of who **you ARE** as a person.
Simply, in society's eye, you **ARE** your sex life.
Person
Sex Act
Society's Perception
I've never heard someone say that!
You've heard of it in action, you just didn't have a name for it before.
Think about the old, traditional ways people used to treat sex, what used to be considered acceptable or not.

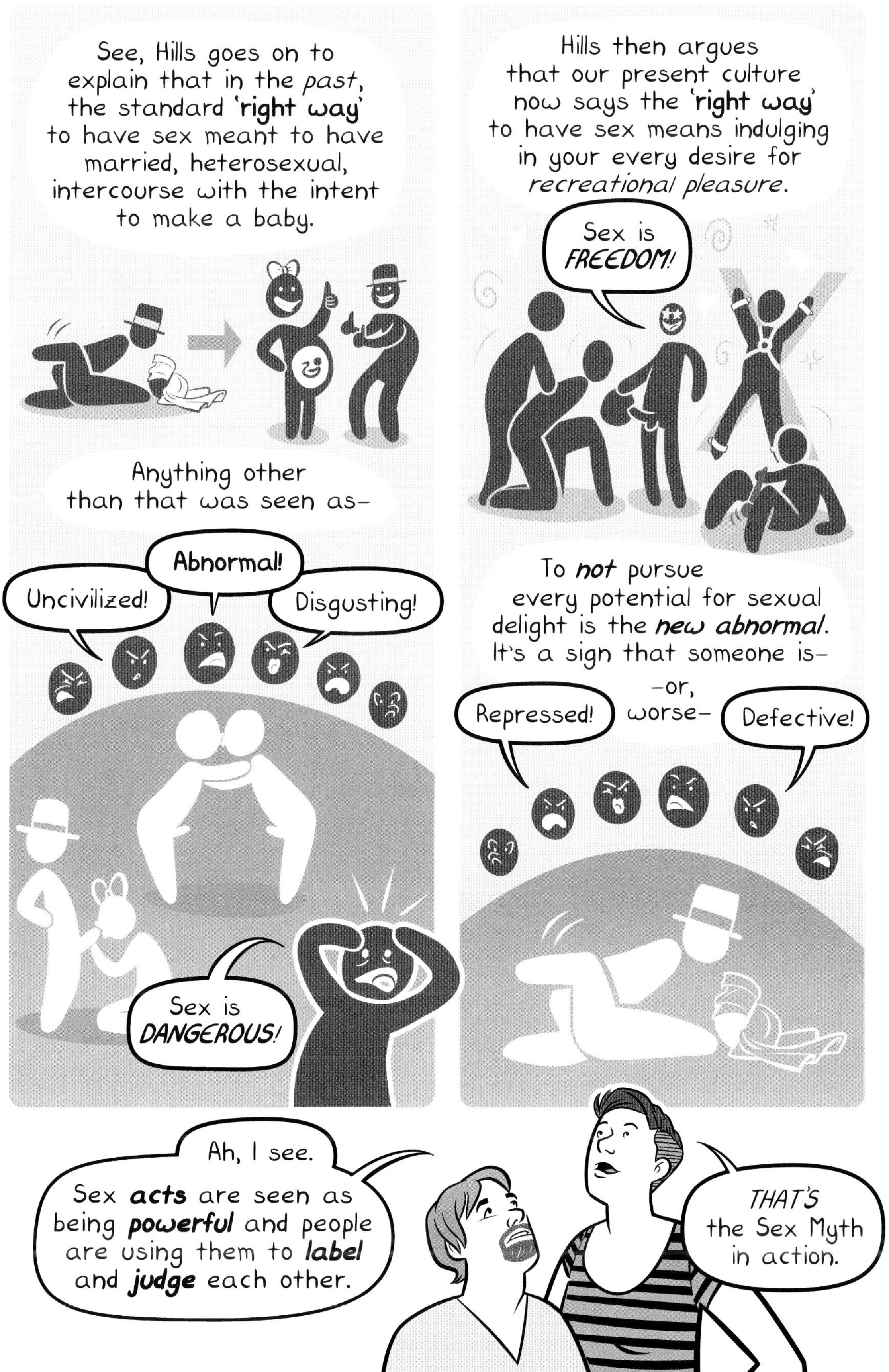

See, Hills goes on to explain that in the *past*, the standard **'right way'** to have sex meant to have married, heterosexual, intercourse with the intent to make a baby.
Anything other than that was seen as–
Uncivilized!
Abnormal!
Disgusting!
Sex is *DANGEROUS!*
Hills then argues that our present culture now says the **'right way'** to have sex means indulging in your every desire for *recreational pleasure*.
Sex is *FREEDOM!*
To ***not*** pursue every potential for sexual delight is the ***new abnormal***. It's a sign that someone is–
Repressed!
–or, worse–
Defective!
Ah, I see.
Sex **acts** are seen as being ***powerful*** and people are using them to ***label*** and ***judge*** each other.
THAT'S the Sex Myth in action.

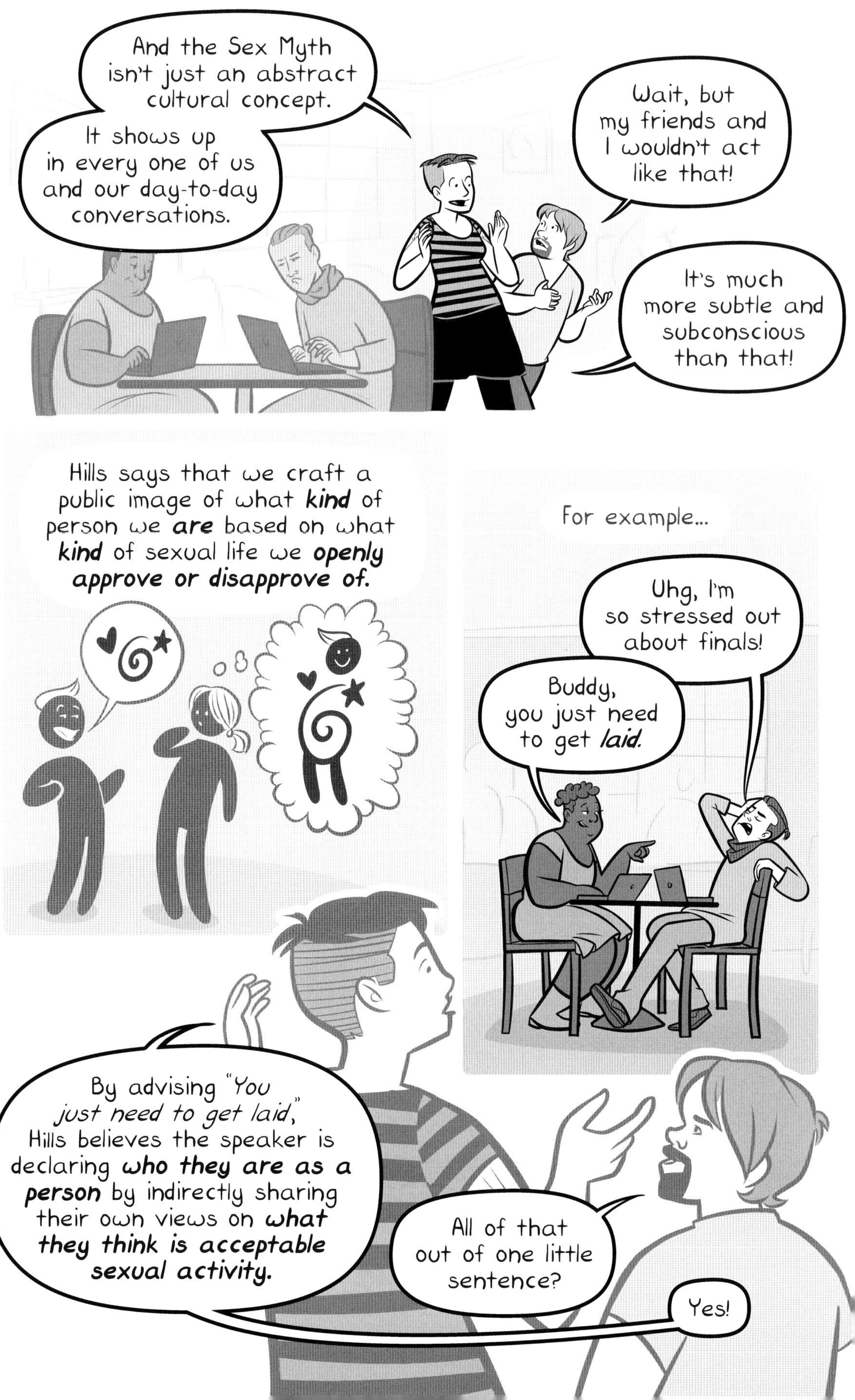
And the Sex Myth isn't just an abstract cultural concept.
It shows up in every one of us and our day-to-day conversations.
Wait, but my friends and I wouldn't act like that!
It's much more subtle and subconscious than that!
Hills says that we craft a public image of what **kind** of person we **are** based on what **kind** of sexual life we **openly approve or disapprove of.**
For example...
Uhg, I'm so stressed out about finals!
Buddy, you just need to get *laid.*
By advising "*You just need to get laid*," Hills believes the speaker is declaring **who they are as a person** by indirectly sharing their own views on **what they think is acceptable sexual activity.**
All of that out of one little sentence?
Yes!

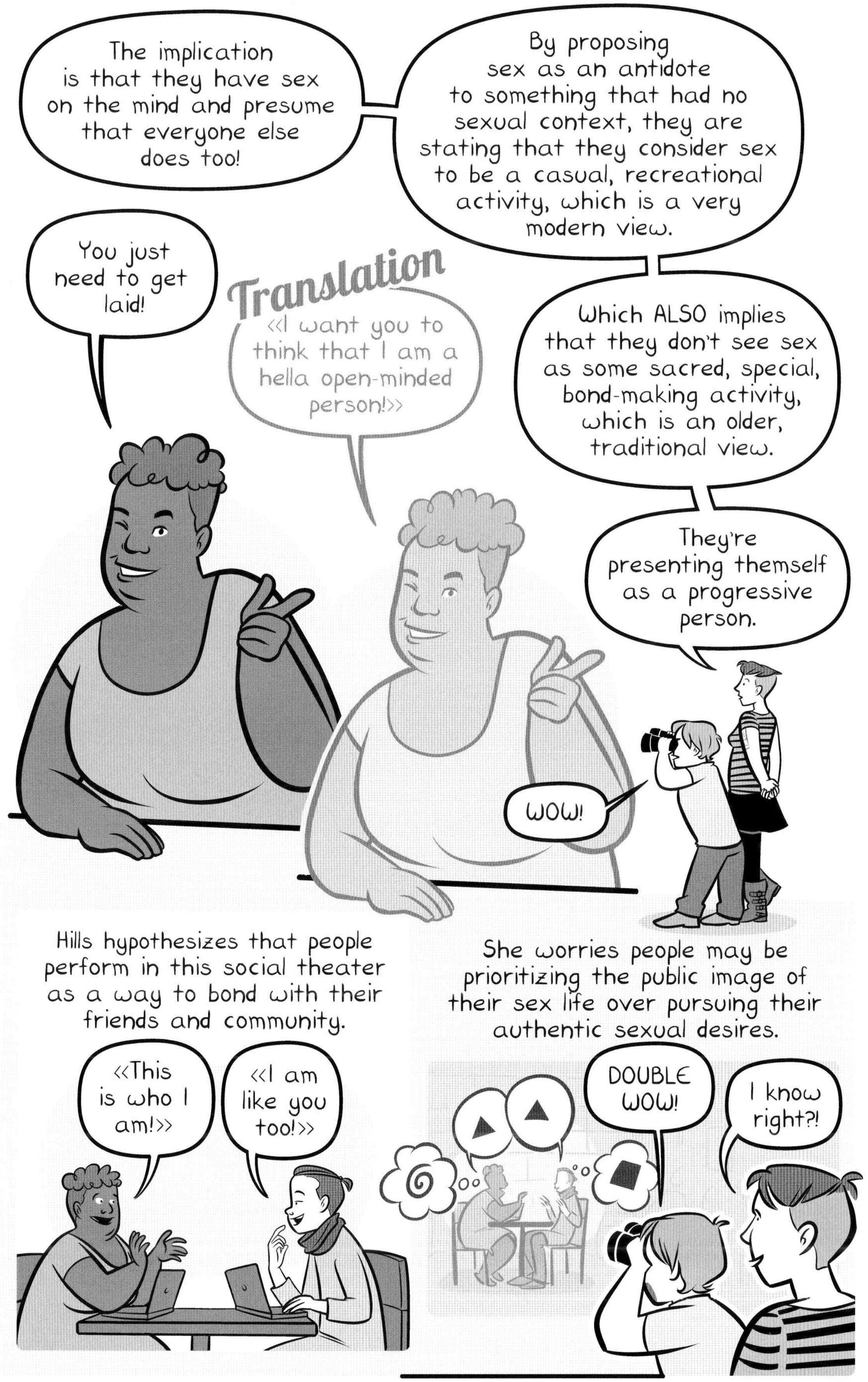
The implication is that they have sex on the mind and presume that everyone else does too!
By proposing sex as an antidote to something that had no sexual context, they are stating that they consider sex to be a casual, recreational activity, which is a very modern view.
You just need to get laid!
Translation
<<I want you to think that I am a hella open-minded person!>>
Which ALSO implies that they don't see sex as some sacred, special, bond-making activity, which is an older, traditional view.
They're presenting themself as a progressive person.
WOW!
Hills hypothesizes that people perform in this social theater as a way to bond with their friends and community.
<<This is who I am!>>
<<I am like you too!>>
She worries people may be prioritizing the public image of their sex life over pursuing their authentic sexual desires.
DOUBLE WOW!
I know right?!

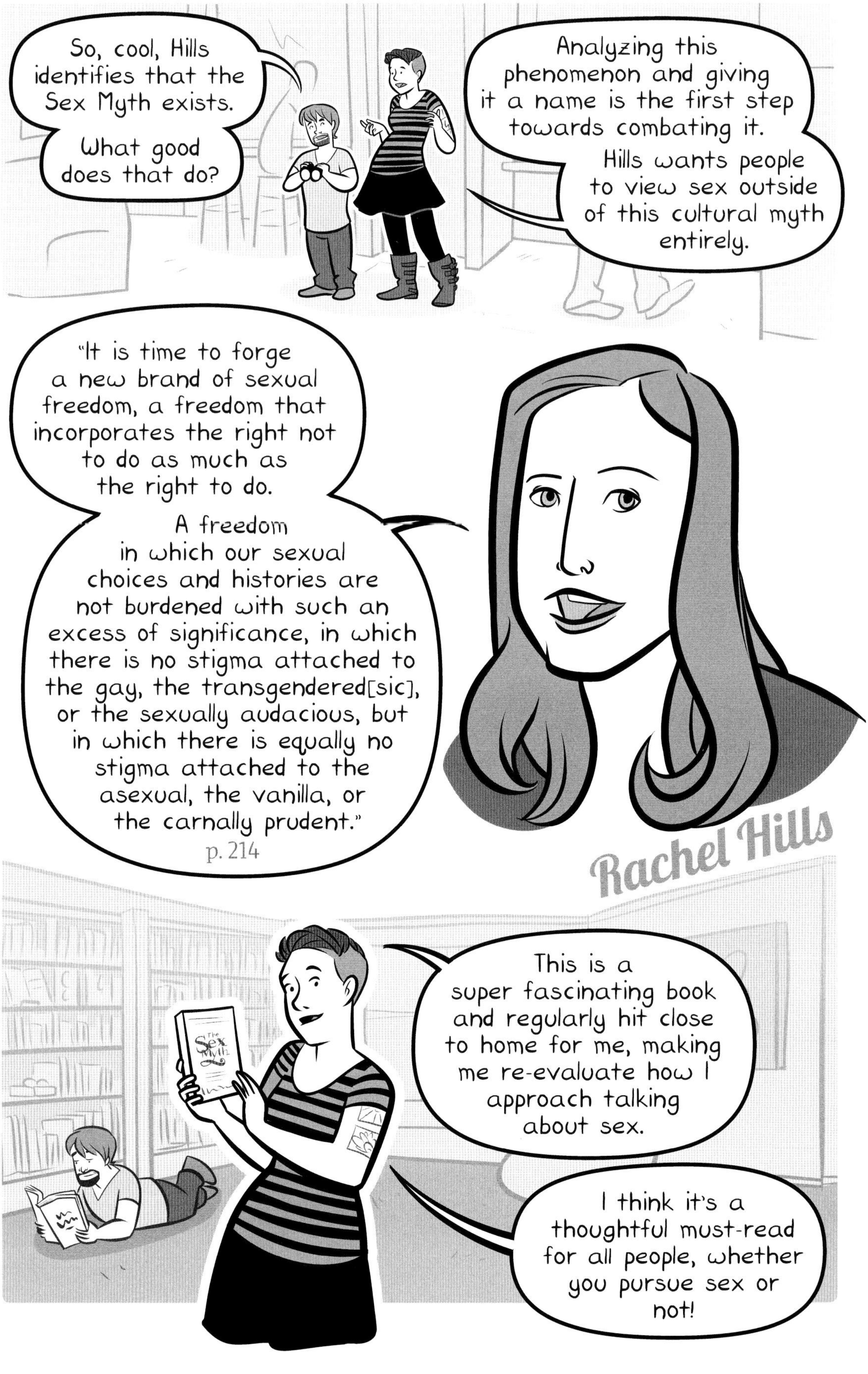
So, cool, Hills identifies that the Sex Myth exists.
What good does that do?
Analyzing this phenomenon and giving it a name is the first step towards combating it.
Hills wants people to view sex outside of this cultural myth entirely.
"It is time to forge a new brand of sexual freedom, a freedom that incorporates the right not to do as much as the right to do.
A freedom in which our sexual choices and histories are not burdened with such an excess of significance, in which there is no stigma attached to the gay, the transgendered[sic], or the sexually audacious, but in which there is equally no stigma attached to the asexual, the vanilla, or the carnally prudent."
p. 214
Rachel Hills
This is a super fascinating book and regularly hit close to home for me, making me re-evaluate how I approach talking about sex.
I think it's a thoughtful must-read for all people, whether you pursue sex or not!

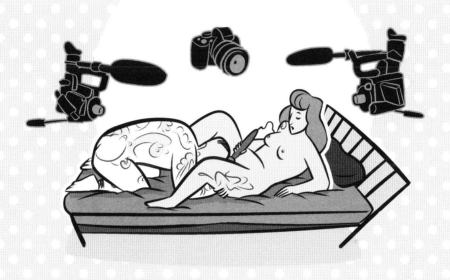

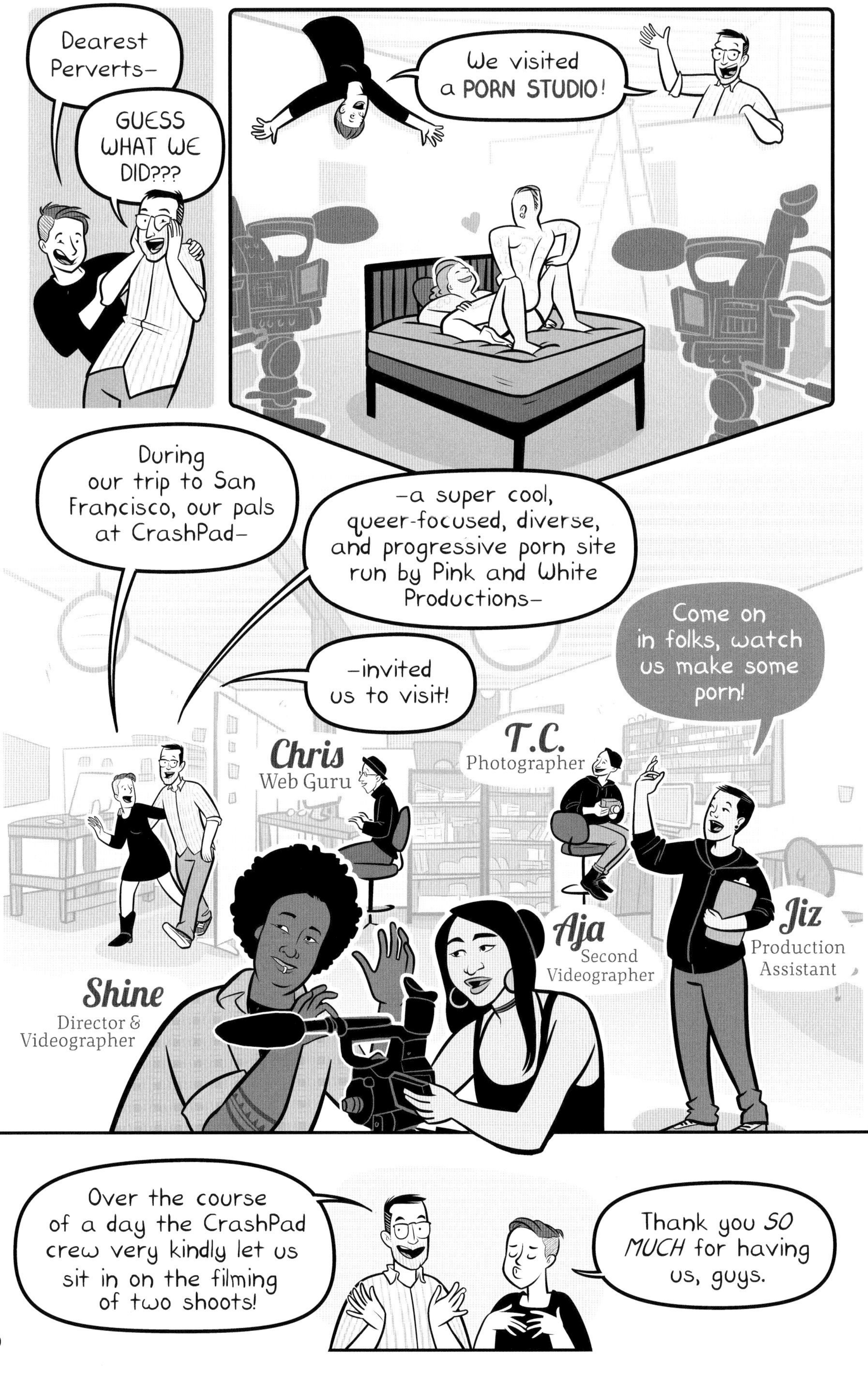
Dearest Perverts–
GUESS WHAT WE DID???
We visited a PORN STUDIO!
During our trip to San Francisco, our pals at CrashPad–
–a super cool, queer-focused, diverse, and progressive porn site run by Pink and White Productions–
–invited us to visit!
Come on in folks, watch us make some porn!
Chris
Web Guru
T.C.
Photographer
Aja
Second Videographer
Jiz
Production Assistant
Shine
Director & Videographer
Over the course of a day the CrashPad crew very kindly let us sit in on the filming of two shoots!
Thank you *SO MUCH* for having us, guys.

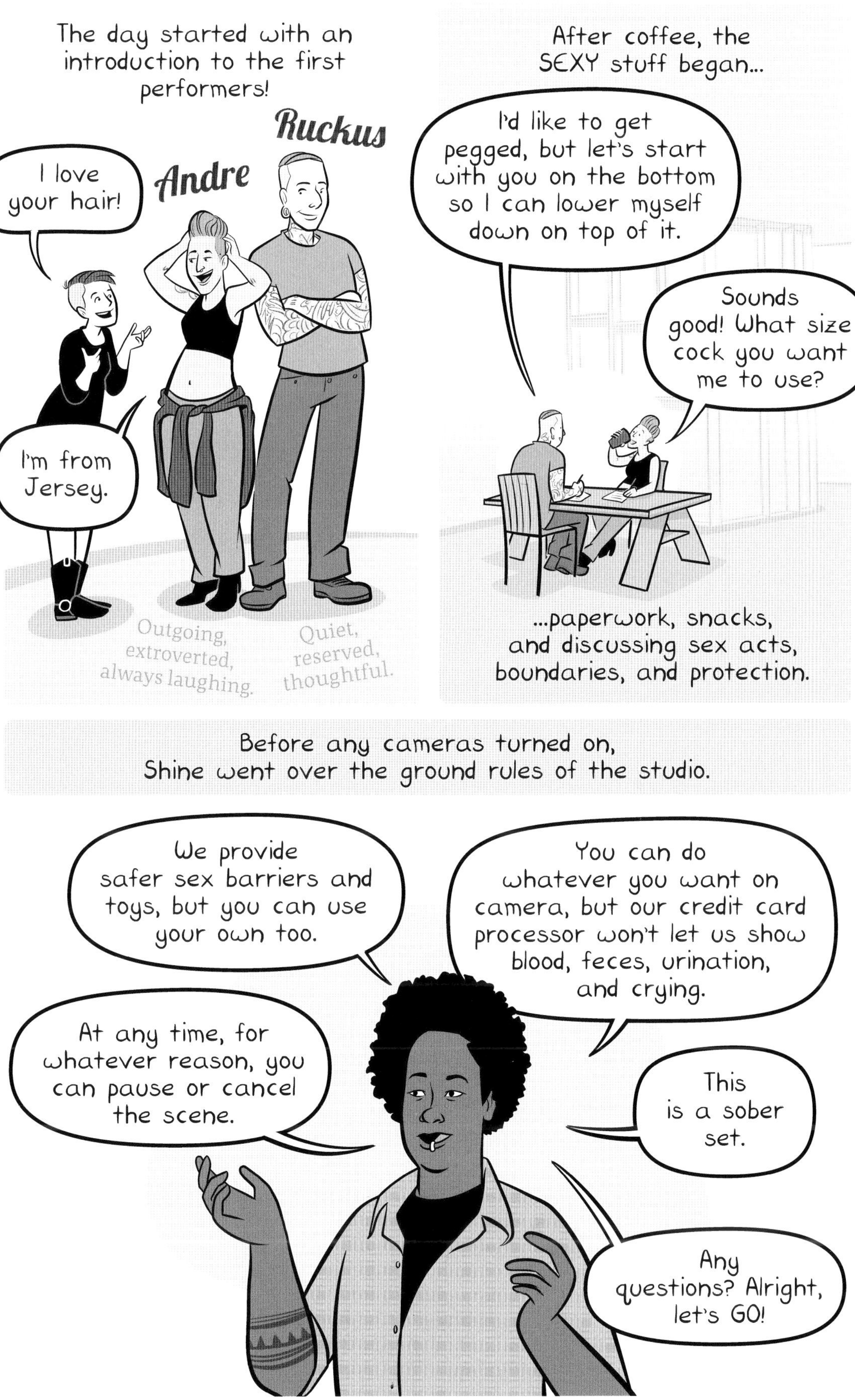
The day started with an introduction to the first performers!
I love your hair!
Andre
Ruckus
I'm from Jersey.
Outgoing, extroverted, always laughing.
Quiet, reserved, thoughtful.
After coffee, the SEXY stuff began...
I'd like to get pegged, but let's start with you on the bottom so I can lower myself down on top of it.
Sounds good! What size cock you want me to use?
...paperwork, snacks, and discussing sex acts, boundaries, and protection.
Before any cameras turned on, Shine went over the ground rules of the studio.
We provide safer sex barriers and toys, but you can use your own too.
You can do whatever you want on camera, but our credit card processor won't let us show blood, feces, urination, and crying.
At any time, for whatever reason, you can pause or cancel the scene.
This is a sober set.
Any questions? Alright, let's GO!

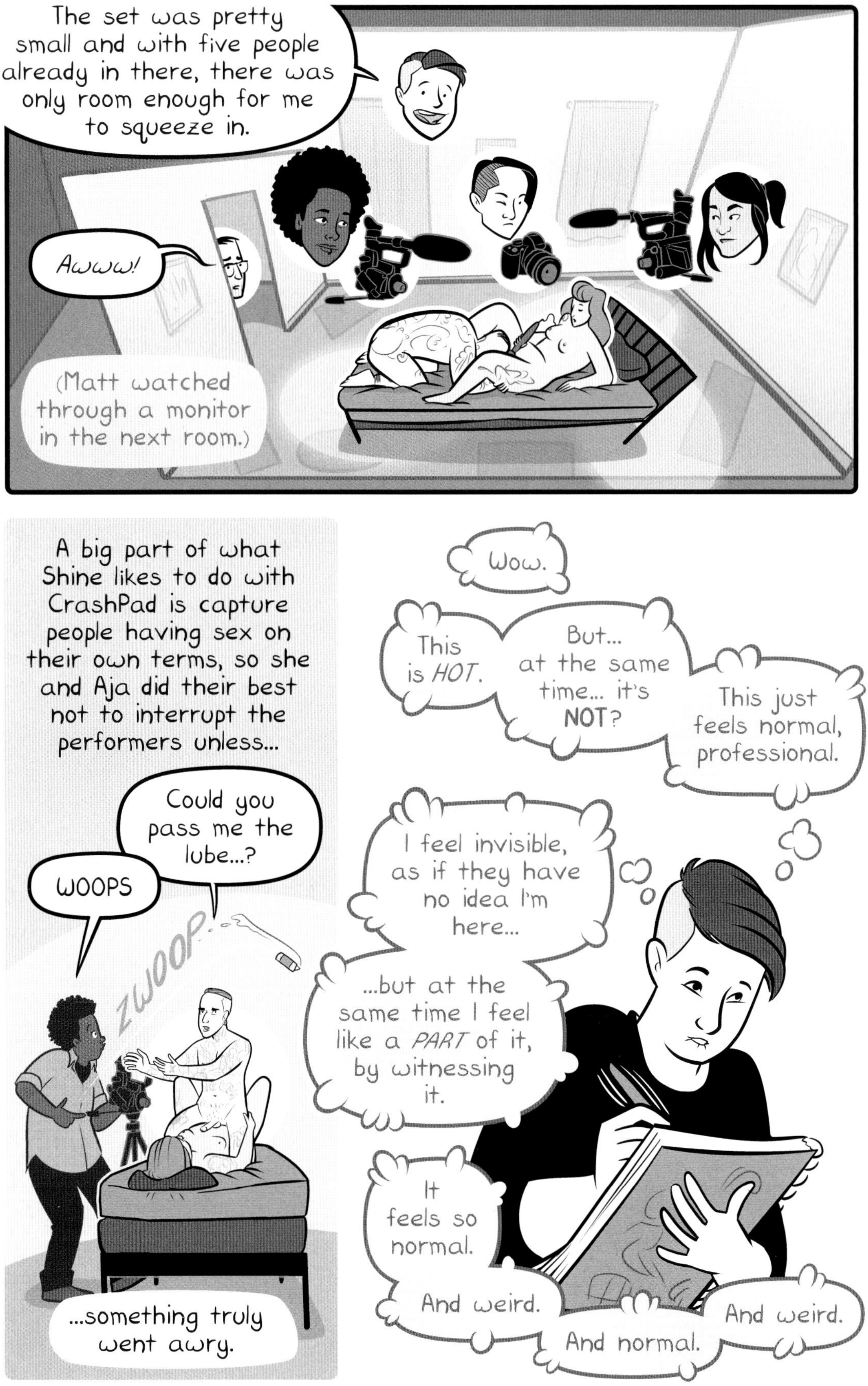

The set was pretty small and with five people already in there, there was only room enough for me to squeeze in.
Awww!
(Matt watched through a monitor in the next room.)
A big part of what Shine likes to do with CrashPad is capture people having sex on their own terms, so she and Aja did their best not to interrupt the performers unless...
Could you pass me the lube...?
WOOPS
ZWOOP
...something truly went awry.
Wow.
This is *HOT*.
But... at the same time... it's **NOT**?
This just feels normal, professional.
I feel invisible, as if they have no idea I'm here...
...but at the same time I feel like a *PART* of it, by witnessing it.
It feels so normal.
And weird.
And normal.
And weird.

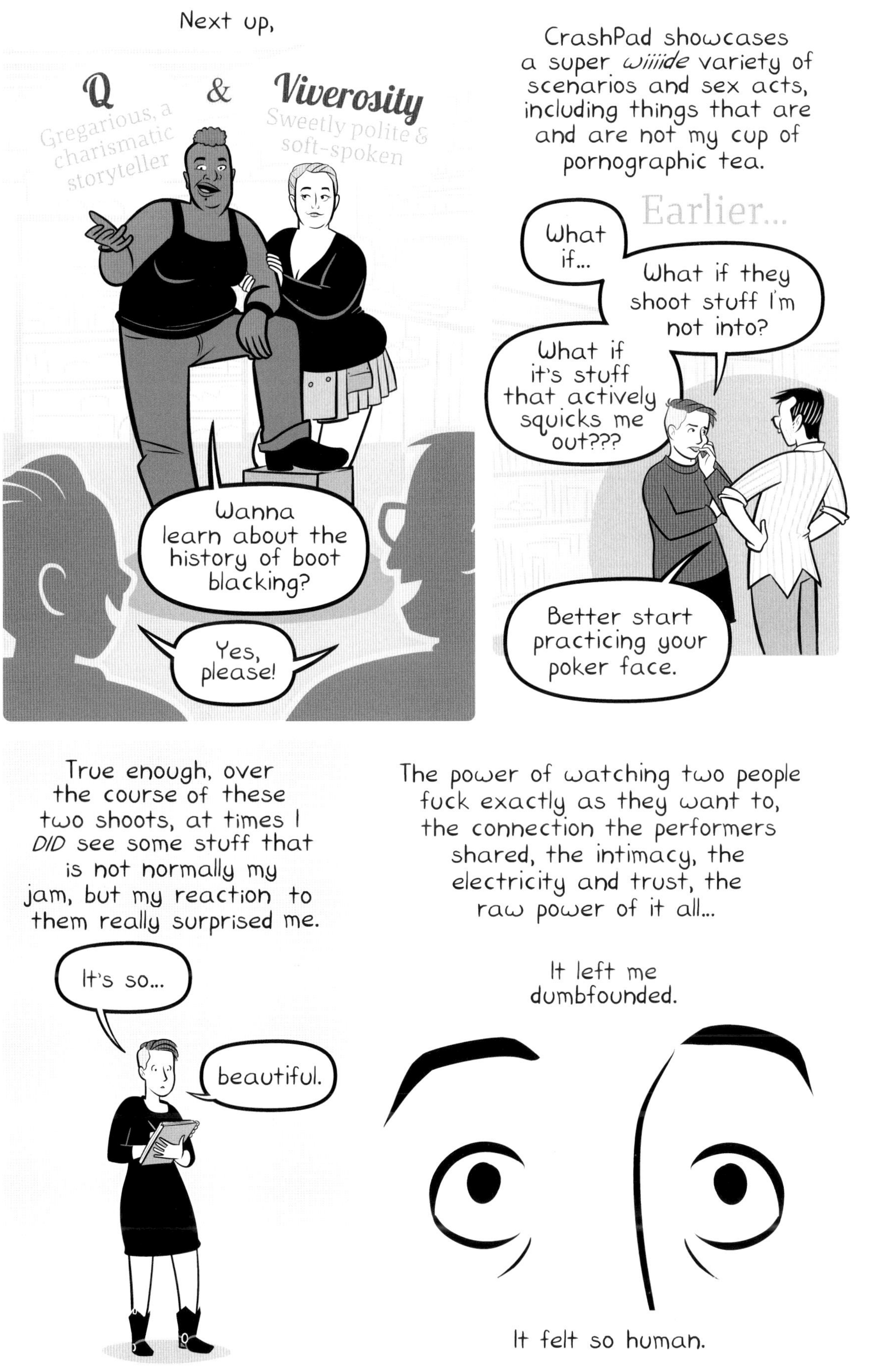
Next up,
Q & Viverosity
Gregarious, a charismatic storyteller
Sweetly polite & soft-spoken
Wanna learn about the history of boot blacking?
Yes, please!
CrashPad showcases a super *wiiiide* variety of scenarios and sex acts, including things that are and are not my cup of pornographic tea.
Earlier...
What if...
What if they shoot stuff I'm not into?
What if it's stuff that actively squicks me out???
Better start practicing your poker face.
True enough, over the course of these two shoots, at times I *DID* see some stuff that is not normally my jam, but my reaction to them really surprised me.
It's so...
beautiful.
The power of watching two people fuck exactly as they want to, the connection the performers shared, the intimacy, the electricity and trust, the raw power of it all...
It left me dumbfounded.
It felt so human.

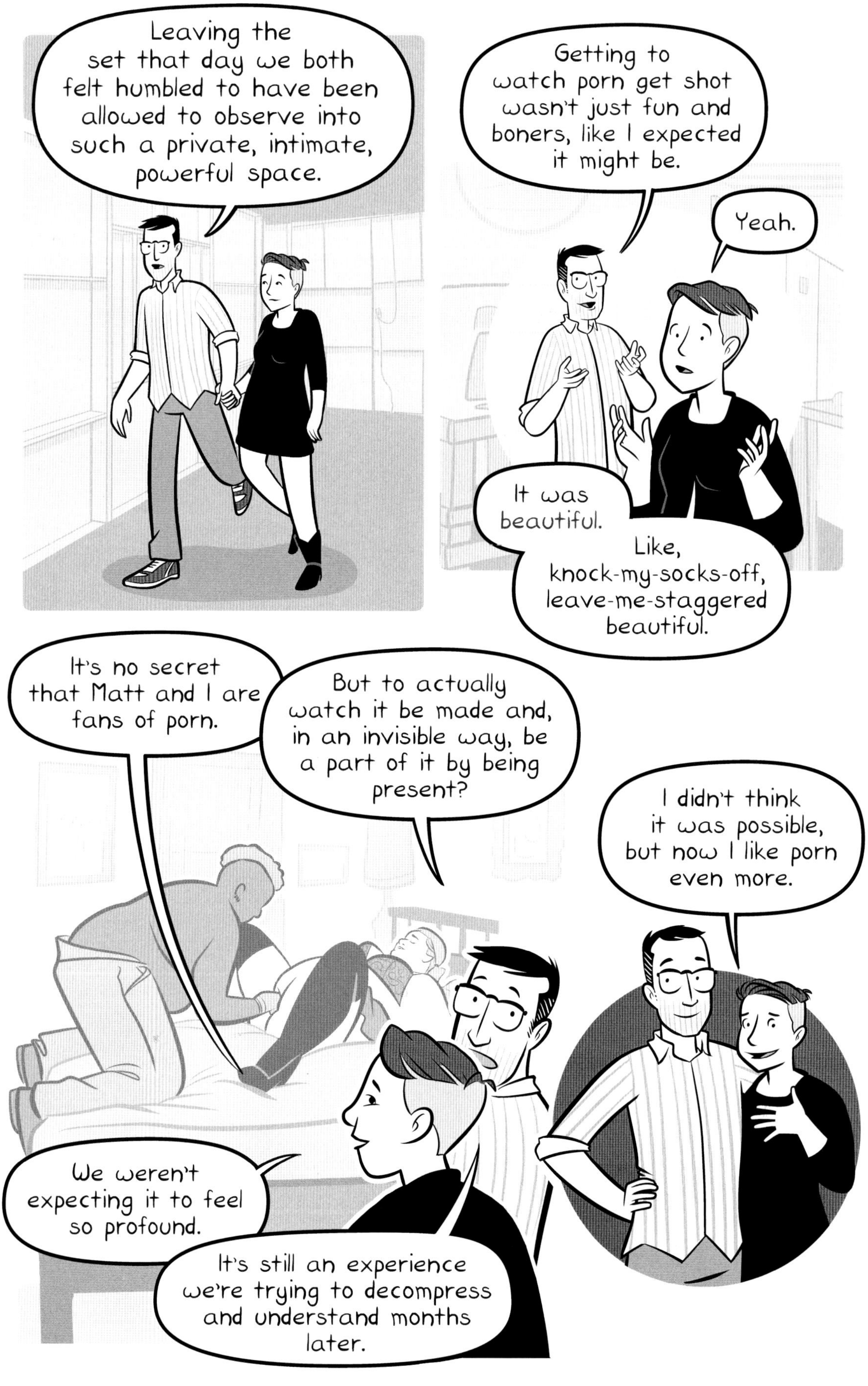
Leaving the set that day we both felt humbled to have been allowed to observe into such a private, intimate, powerful space.
Getting to watch porn get shot wasn't just fun and boners, like I expected it might be.
Yeah.
It was beautiful.
Like, knock-my-socks-off, leave-me-staggered beautiful.
It's no secret that Matt and I are fans of porn.
But to actually watch it be made and, in an invisible way, be a part of it by being present?
I didn't think it was possible, but now I like porn even more.
We weren't expecting it to feel so profound.
It's still an experience we're trying to decompress and understand months later.

Oh Joy Sex Toy
vol 2
2

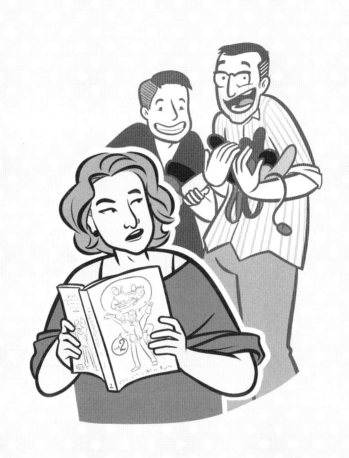

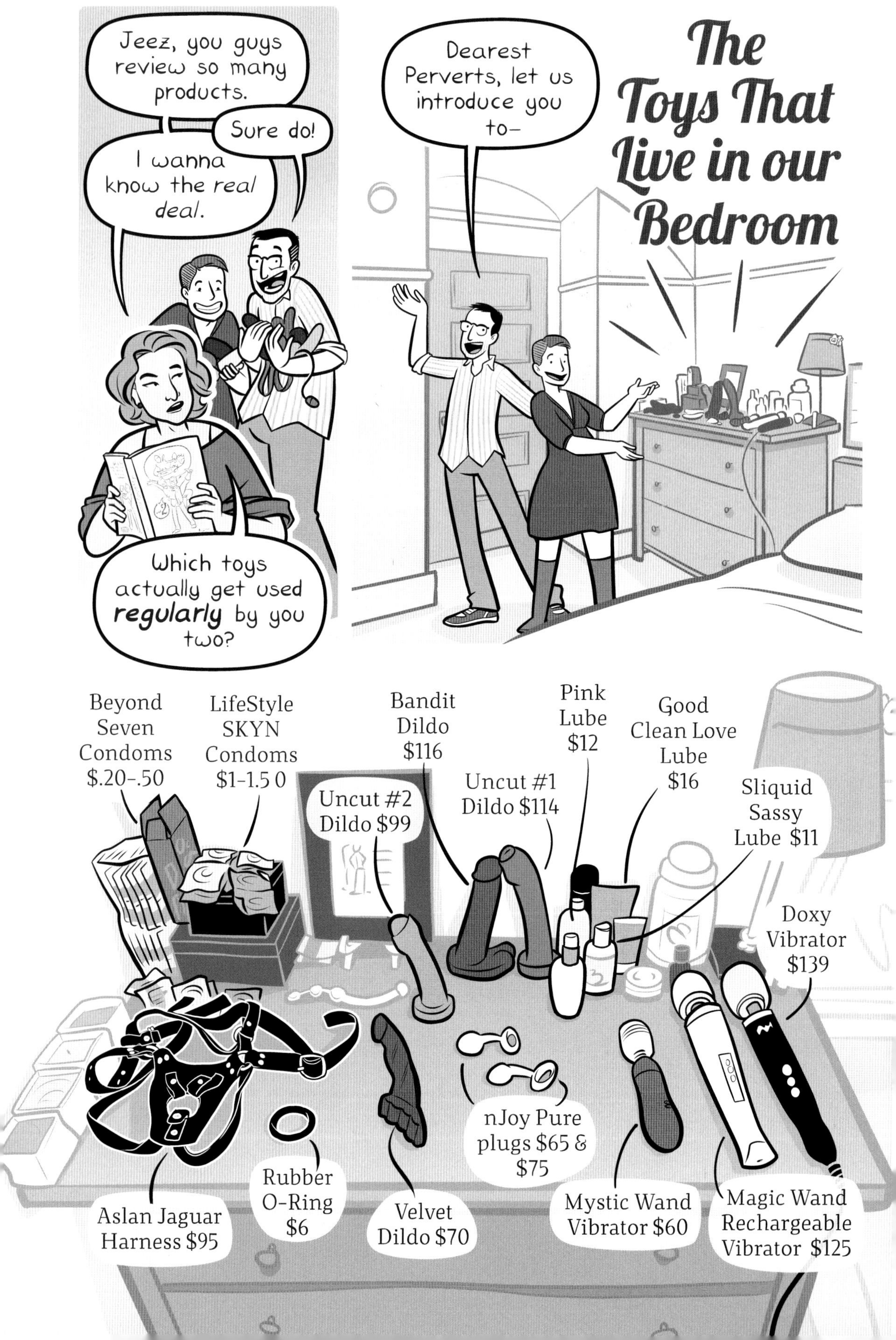
Jeez, you guys review so many products.
Sure do!
I wanna know the real deal.
Which toys actually get used **regularly** by you two?
Dearest Perverts, let us introduce you to–
The Toys That Live in our Bedroom
Beyond Seven Condoms $.20-.50
LifeStyle SKYN Condoms $1-1.5 0
Bandit Dildo $116
Pink Lube $12
Good Clean Love Lube $16
Uncut #1 Dildo $114
Uncut #2 Dildo $99
Sliquid Sassy Lube $11
Doxy Vibrator $139
nJoy Pure plugs $65 & $75
Aslan Jaguar Harness $95
Rubber O-Ring $6
Velvet Dildo $70
Mystic Wand Vibrator $60
Magic Wand Rechargeable Vibrator $125

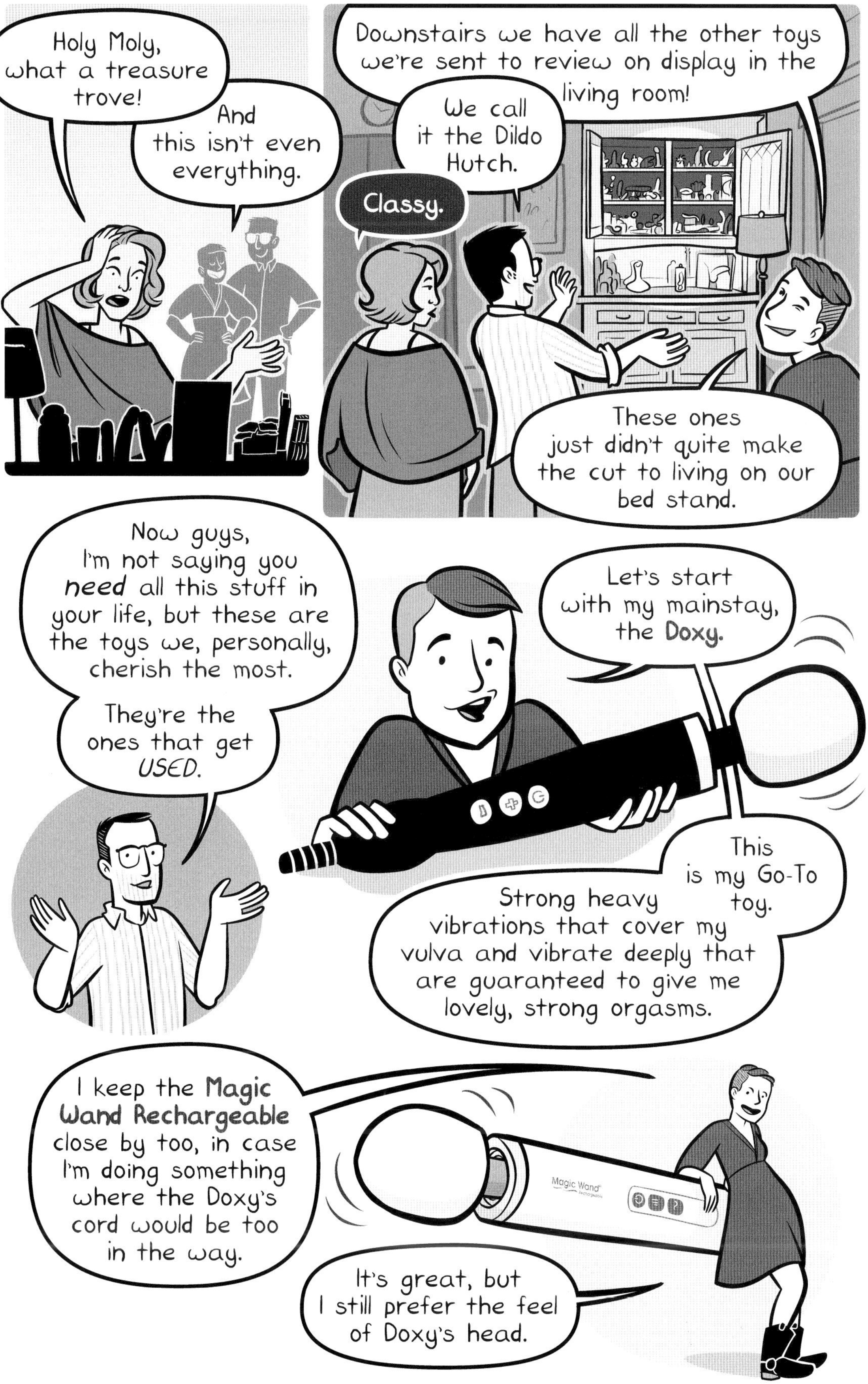

Holy Moly, what a treasure trove!
And this isn't even everything.
Downstairs we have all the other toys we're sent to review on display in the living room!
We call it the Dildo Hutch.
Classy.
These ones just didn't quite make the cut to living on our bed stand.
Now guys, I'm not saying you *need* all this stuff in your life, but these are the toys we, personally, cherish the most.
They're the ones that get *USED.*
Let's start with my mainstay, the **Doxy.**
This is my Go-To toy.
Strong heavy vibrations that cover my vulva and vibrate deeply that are guaranteed to give me lovely, strong orgasms.
I keep the **Magic Wand Rechargeable** close by too, in case I'm doing something where the Doxy's cord would be too in the way.
Magic Wand
It's great, but I still prefer the feel of Doxy's head.

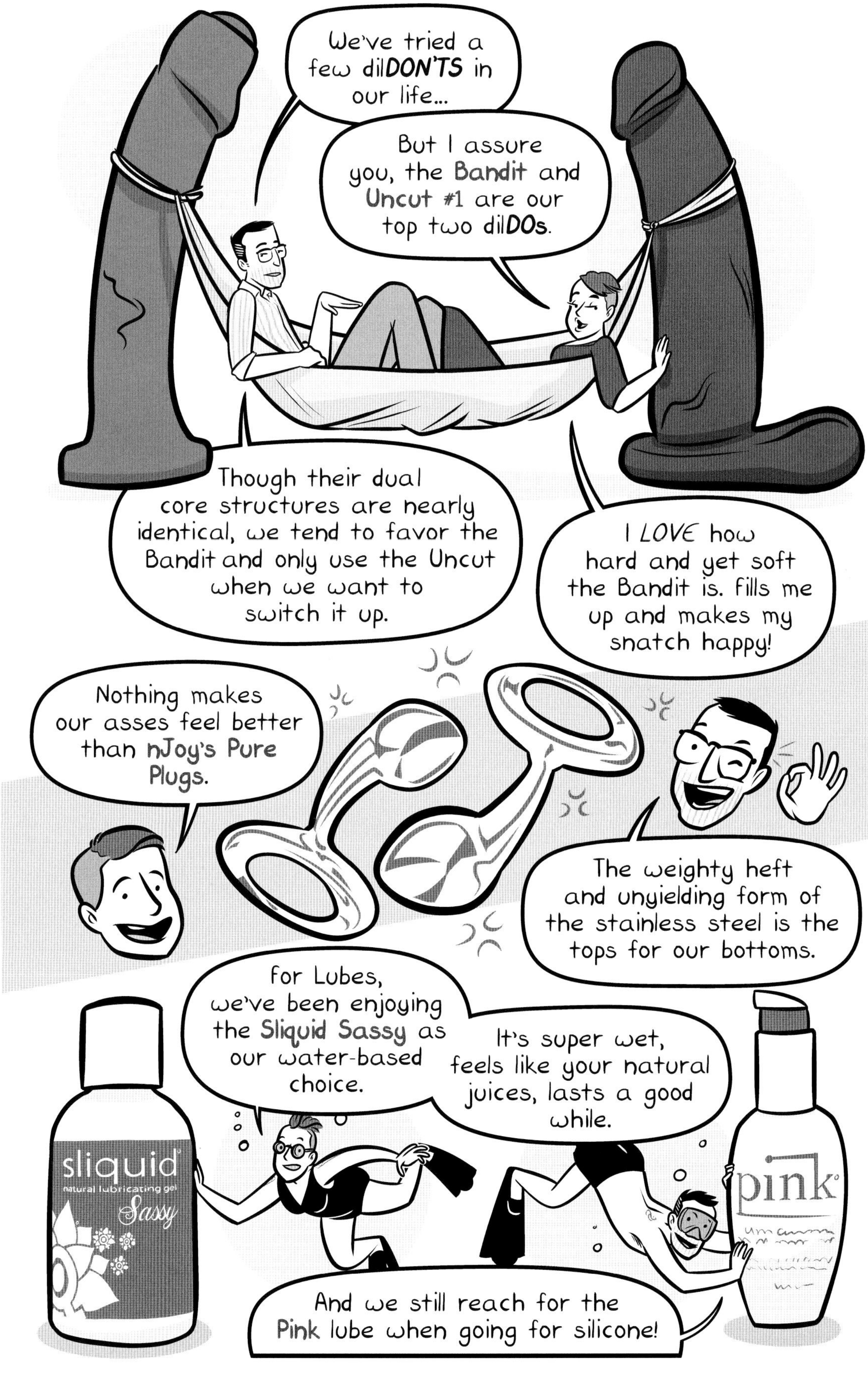

We've tried a few dilDON'TS in our life...
But I assure you, the Bandit and Uncut #1 are our top two dilDOs.
Though their dual core structures are nearly identical, we tend to favor the Bandit and only use the Uncut when we want to switch it up.
I LOVE how hard and yet soft the Bandit is. Fills me up and makes my snatch happy!
Nothing makes our asses feel better than nJoy's Pure Plugs.
The weighty heft and unyielding form of the stainless steel is the tops for our bottoms.
For Lubes, we've been enjoying the Sliquid Sassy as our water-based choice.
It's super wet, feels like your natural juices, lasts a good while.
sliquid
natural lubricating gel
Sassy
pink
And we still reach for the Pink lube when going for silicone!

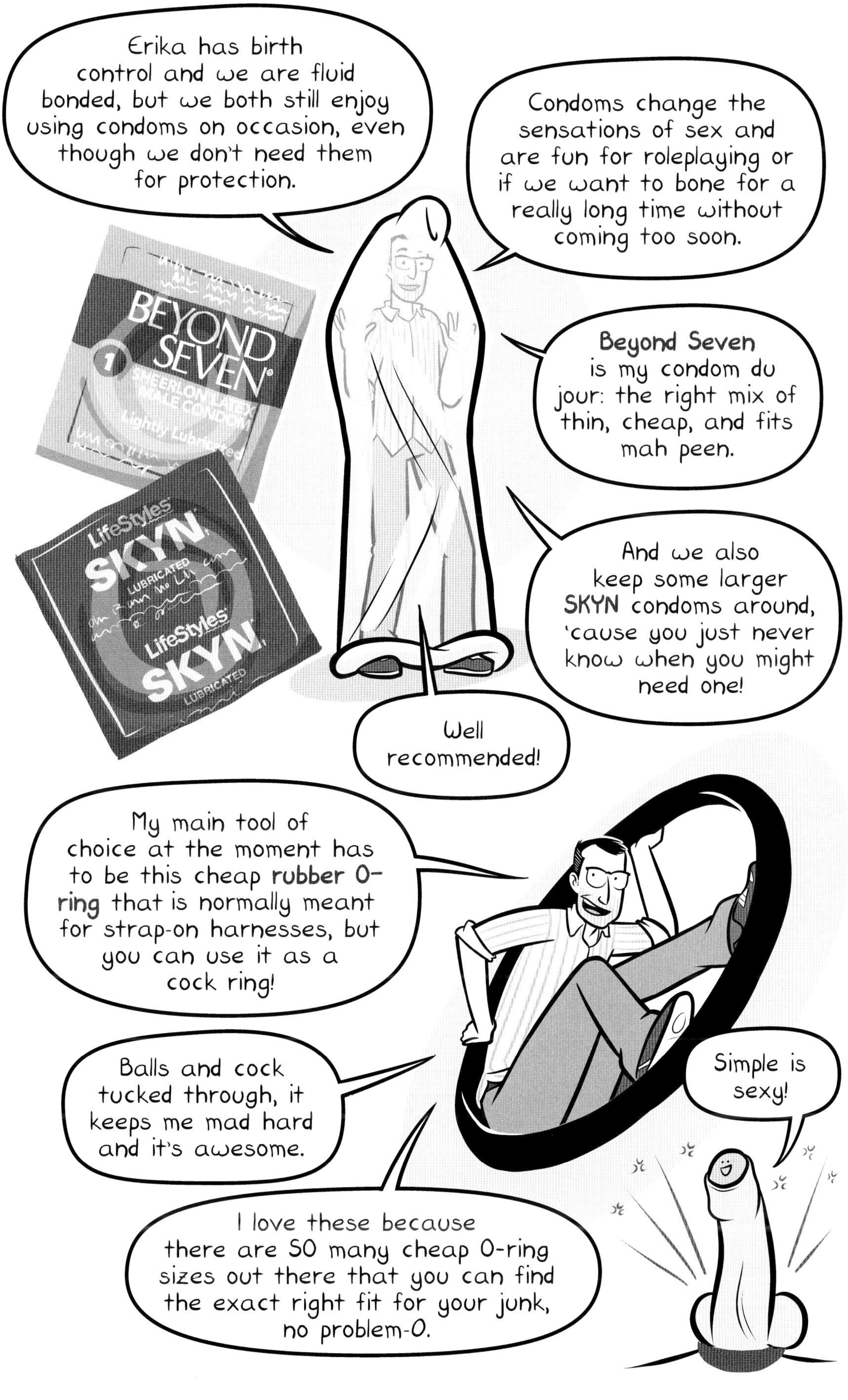
Erika has birth control and we are fluid bonded, but we both still enjoy using condoms on occasion, even though we don't need them for protection.
Condoms change the sensations of sex and are fun for roleplaying or if we want to bone for a really long time without coming too soon.
BEYOND SEVEN
SHEERLON LATEX MALE CONDOM
Lightly Lubricated
Beyond Seven is my condom du jour: the right mix of thin, cheap, and fits mah peen.
LifeStyles SKYN
LUBRICATED
And we also keep some larger SKYN condoms around, 'cause you just never know when you might need one!
Well recommended!
My main tool of choice at the moment has to be this cheap rubber O-ring that is normally meant for strap-on harnesses, but you can use it as a cock ring!
Balls and cock tucked through, it keeps me mad hard and it's awesome.
Simple is sexy!
I love these because there are SO many cheap O-ring sizes out there that you can find the exact right fit for your junk, no problem-O.

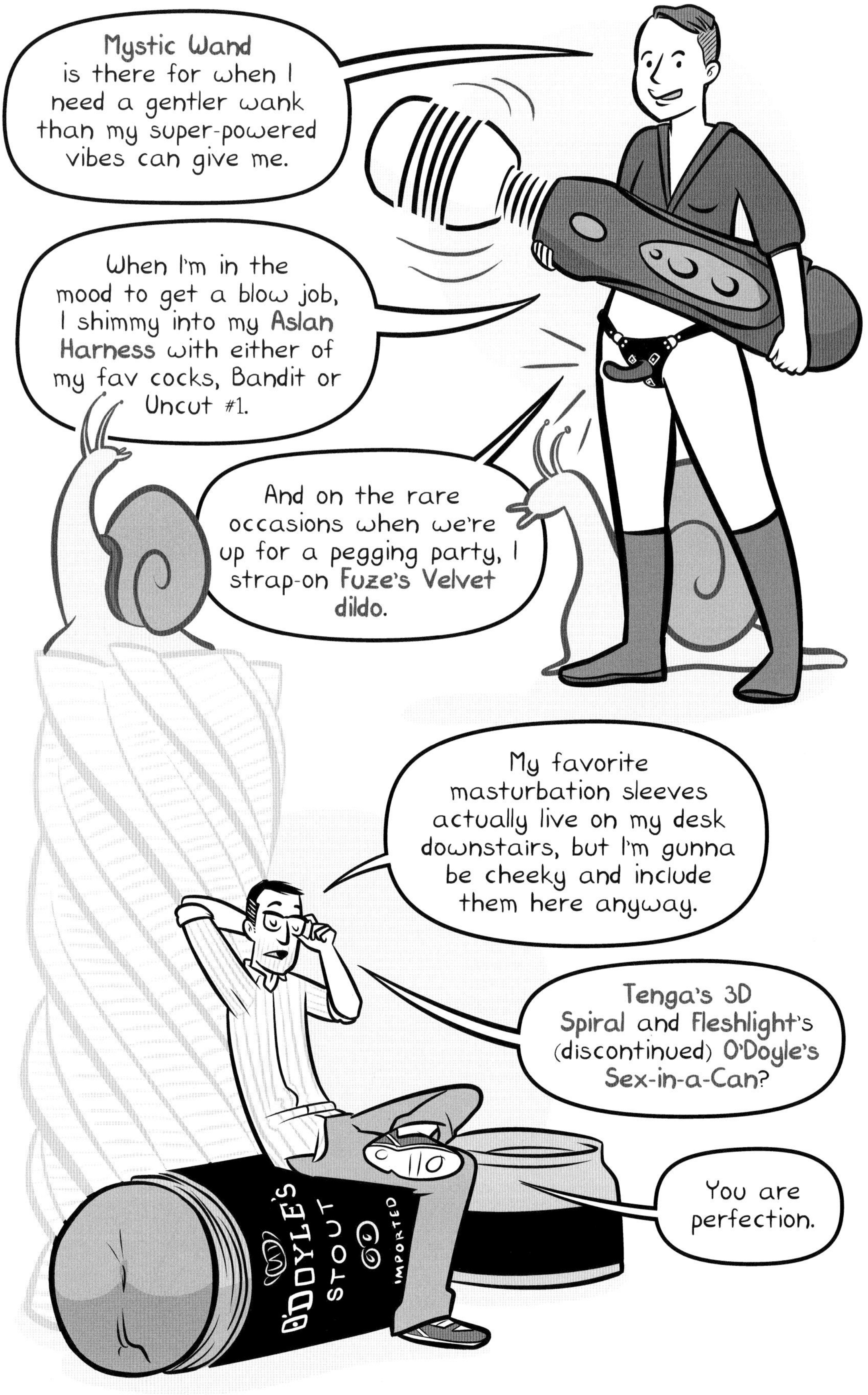
Mystic Wand is there for when I need a gentler wank than my super-powered vibes can give me.
When I'm in the mood to get a blow job, I shimmy into my Aslan Harness with either of my fav cocks, Bandit or Uncut #1.
And on the rare occasions when we're up for a pegging party, I strap-on Fuze's Velvet dildo.
My favorite masturbation sleeves actually live on my desk downstairs, but I'm gunna be cheeky and include them here anyway.
Tenga's 3D Spiral and Fleshlight's (discontinued) O'Doyle's Sex-in-a-Can?
You are perfection.
O'DOYLE'S STOUT
IMPORTED

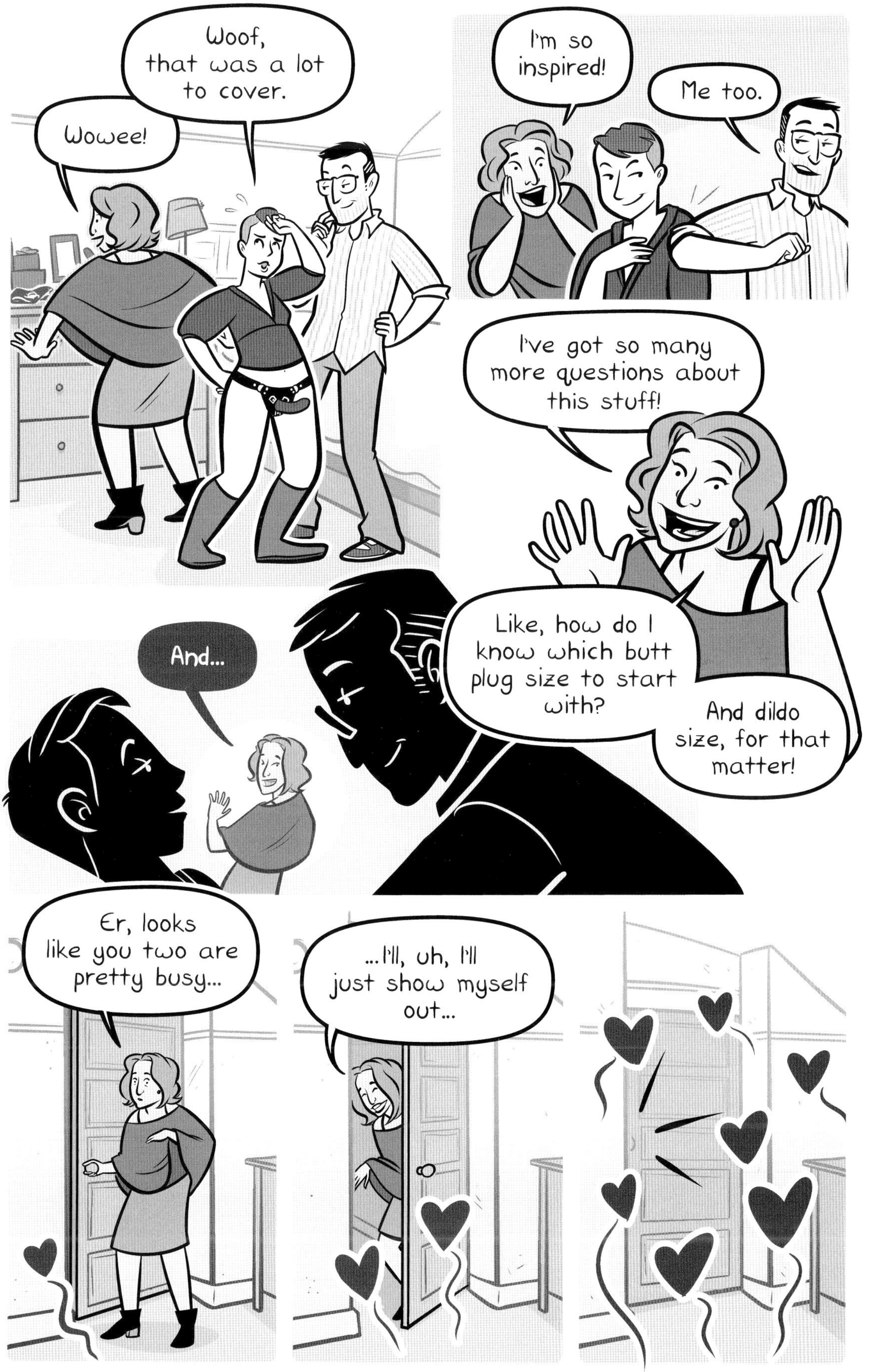
Wowee!
Woof, that was a lot to cover.
I'm so inspired!
Me too.
I've got so many more questions about this stuff!
Like, how do I know which butt plug size to start with?
And dildo size, for that matter!
And...
Er, looks like you two are pretty busy...
...I'll, uh, I'll just show myself out...

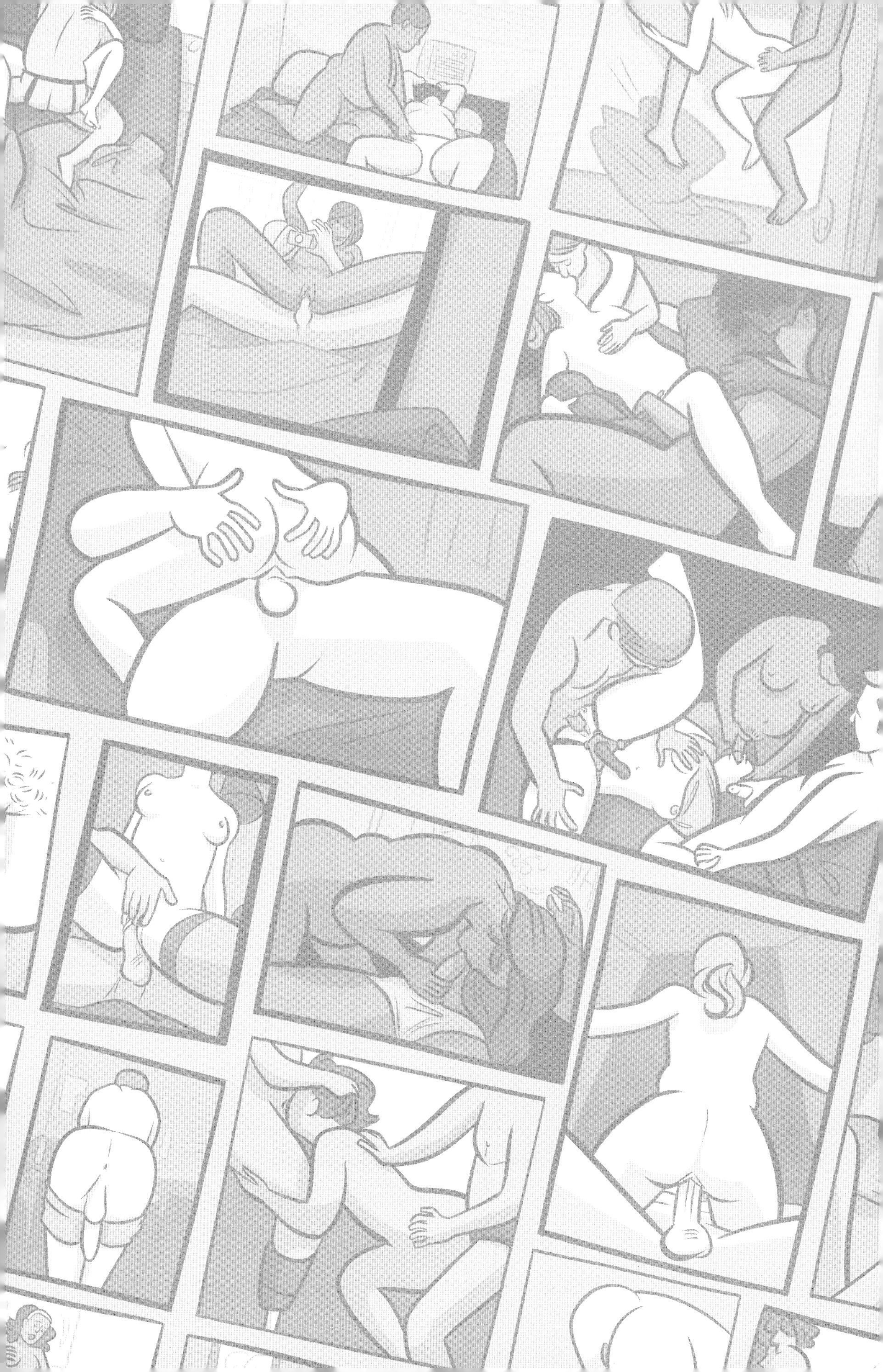

Thanks for reading Perverts!

Fin

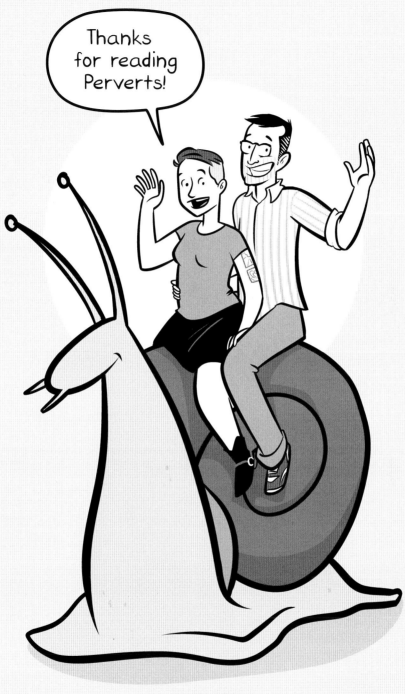

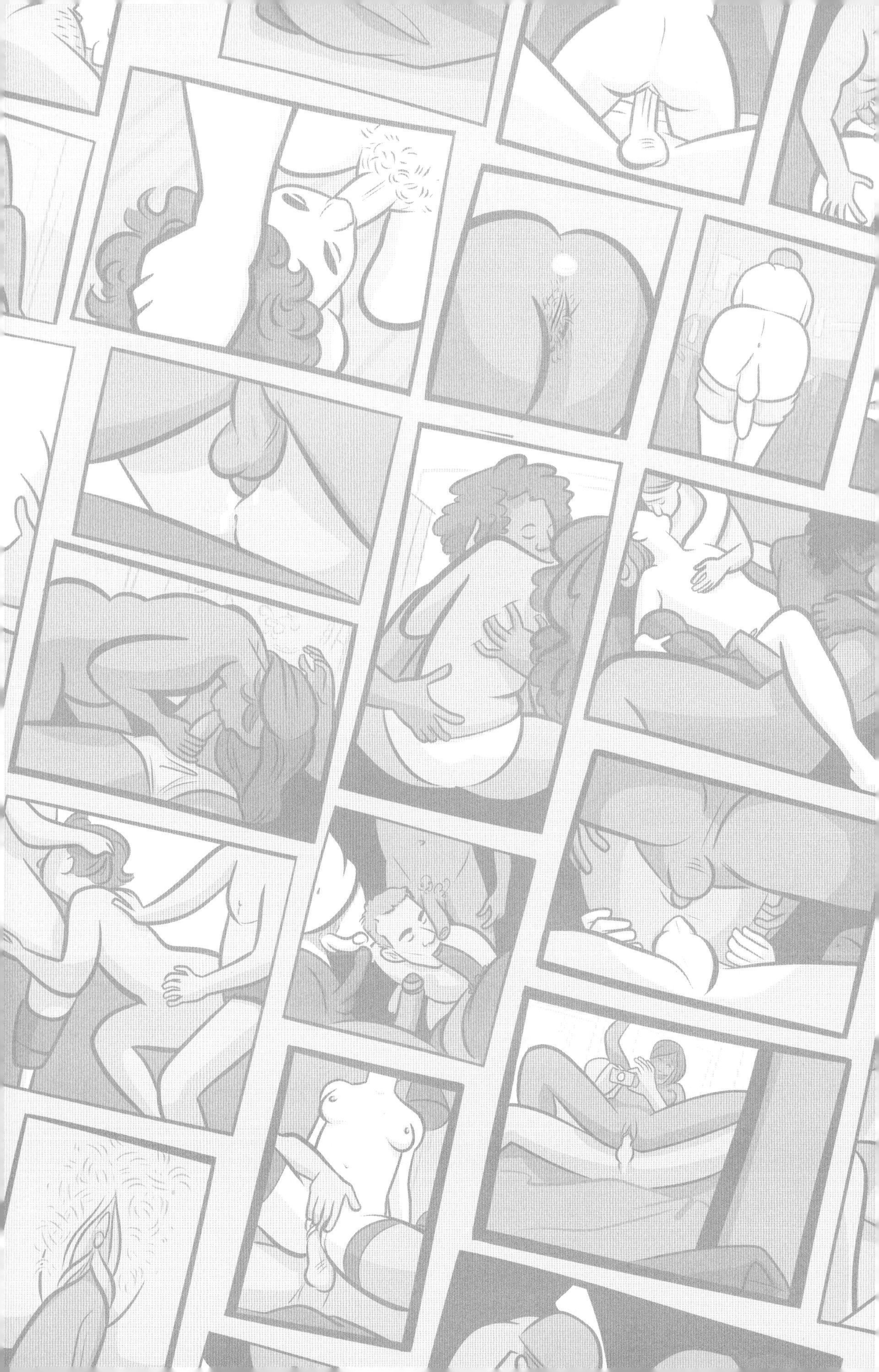

Guest Strips

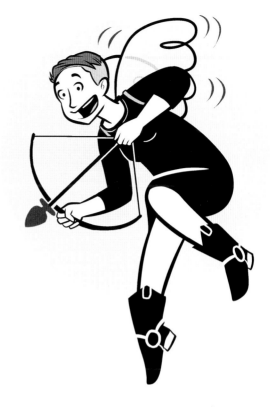

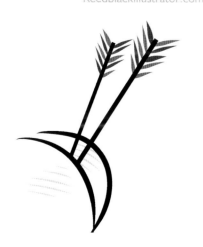

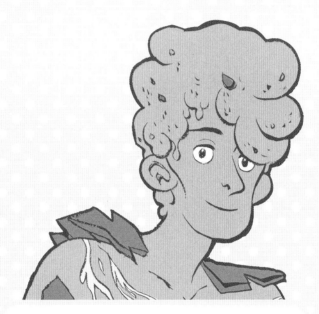

CREAM FOR YOU
by Donut

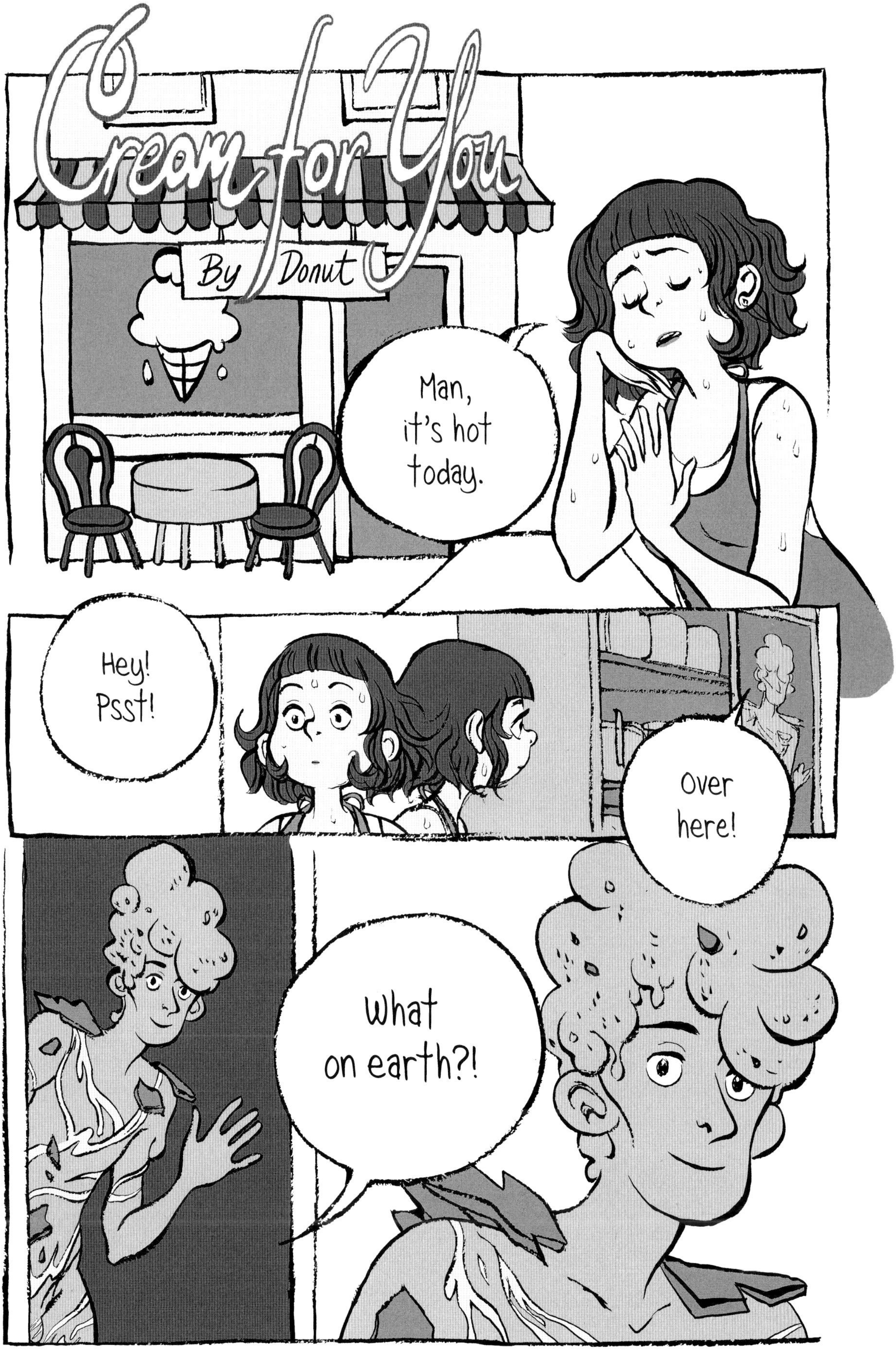
Cream for You
By Donut
Man, it's hot today.
Hey! Psst!
Over here!
What on earth?!

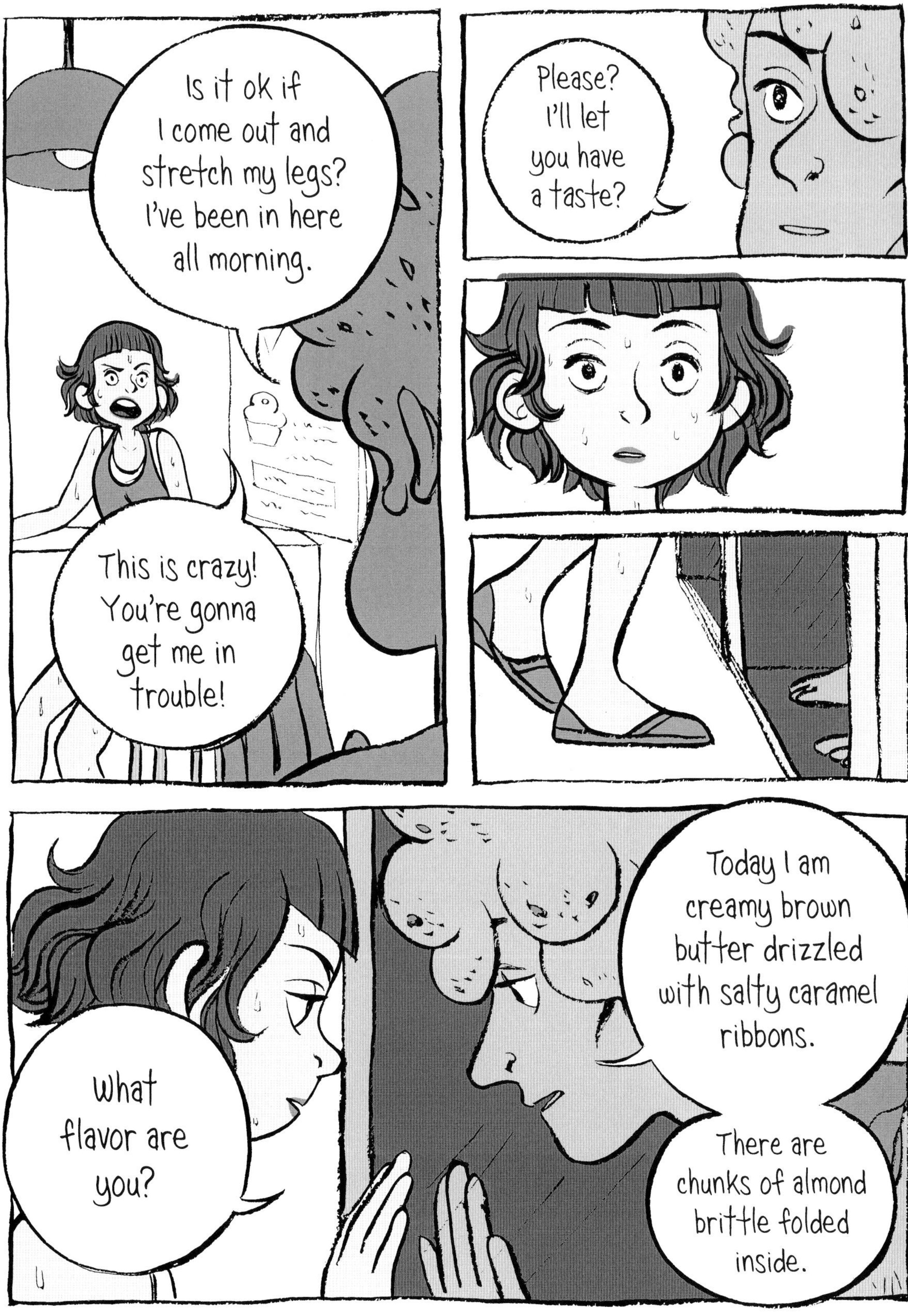
Is it ok if I come out and stretch my legs? I've been in here all morning.
This is crazy! You're gonna get me in trouble!
Please? I'll let you have a taste?
What flavor are you?
Today I am creamy brown butter drizzled with salty caramel ribbons.
There are chunks of almond brittle folded inside.

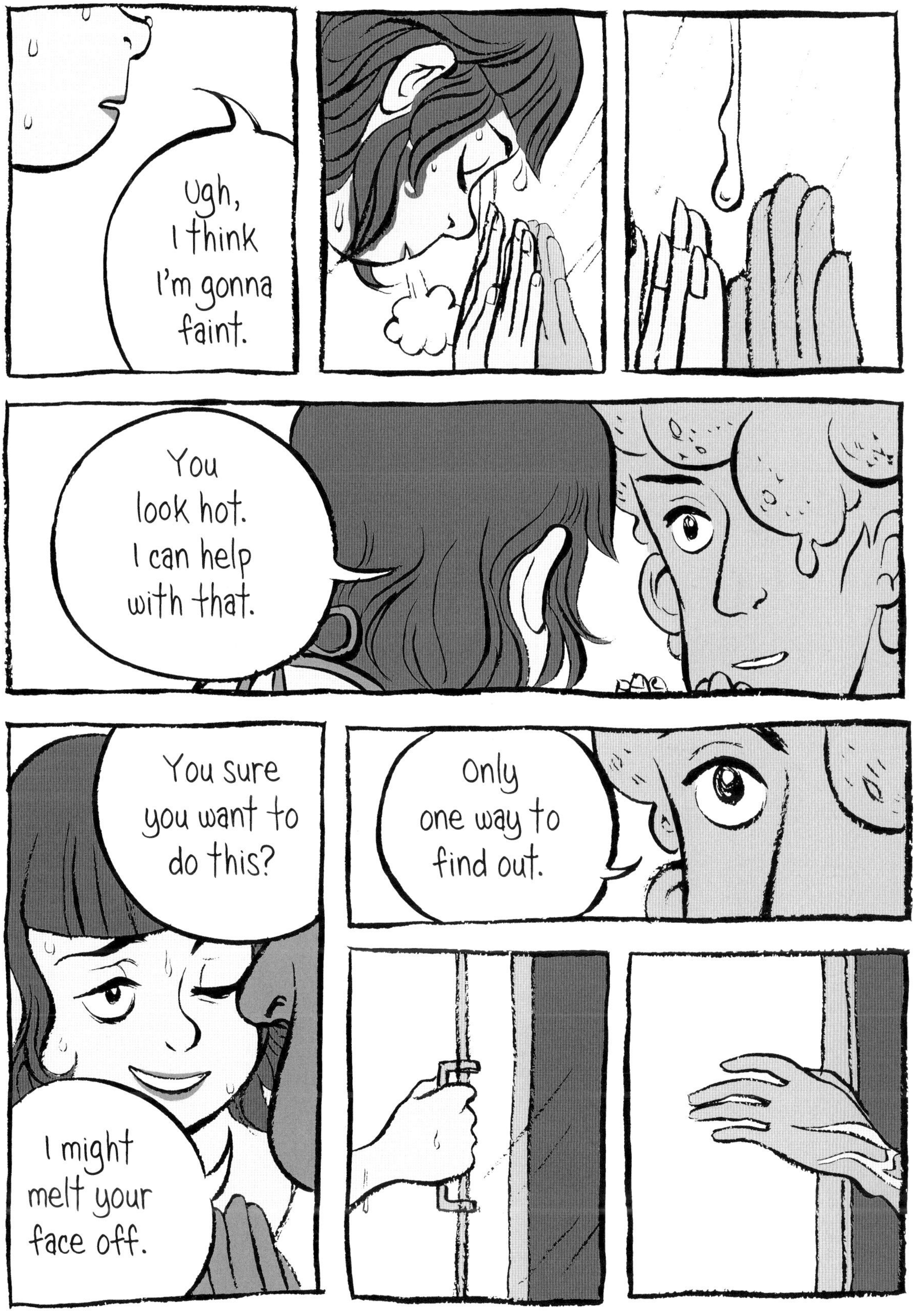
Ugh, I think I'm gonna faint.
You look hot. I can help with that.
You sure you want to do this?
I might melt your face off.
Only one way to find out.

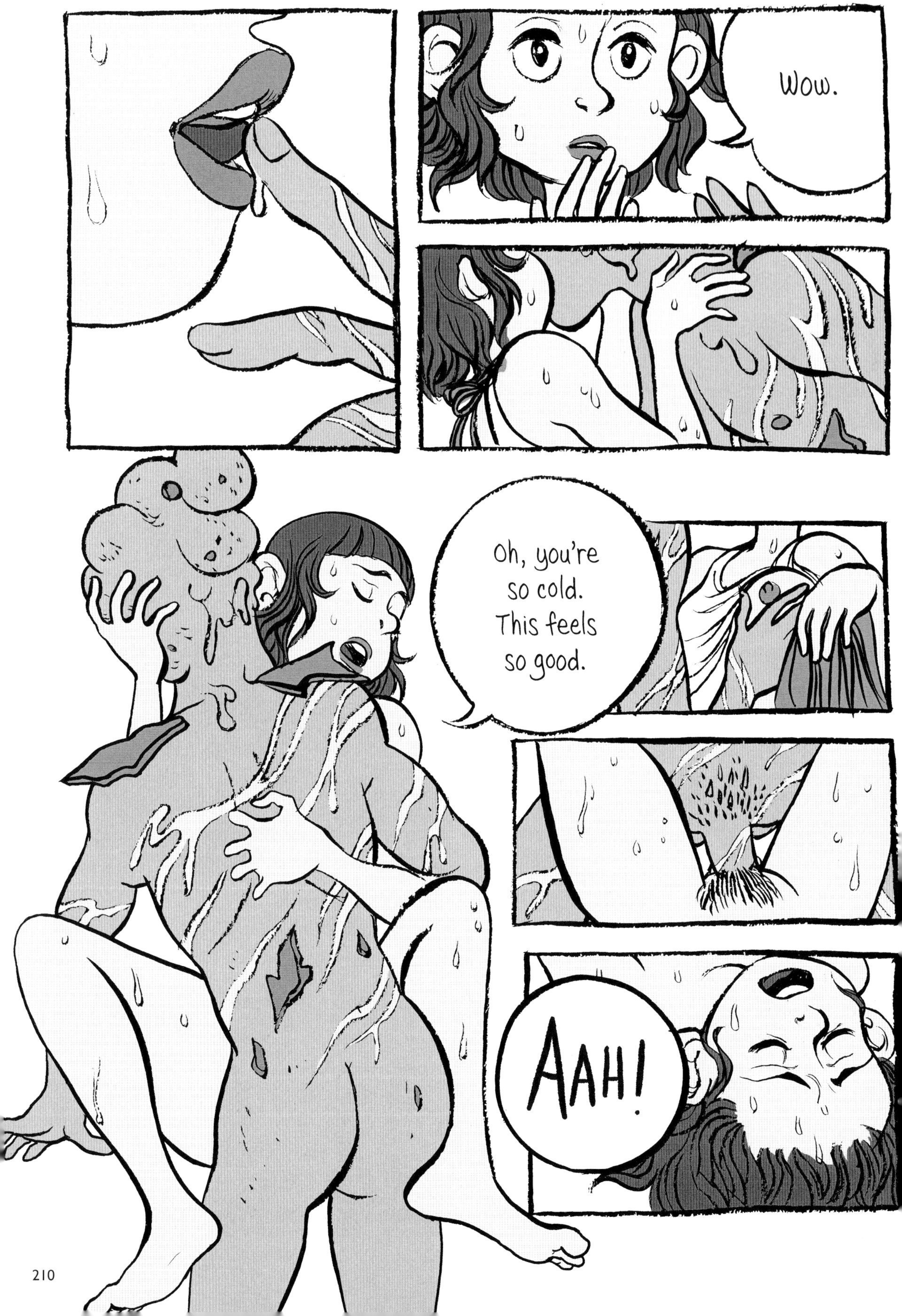
Wow.
Oh, you're so cold. This feels so good.
AAH!

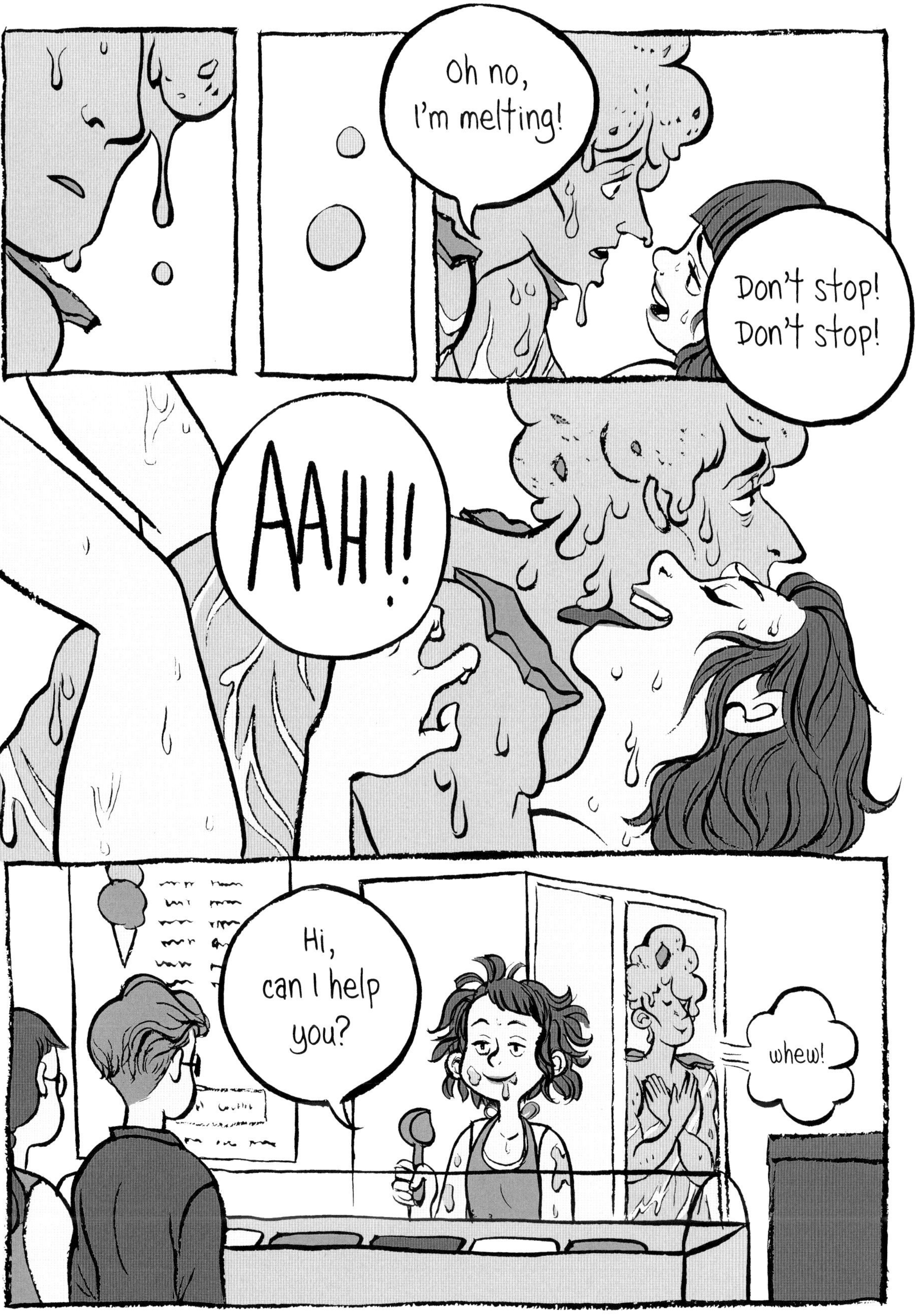
Oh no, I'm melting!
Don't stop! Don't stop!
AAH!!
Hi, can I help you?
whew!

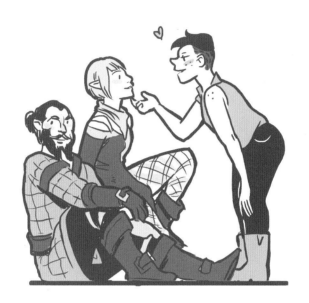

DRAGON AGE
by Molly Ostertag
Mollyostertag.com

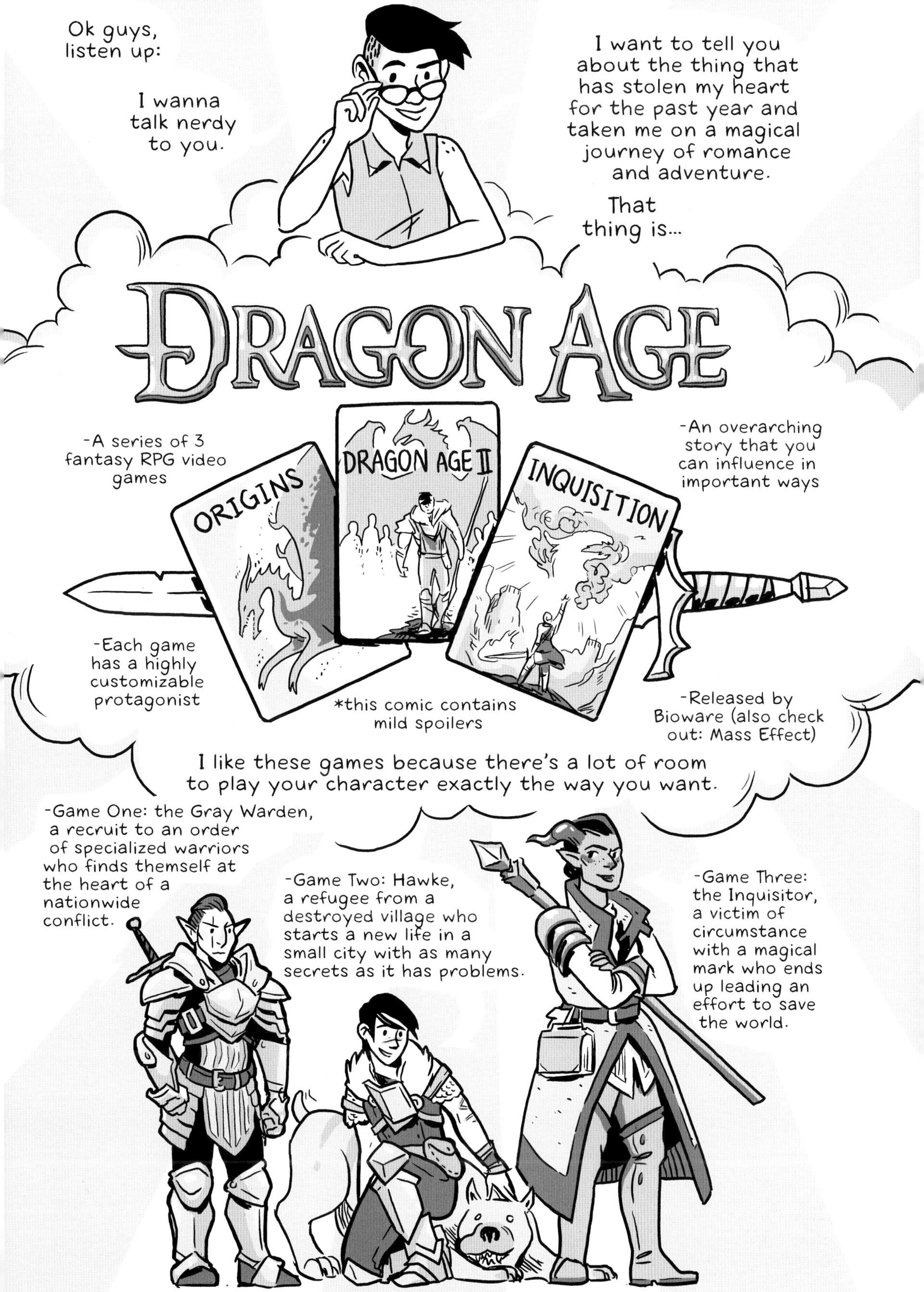

Ok guys, listen up:
I wanna talk nerdy to you.
I want to tell you about the thing that has stolen my heart for the past year and taken me on a magical journey of romance and adventure.
That thing is...
DRAGON AGE
-A series of 3 fantasy RPG video games
ORIGINS
DRAGON AGE II
INQUISITION
-An overarching story that you can influence in important ways
-Each game has a highly customizable protagonist
*this comic contains mild spoilers
-Released by Bioware (also check out: Mass Effect)
I like these games because there's a lot of room to play your character exactly the way you want.
-Game One: the Gray Warden, a recruit to an order of specialized warriors who finds themself at the heart of a nationwide conflict.
-Game Two: Hawke, a refugee from a destroyed village who starts a new life in a small city with as many secrets as it has problems.
-Game Three: the Inquisitor, a victim of circumstance with a magical mark who ends up leading an effort to save the world.

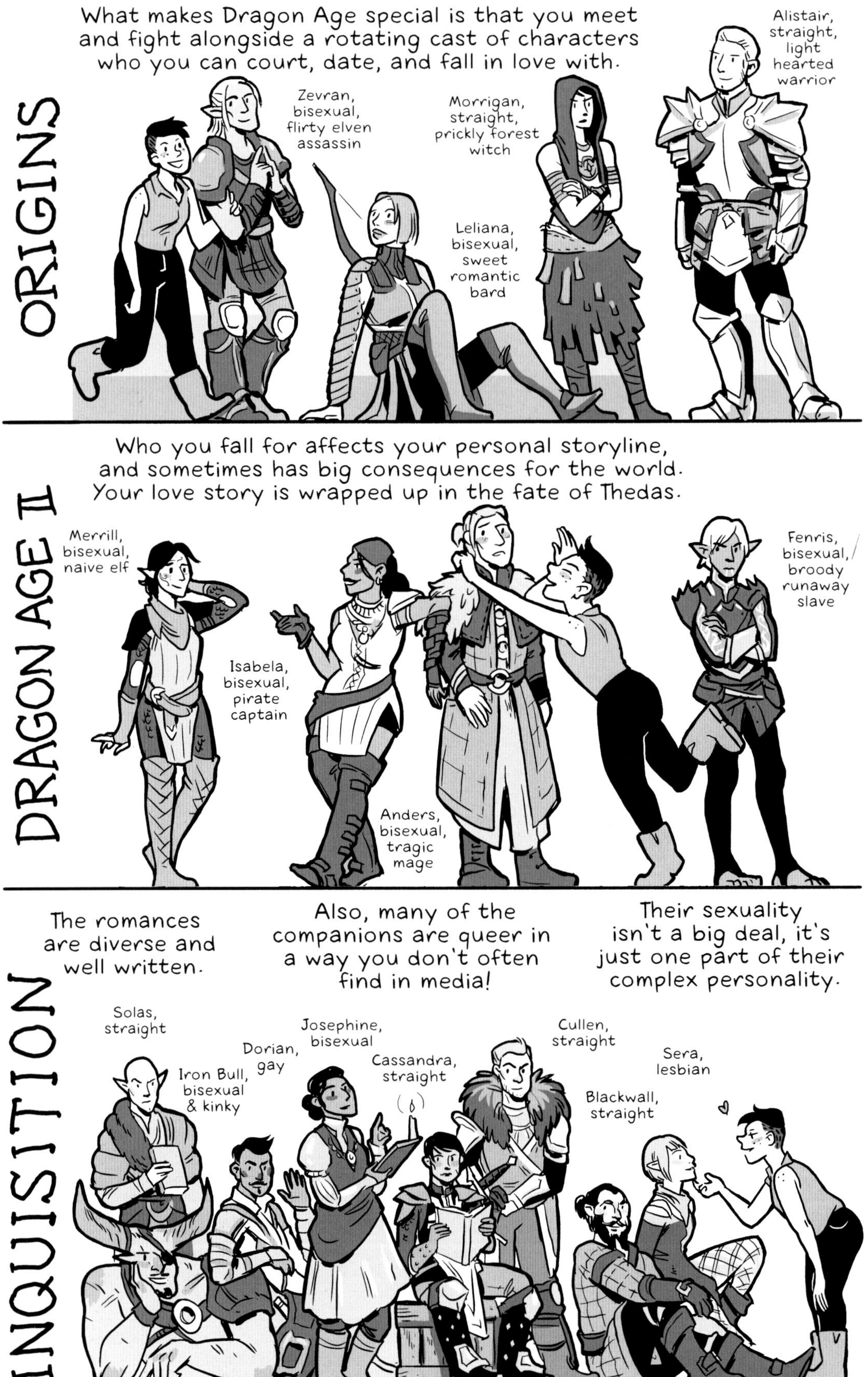
What makes Dragon Age special is that you meet and fight alongside a rotating cast of characters who you can court, date, and fall in love with.
ORIGINS
Zevran, bisexual, flirty elven assassin
Leliana, bisexual, sweet romantic bard
Morrigan, straight, prickly forest witch
Alistair, straight, light hearted warrior
Who you fall for affects your personal storyline, and sometimes has big consequences for the world. Your love story is wrapped up in the fate of Thedas.
DRAGON AGE II
Merrill, bisexual, naive elf
Isabela, bisexual, pirate captain
Anders, bisexual, tragic mage
Fenris, bisexual, broody runaway slave
INQUISITION
The romances are diverse and well written.
Also, many of the companions are queer in a way you don't often find in media!
Their sexuality isn't a big deal, it's just one part of their complex personality.
Solas, straight
Iron Bull, bisexual & kinky
Dorian, gay
Josephine, bisexual
Cassandra, straight
Cullen, straight
Blackwall, straight
Sera, lesbian

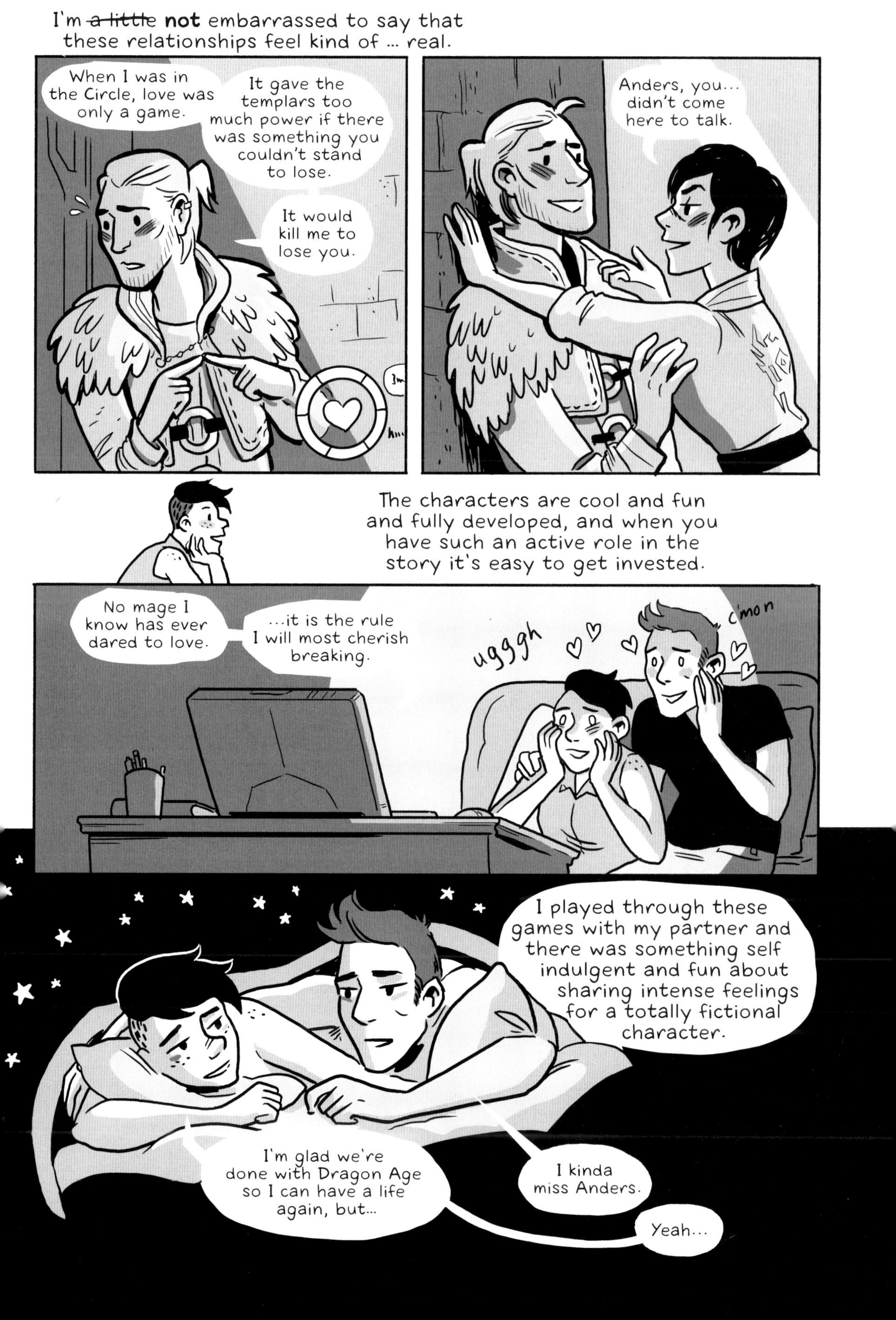
I'm ~~a little~~ **not** embarrassed to say that these relationships feel kind of ... real.
When I was in the Circle, love was only a game.
It gave the templars too much power if there was something you couldn't stand to lose.
It would kill me to lose you.
Anders, you... didn't come here to talk.
The characters are cool and fun and fully developed, and when you have such an active role in the story it's easy to get invested.
No mage I know has ever dared to love.
...it is the rule I will most cherish breaking.
uggghh
c'mon
I played through these games with my partner and there was something self indulgent and fun about sharing intense feelings for a totally fictional character.
I'm glad we're done with Dragon Age so I can have a life again, but...
I kinda miss Anders.
Yeah...

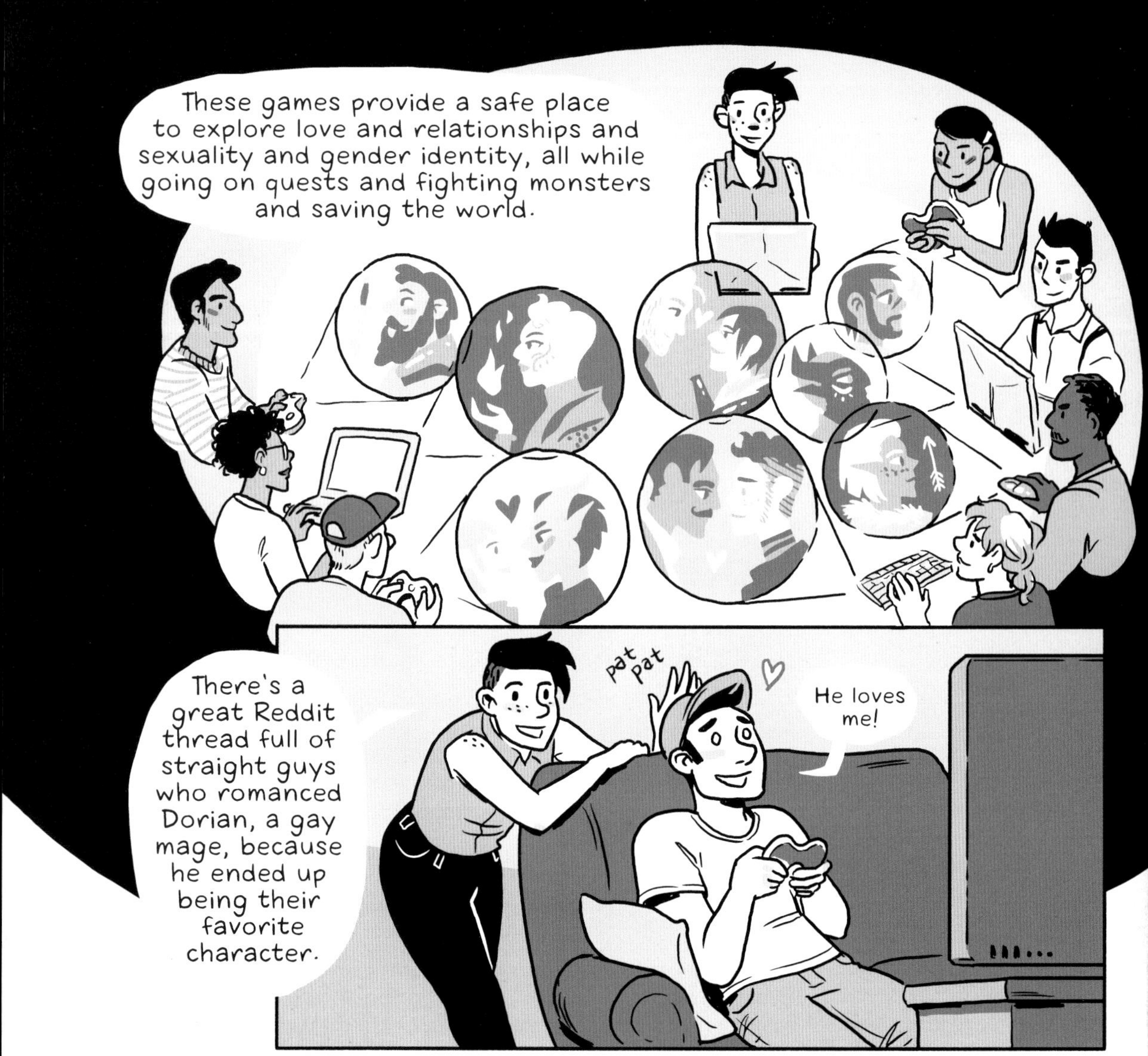
These games provide a safe place to explore love and relationships and sexuality and gender identity, all while going on quests and fighting monsters and saving the world.
There's a great Reddit thread full of straight guys who romanced Dorian, a gay mage, because he ended up being their favorite character.
pat pat
He loves me!

Another character is trans, and after getting to know him you can learn about his gender identity.

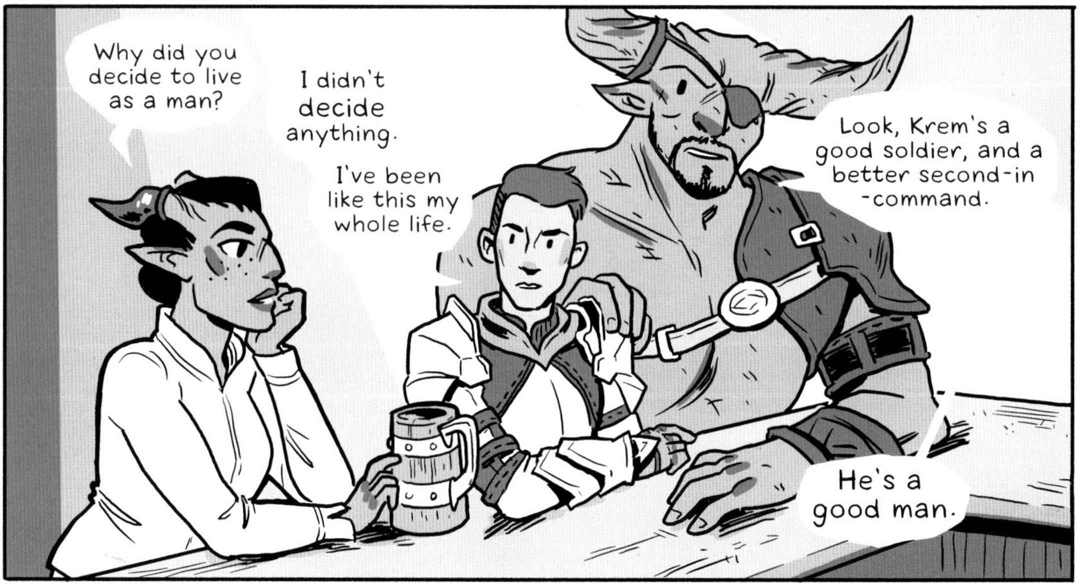
Why did you decide to live as a man?
I didn't decide anything.
I've been like this my whole life.
Look, Krem's a good soldier, and a better second-in-command.
He's a good man.

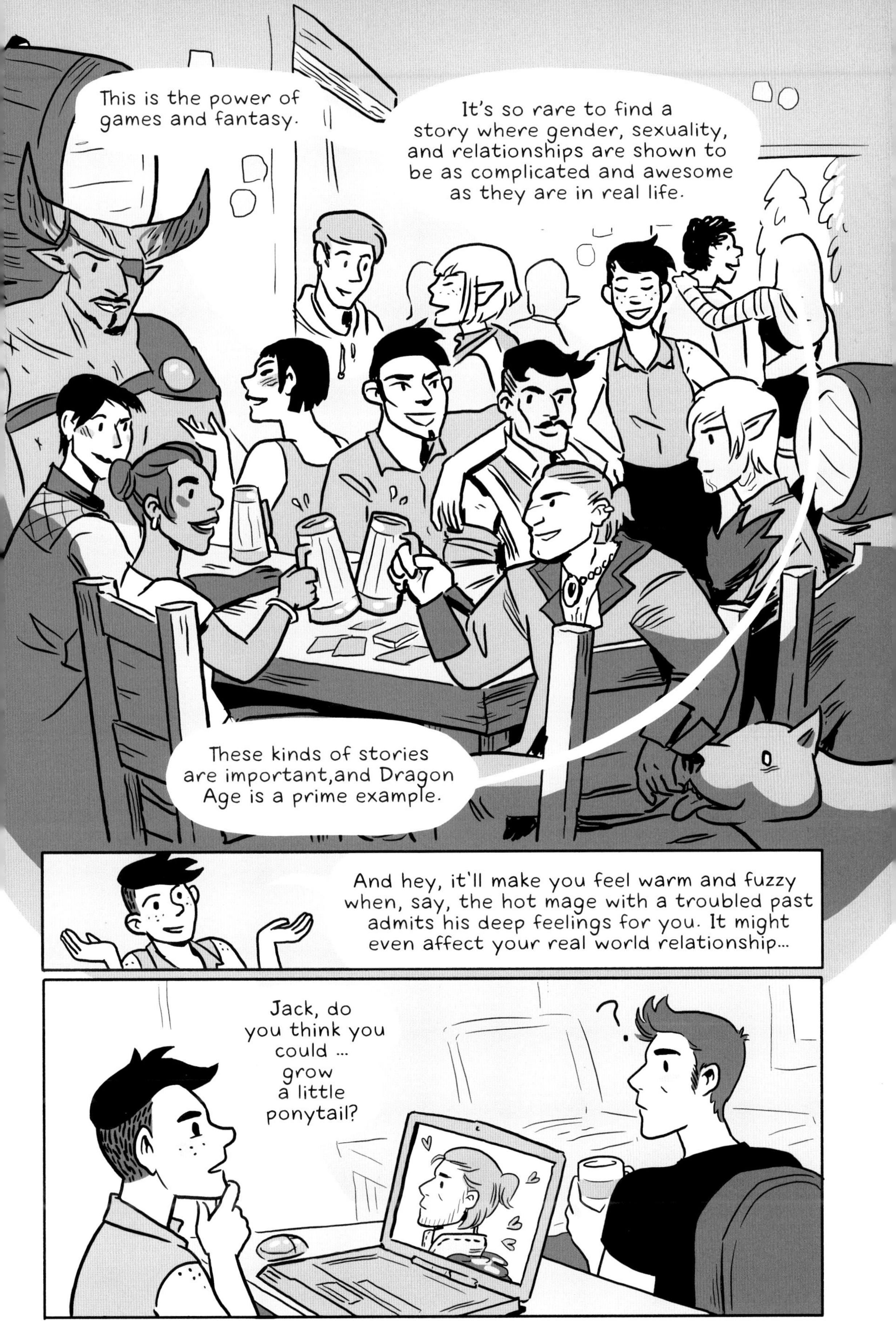

This is the power of games and fantasy.
It's so rare to find a story where gender, sexuality, and relationships are shown to be as complicated and awesome as they are in real life.
These kinds of stories are important,and Dragon Age is a prime example.
And hey, it'll make you feel warm and fuzzy when, say, the hot mage with a troubled past admits his deep feelings for you. It might even affect your real world relationship...
Jack, do you think you could ... grow a little ponytail?
?

WATERSPORTS

by Sicklyhypnos

Furaffinity.net/user/sicklyhypnos

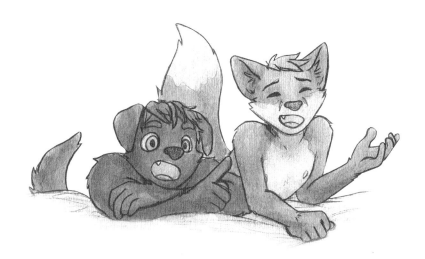

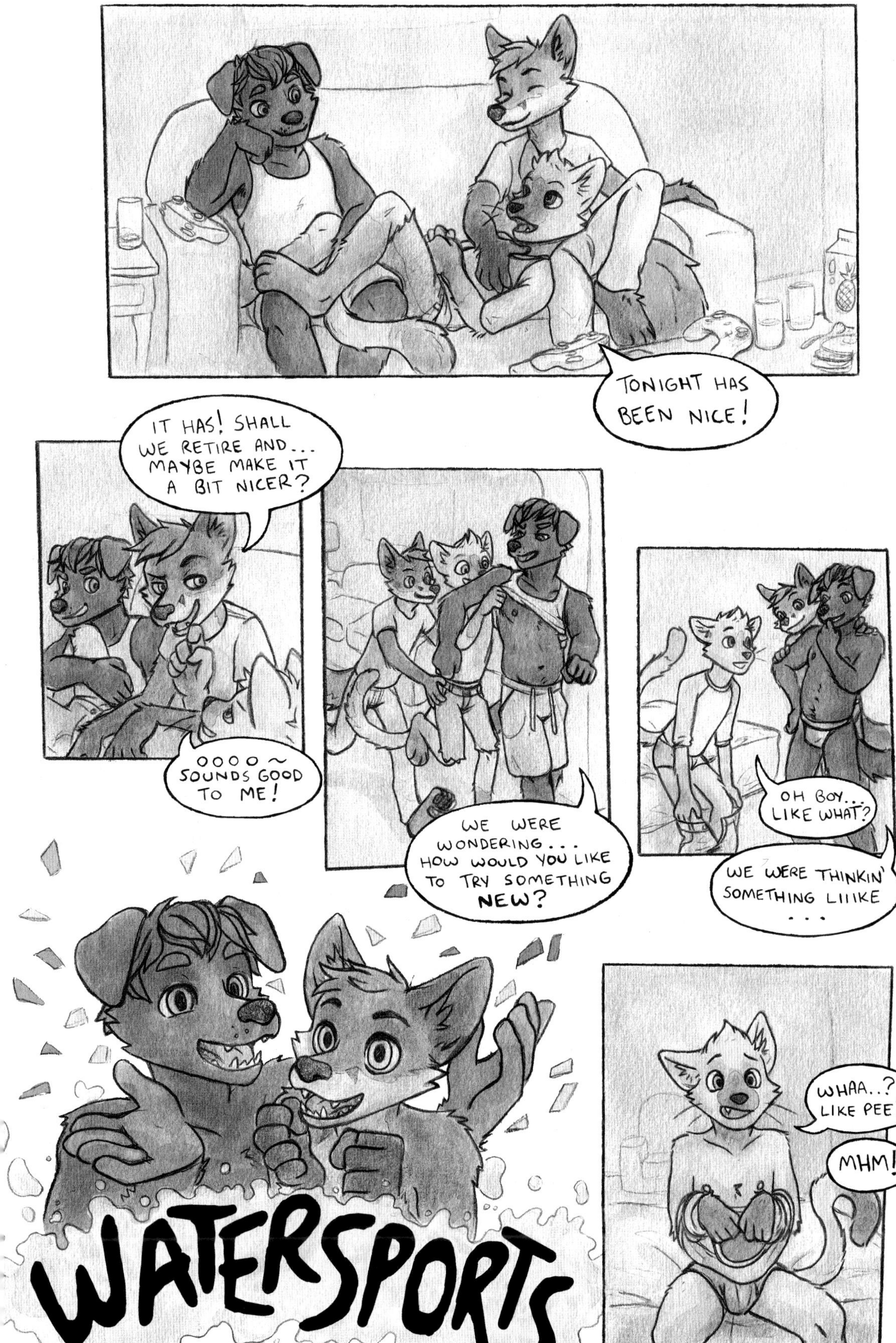
TONIGHT HAS BEEN NICE!
IT HAS! SHALL WE RETIRE AND... MAYBE MAKE IT A BIT NICER?
OOOO~ SOUNDS GOOD TO ME!
WE WERE WONDERING... HOW WOULD YOU LIKE TO TRY SOMETHING NEW?
OH BOY... LIKE WHAT?
WE WERE THINKIN' SOMETHING LIIIKE ...
WATERSPORTS
WHAA..? LIKE PEE?
MHM!

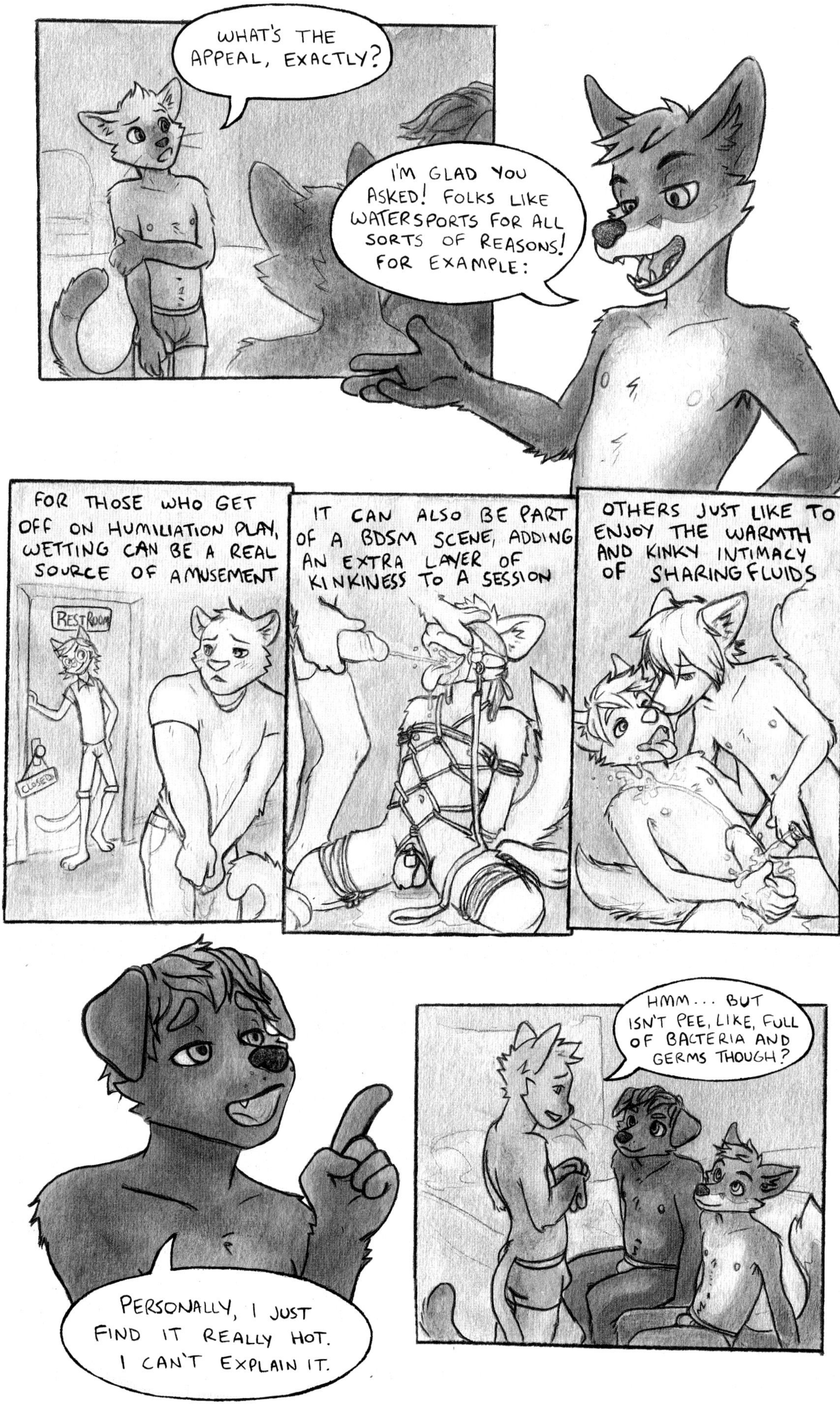
WHAT'S THE APPEAL, EXACTLY?
I'M GLAD YOU ASKED! FOLKS LIKE WATERSPORTS FOR ALL SORTS OF REASONS! FOR EXAMPLE:
FOR THOSE WHO GET OFF ON HUMILIATION PLAY, WETTING CAN BE A REAL SOURCE OF AMUSEMENT
RESTROOM
CLOSED
IT CAN ALSO BE PART OF A BDSM SCENE, ADDING AN EXTRA LAYER OF KINKINESS TO A SESSION
OTHERS JUST LIKE TO ENJOY THE WARMTH AND KINKY INTIMACY OF SHARING FLUIDS
PERSONALLY, I JUST FIND IT REALLY HOT. I CAN'T EXPLAIN IT.
HMM... BUT ISN'T PEE, LIKE, FULL OF BACTERIA AND GERMS THOUGH?

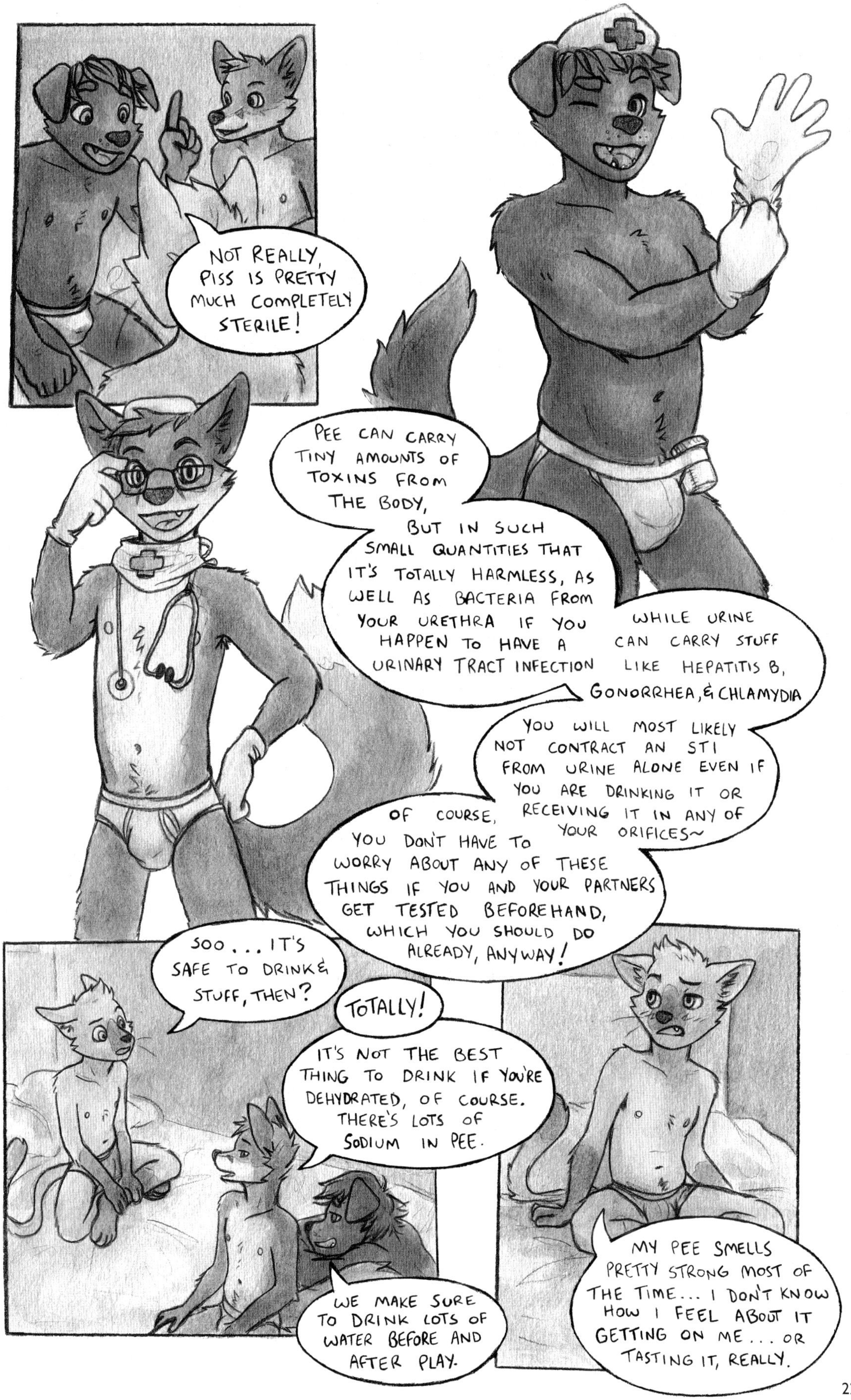
NOT REALLY, PISS IS PRETTY MUCH COMPLETELY STERILE!
PEE CAN CARRY TINY AMOUNTS OF TOXINS FROM THE BODY, BUT IN SUCH SMALL QUANTITIES THAT IT'S TOTALLY HARMLESS, AS WELL AS BACTERIA FROM YOUR URETHRA IF YOU HAPPEN TO HAVE A URINARY TRACT INFECTION
WHILE URINE CAN CARRY STUFF LIKE HEPATITIS B, GONORRHEA, & CHLAMYDIA
YOU WILL MOST LIKELY NOT CONTRACT AN STI FROM URINE ALONE EVEN IF YOU ARE DRINKING IT OR RECEIVING IT IN ANY OF YOUR ORIFICES~
OF COURSE, YOU DON'T HAVE TO WORRY ABOUT ANY OF THESE THINGS IF YOU AND YOUR PARTNERS GET TESTED BEFOREHAND, WHICH YOU SHOULD DO ALREADY, ANYWAY!
SOO... IT'S SAFE TO DRINK & STUFF, THEN?
TOTALLY!
IT'S NOT THE BEST THING TO DRINK IF YOU'RE DEHYDRATED, OF COURSE. THERE'S LOTS OF SODIUM IN PEE.
WE MAKE SURE TO DRINK LOTS OF WATER BEFORE AND AFTER PLAY.
MY PEE SMELLS PRETTY STRONG MOST OF THE TIME... I DON'T KNOW HOW I FEEL ABOUT IT GETTING ON ME... OR TASTING IT, REALLY.

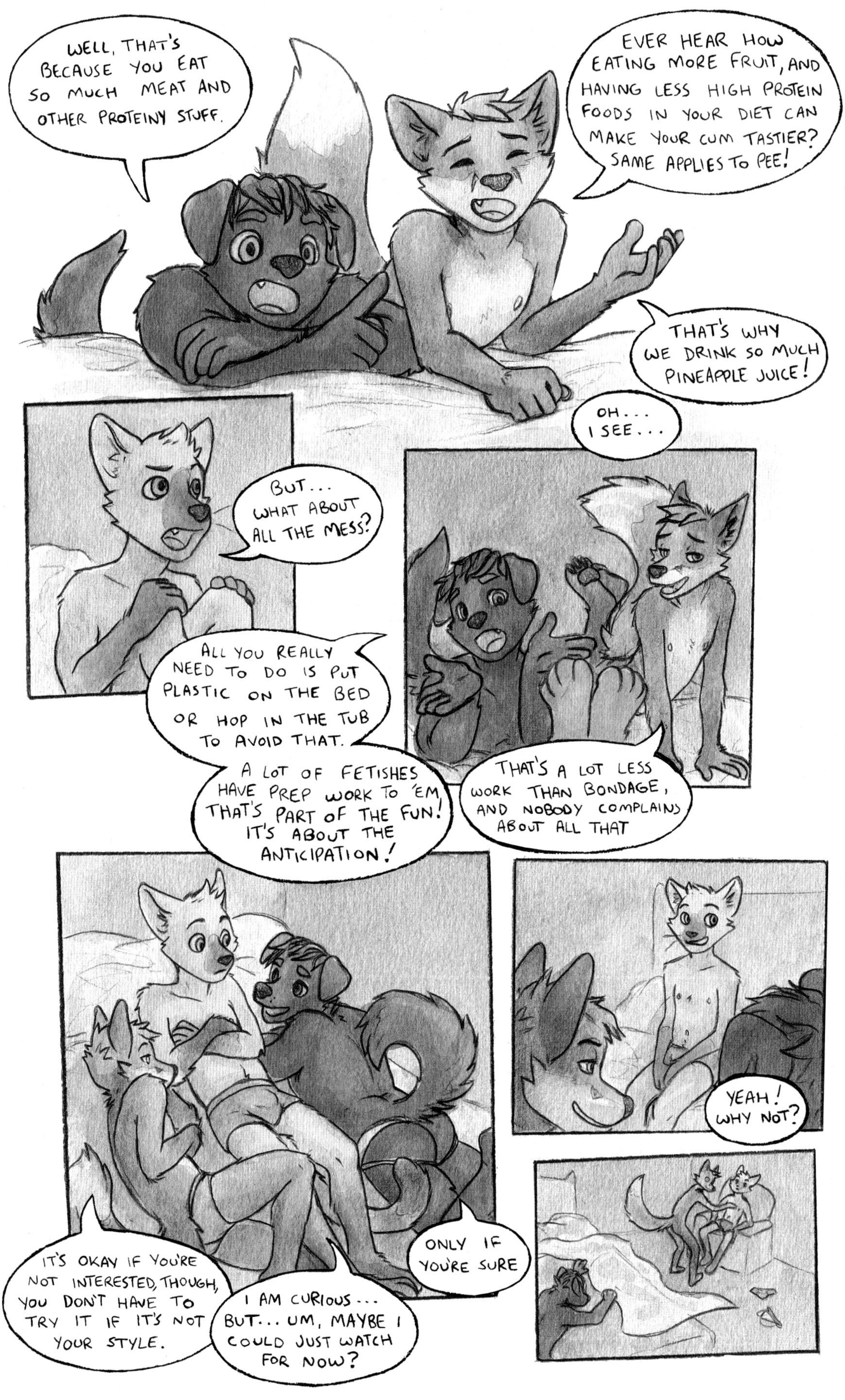
WELL, THAT'S BECAUSE YOU EAT SO MUCH MEAT AND OTHER PROTEINY STUFF.
EVER HEAR HOW EATING MORE FRUIT, AND HAVING LESS HIGH PROTEIN FOODS IN YOUR DIET CAN MAKE YOUR CUM TASTIER? SAME APPLIES TO PEE!
THAT'S WHY WE DRINK SO MUCH PINEAPPLE JUICE!
OH... I SEE...
BUT... WHAT ABOUT ALL THE MESS?
ALL YOU REALLY NEED TO DO IS PUT PLASTIC ON THE BED OR HOP IN THE TUB TO AVOID THAT.
A LOT OF FETISHES HAVE PREP WORK TO 'EM. THAT'S PART OF THE FUN! IT'S ABOUT THE ANTICIPATION!
THAT'S A LOT LESS WORK THAN BONDAGE, AND NOBODY COMPLAINS ABOUT ALL THAT
YEAH! WHY NOT?
IT'S OKAY IF YOU'RE NOT INTERESTED, THOUGH, YOU DON'T HAVE TO TRY IT IF IT'S NOT YOUR STYLE.
I AM CURIOUS... BUT... UM, MAYBE I COULD JUST WATCH FOR NOW?
ONLY IF YOU'RE SURE

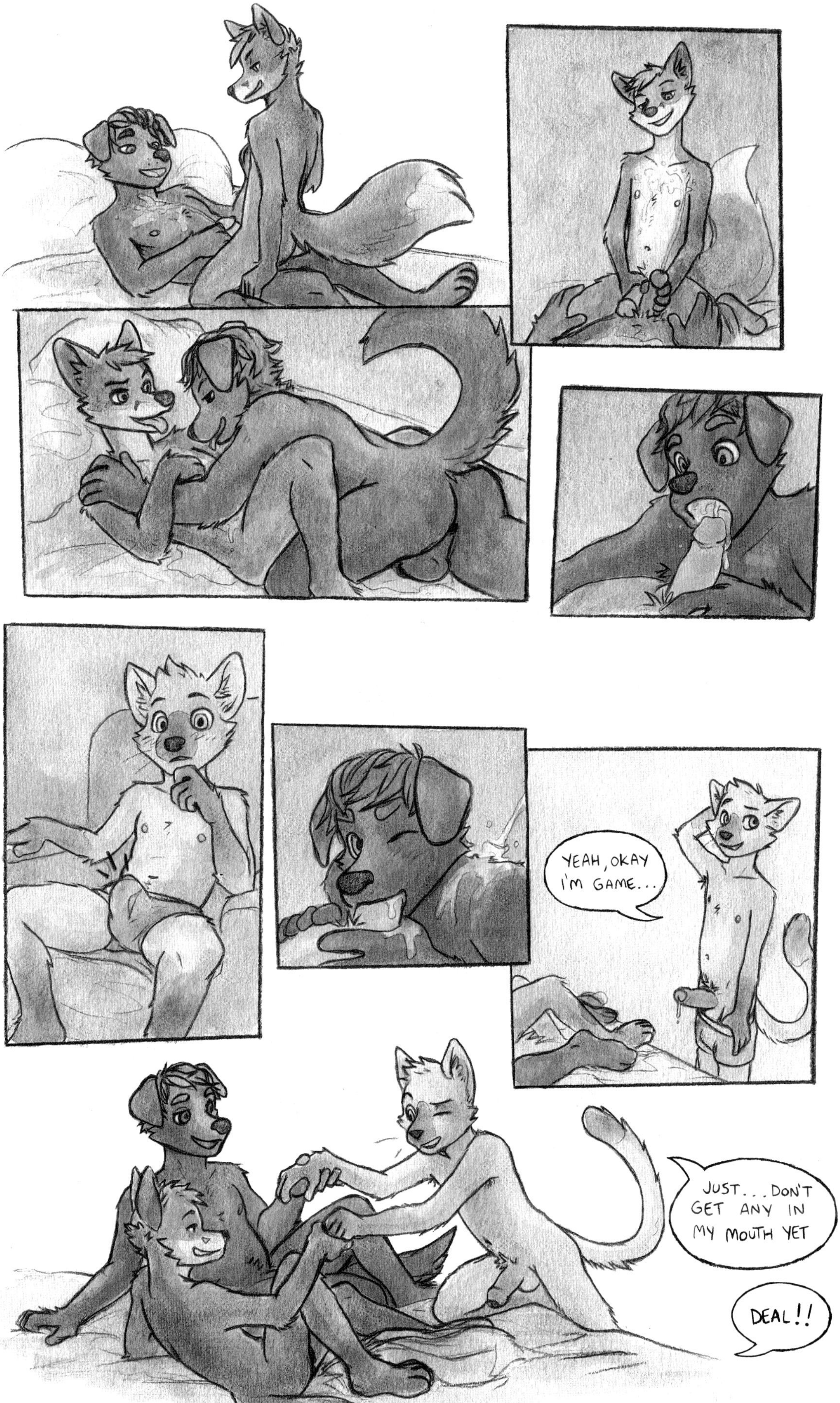
YEAH, OKAY I'M GAME...
JUST...DON'T GET ANY IN MY MOUTH YET
DEAL!!

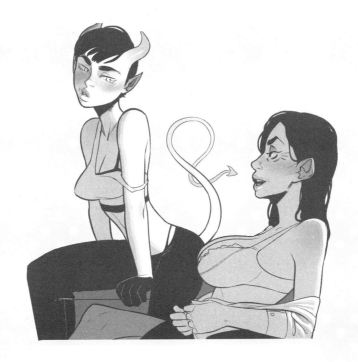

DEVILISH DEAL

by Incase

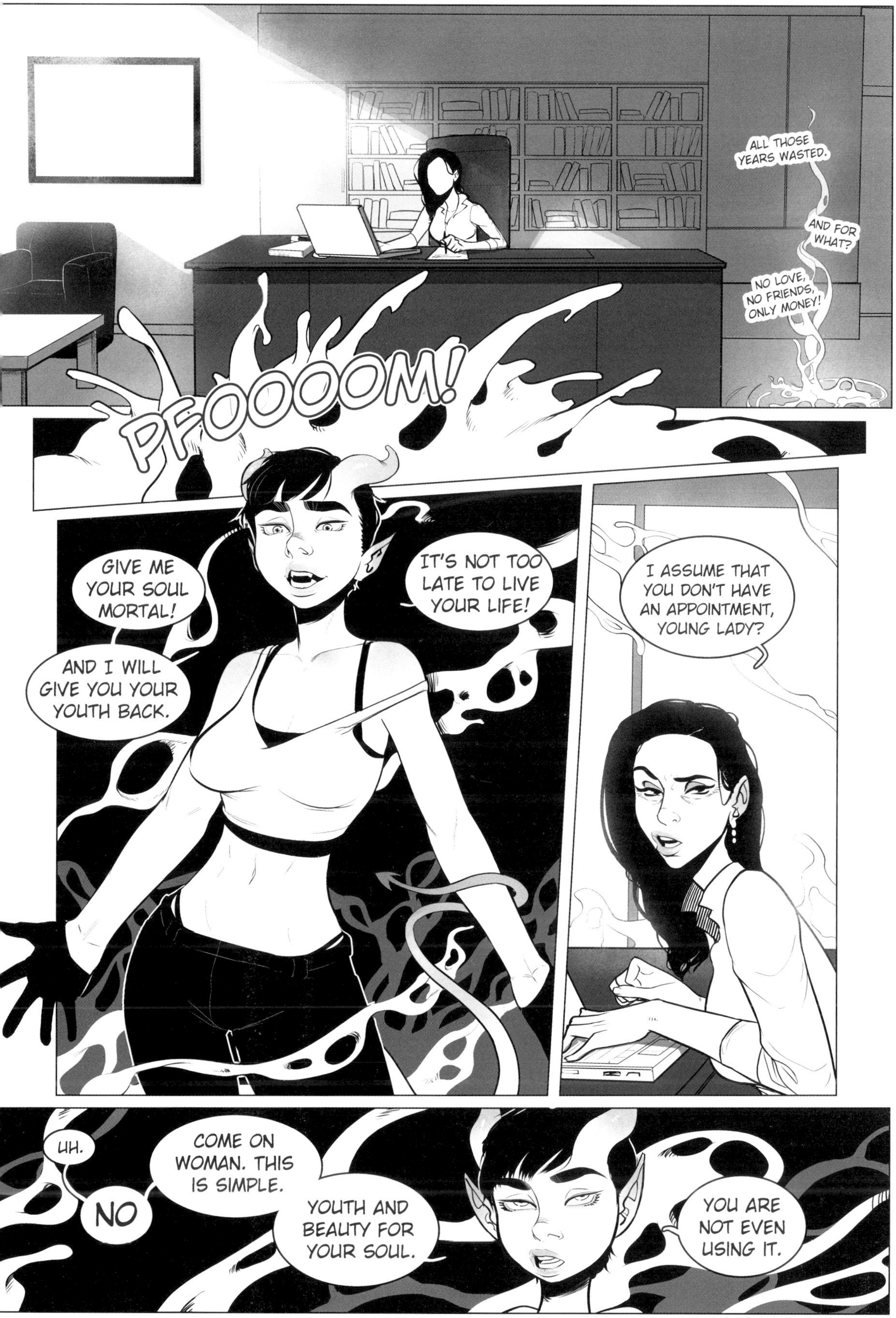
ALL THOSE YEARS WASTED.
AND FOR WHAT?
NO LOVE, NO FRIENDS, ONLY MONEY!
PFOOOOM!
GIVE ME YOUR SOUL MORTAL!
AND I WILL GIVE YOU YOUR YOUTH BACK.
IT'S NOT TOO LATE TO LIVE YOUR LIFE!
I ASSUME THAT YOU DON'T HAVE AN APPOINTMENT, YOUNG LADY?
UH.
NO
COME ON WOMAN. THIS IS SIMPLE.
YOUTH AND BEAUTY FOR YOUR SOUL.
YOU ARE NOT EVEN USING IT.

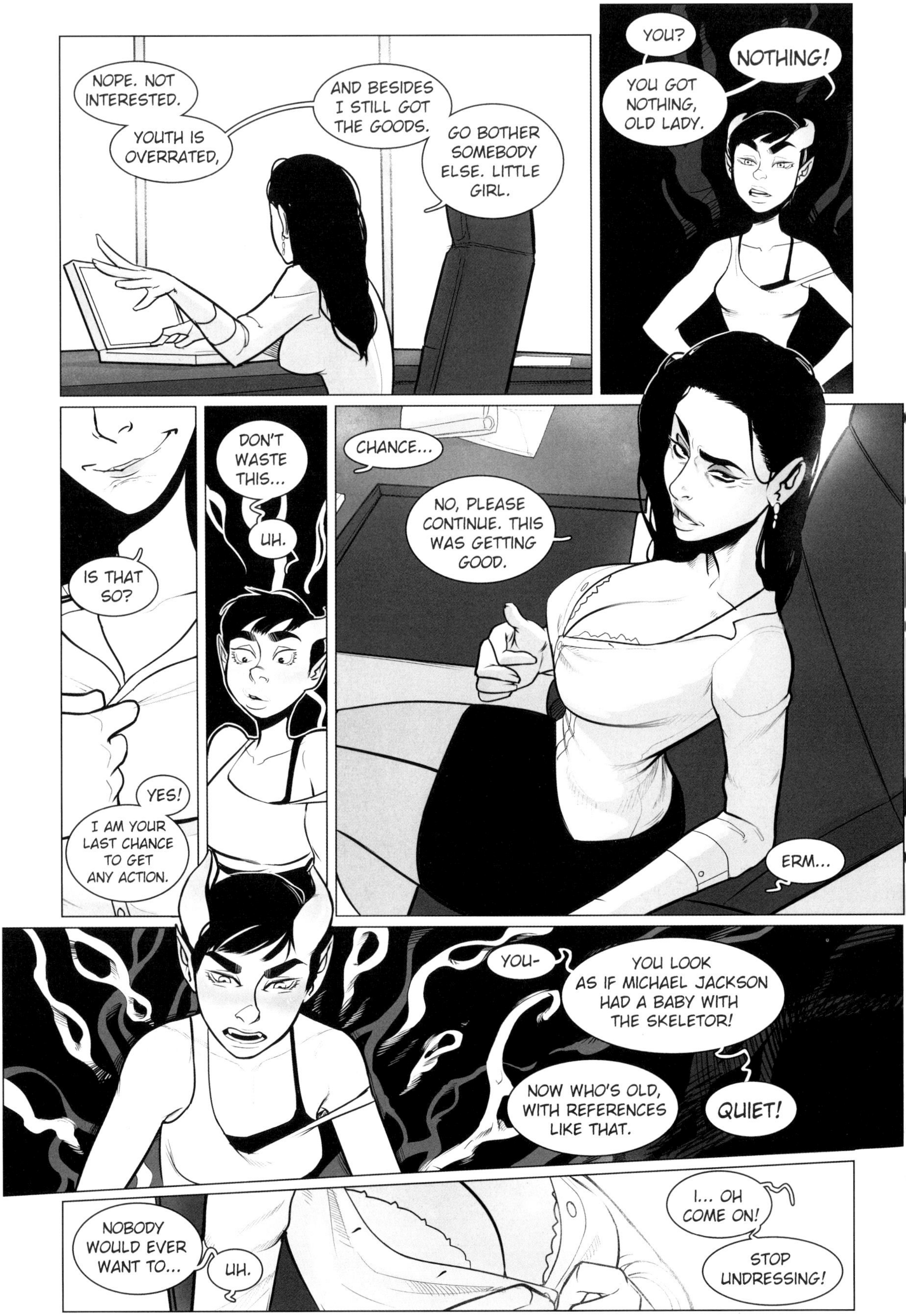

NOPE. NOT INTERESTED.
YOUTH IS OVERRATED,
AND BESIDES I STILL GOT THE GOODS.
GO BOTHER SOMEBODY ELSE. LITTLE GIRL.
YOU?
YOU GOT NOTHING, OLD LADY.
NOTHING!
IS THAT SO?
YES!
I AM YOUR LAST CHANCE TO GET ANY ACTION.
DON'T WASTE THIS...
UH.
CHANCE...
NO, PLEASE CONTINUE. THIS WAS GETTING GOOD.
ERM...
YOU-
YOU LOOK AS IF MICHAEL JACKSON HAD A BABY WITH THE SKELETOR!
NOW WHO'S OLD, WITH REFERENCES LIKE THAT.
QUIET!
NOBODY WOULD EVER WANT TO...
UH.
I... OH COME ON!
STOP UNDRESSING!

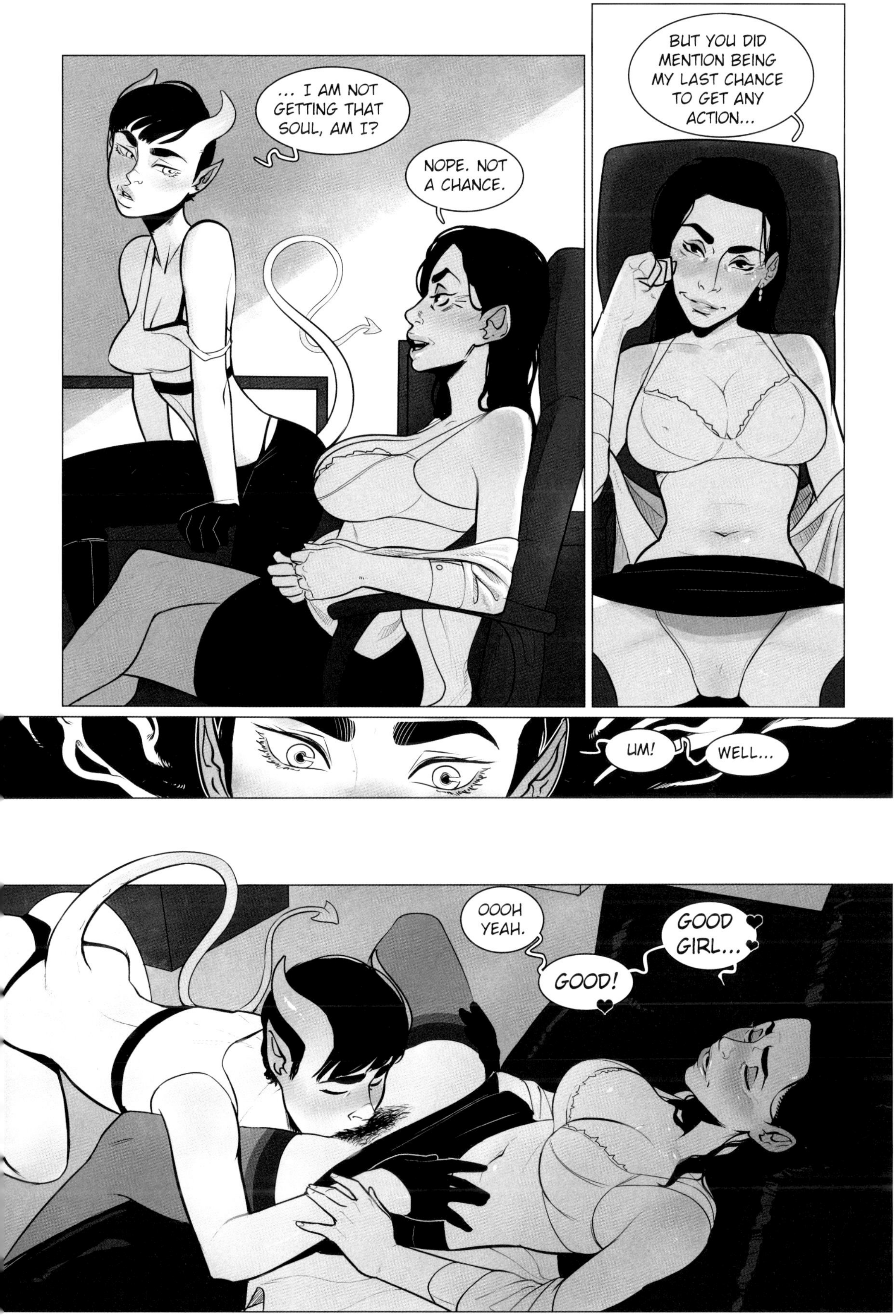

... I AM NOT GETTING THAT SOUL, AM I?
NOPE. NOT A CHANCE.
BUT YOU DID MENTION BEING MY LAST CHANCE TO GET ANY ACTION...
UM!
WELL...
OOOH YEAH.
GOOD!
GOOD GIRL...

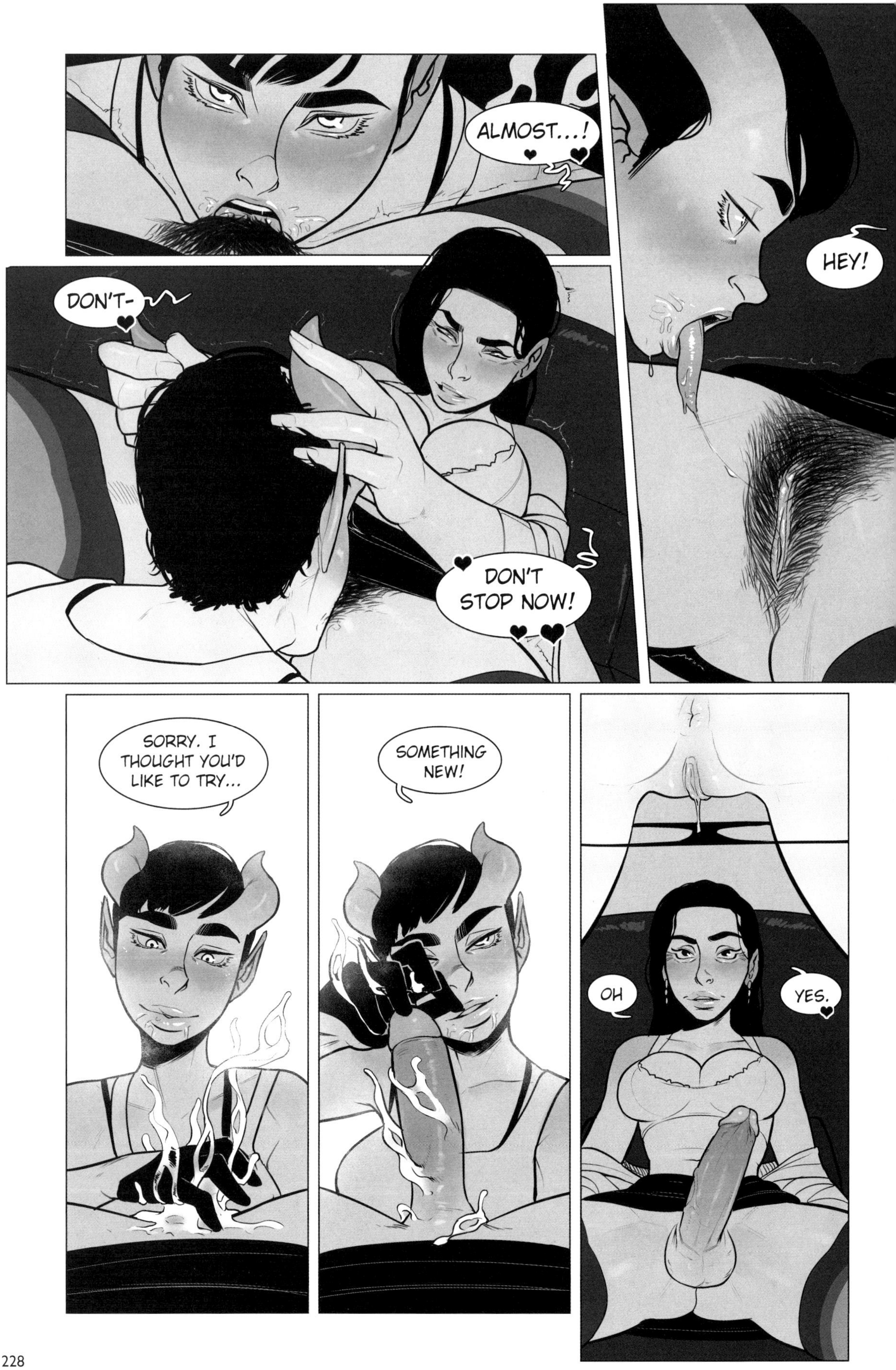
ALMOST...!
DON'T-
DON'T STOP NOW!
HEY!
SORRY. I THOUGHT YOU'D LIKE TO TRY...
SOMETHING NEW!
OH
YES.

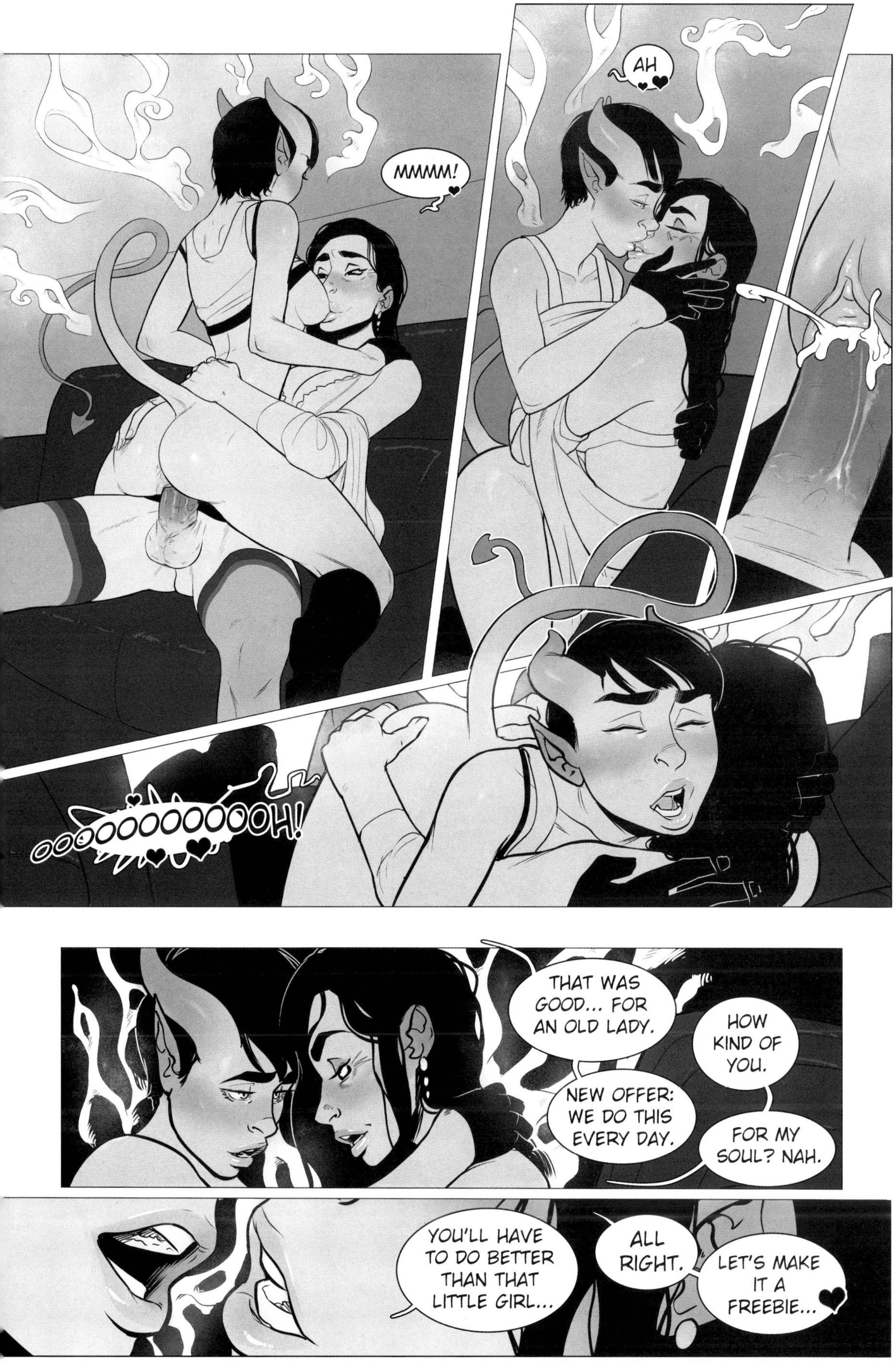
MMMM!
AH
OOOOOOOOOOOOOH!
THAT WAS GOOD... FOR AN OLD LADY.
HOW KIND OF YOU.
NEW OFFER: WE DO THIS EVERY DAY.
FOR MY SOUL? NAH.
YOU'LL HAVE TO DO BETTER THAN THAT LITTLE GIRL...
ALL RIGHT.
LET'S MAKE IT A FREEBIE...

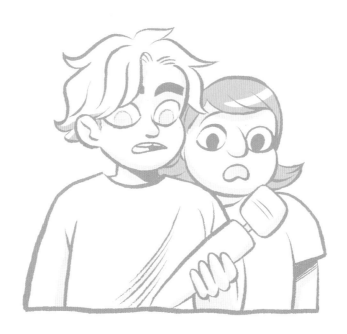

SHORT STORIES

by Kelly Bastow

Kellybastow.com

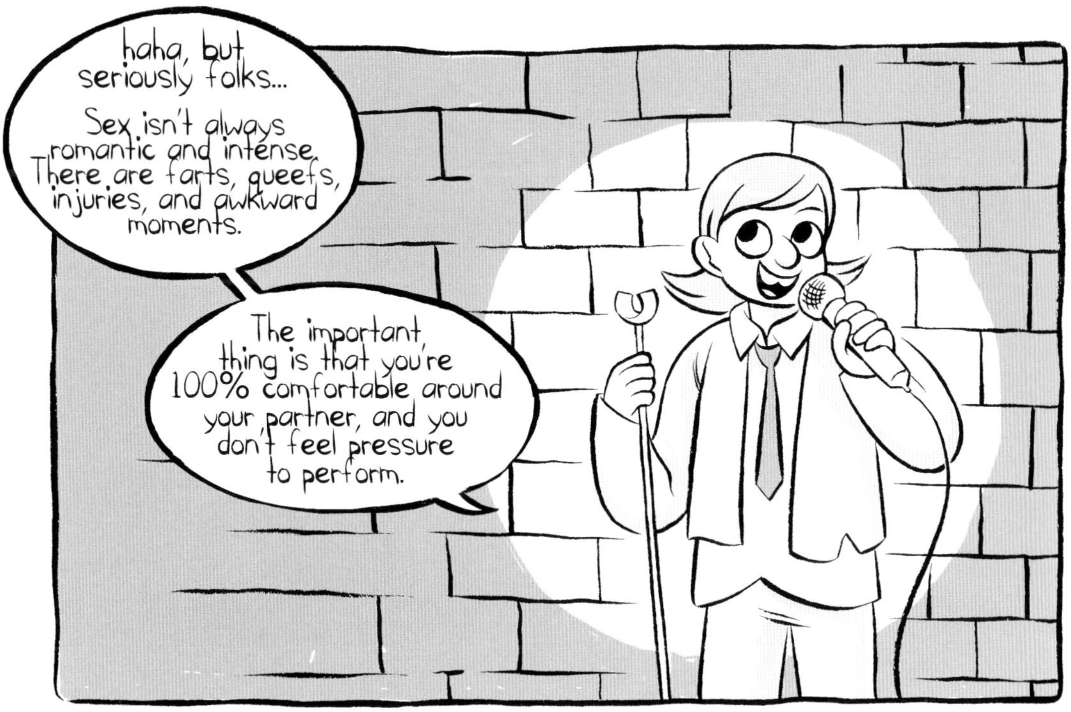
haha, but seriously folks...
Sex isn't always romantic and intense. There are farts, queefs, injuries, and awkward moments.
The important thing is that you're 100% comfortable around your partner, and you don't feel pressure to perform.

DIRTY TALK

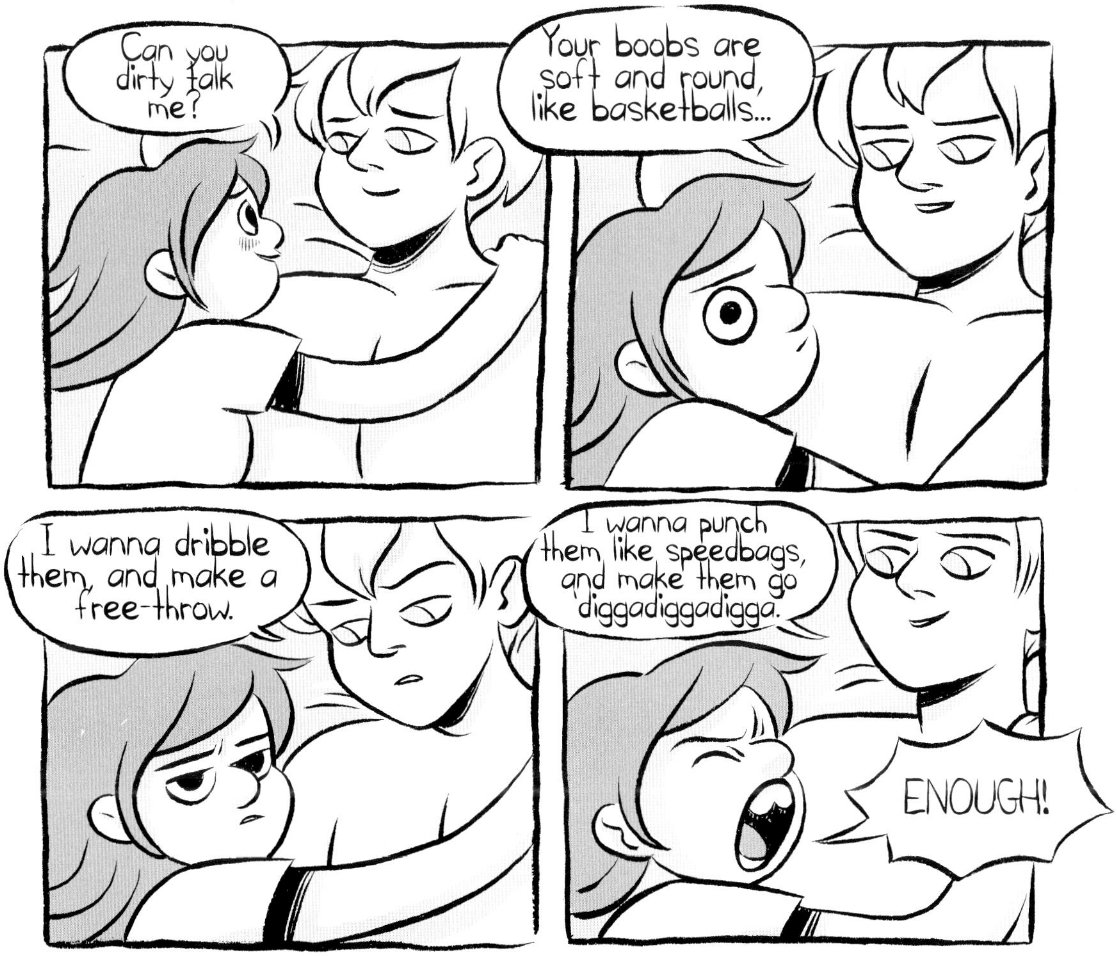
Can you dirty talk me?
Your boobs are soft and round, like basketballs...
I wanna dribble them, and make a free-throw.
I wanna punch them like speedbags, and make them go diggadiggadigga.
ENOUGH!

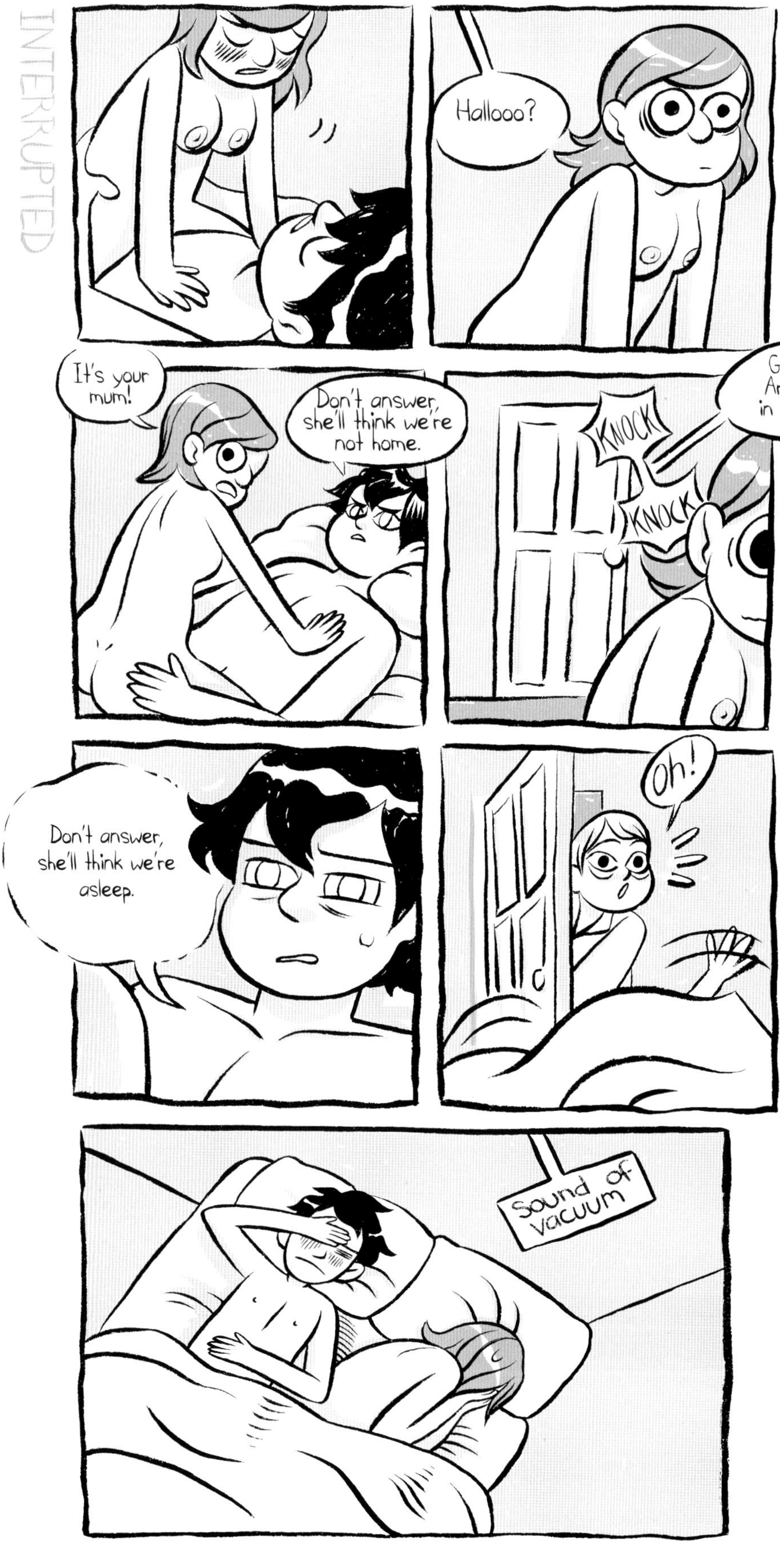
Hallooo?
It's your mum!
Don't answer, she'll think we're not home.
KNOCK
KNOCK
Guys? Are you in there?
Don't answer, she'll think we're asleep.
Oh!
Sound of vacuum

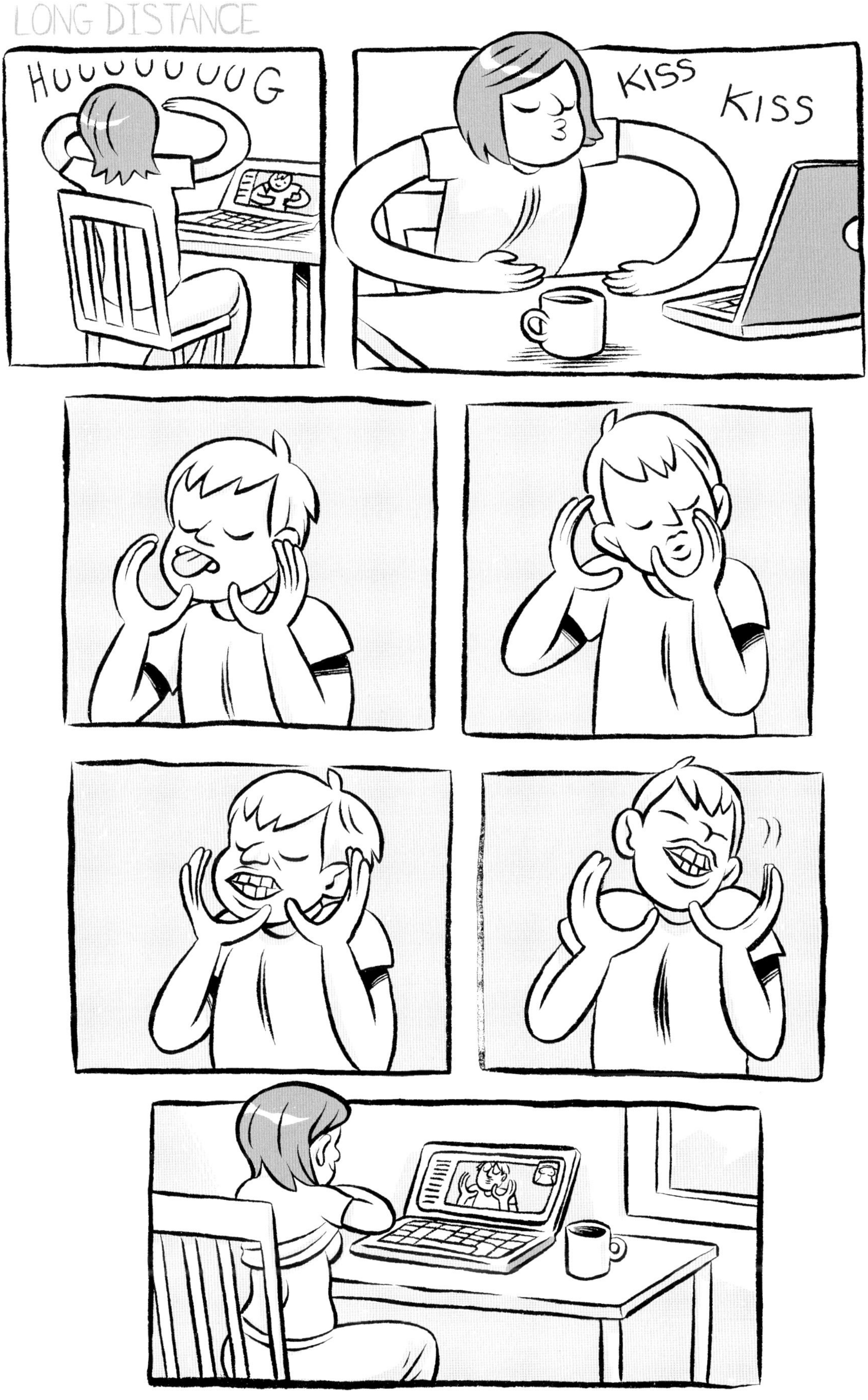
LONG DISTANCE
HUUUUUUUG
KISS
KISS

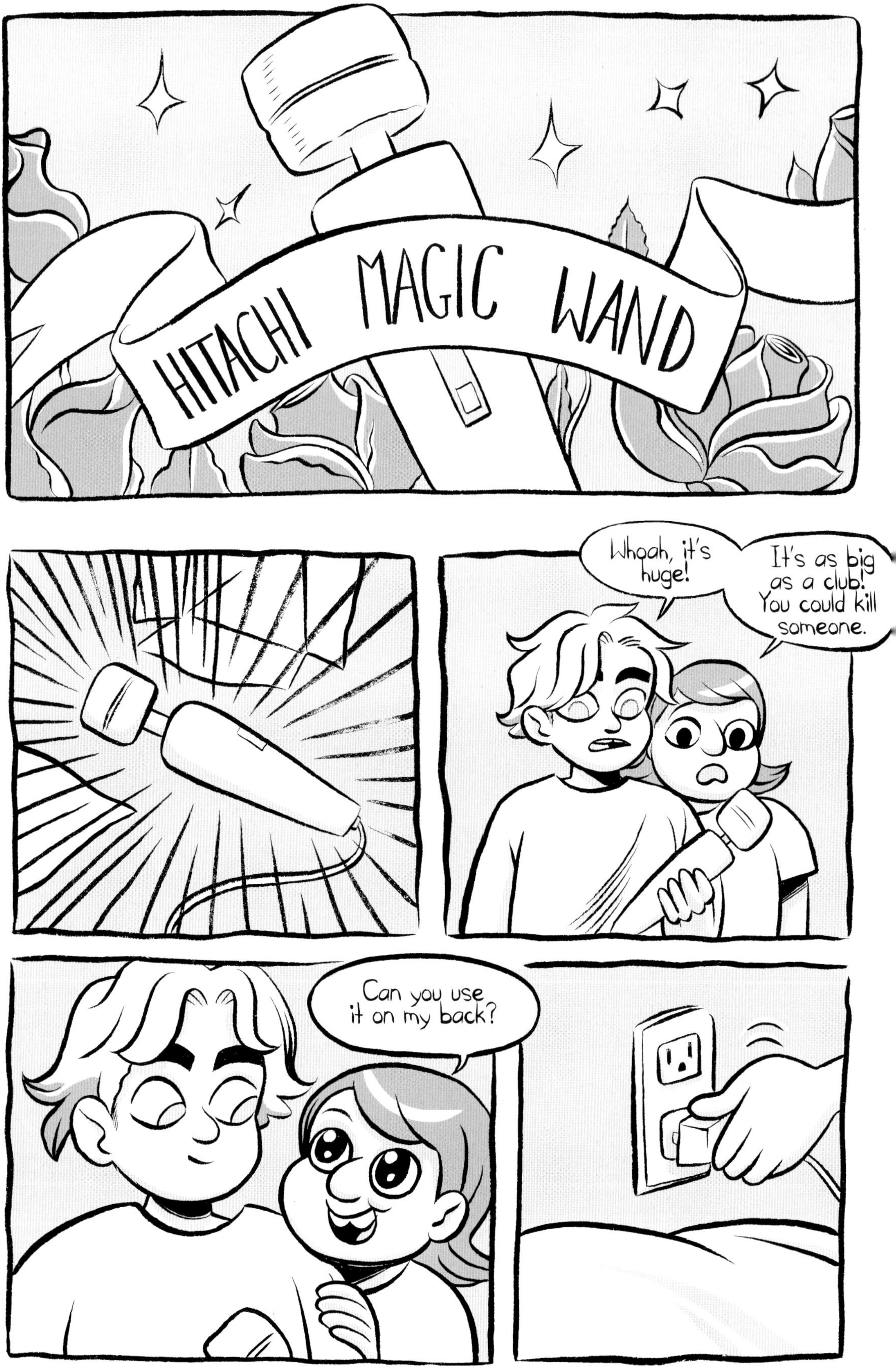
HITACHI MAGIC WAND
Whoah, it's huge!
It's as big as a club! You could kill someone.
Can you use it on my back?

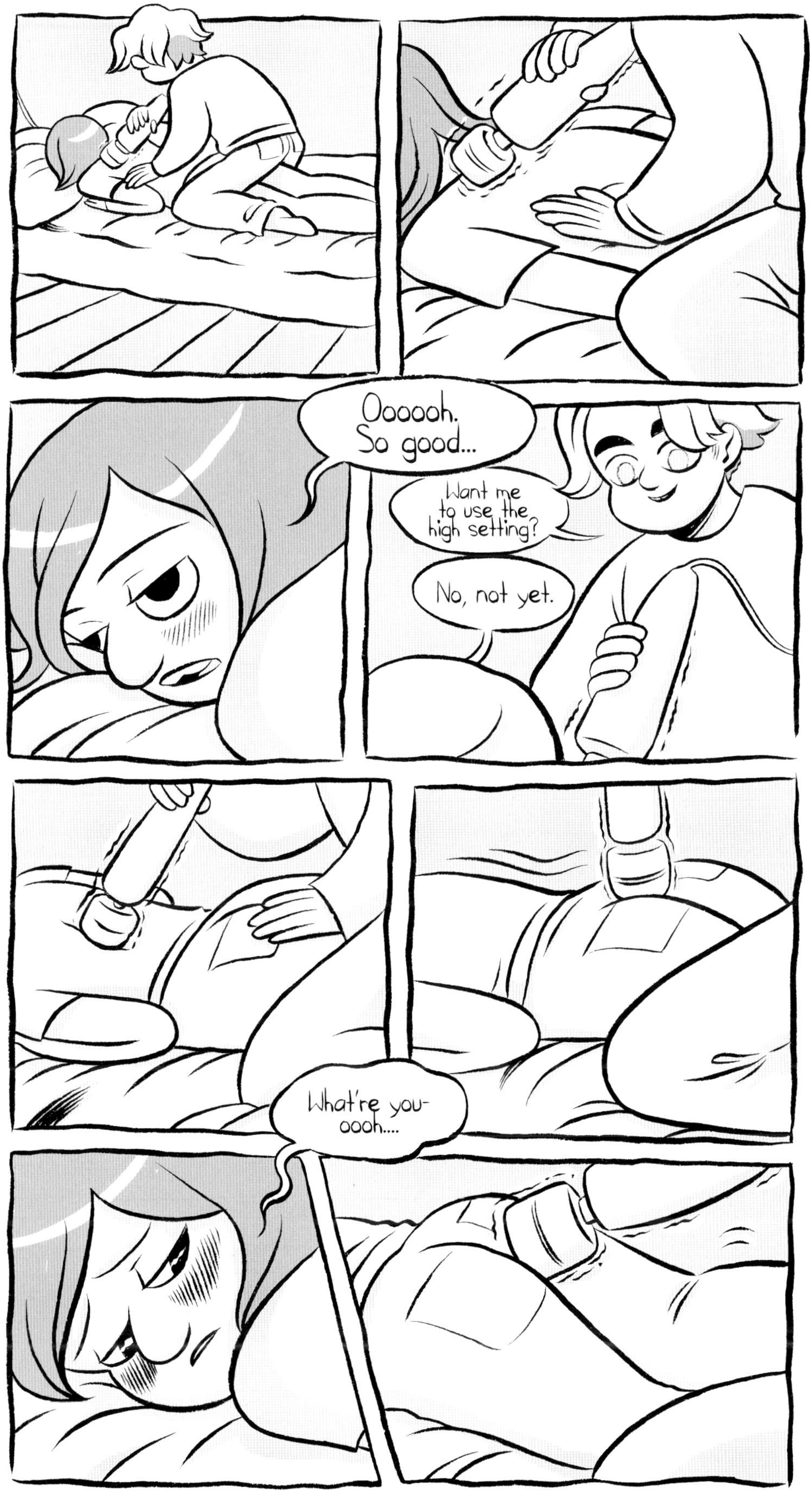
Oooooh.
So good...
Want me to use the high setting?
No, not yet.
What're you-oooh....

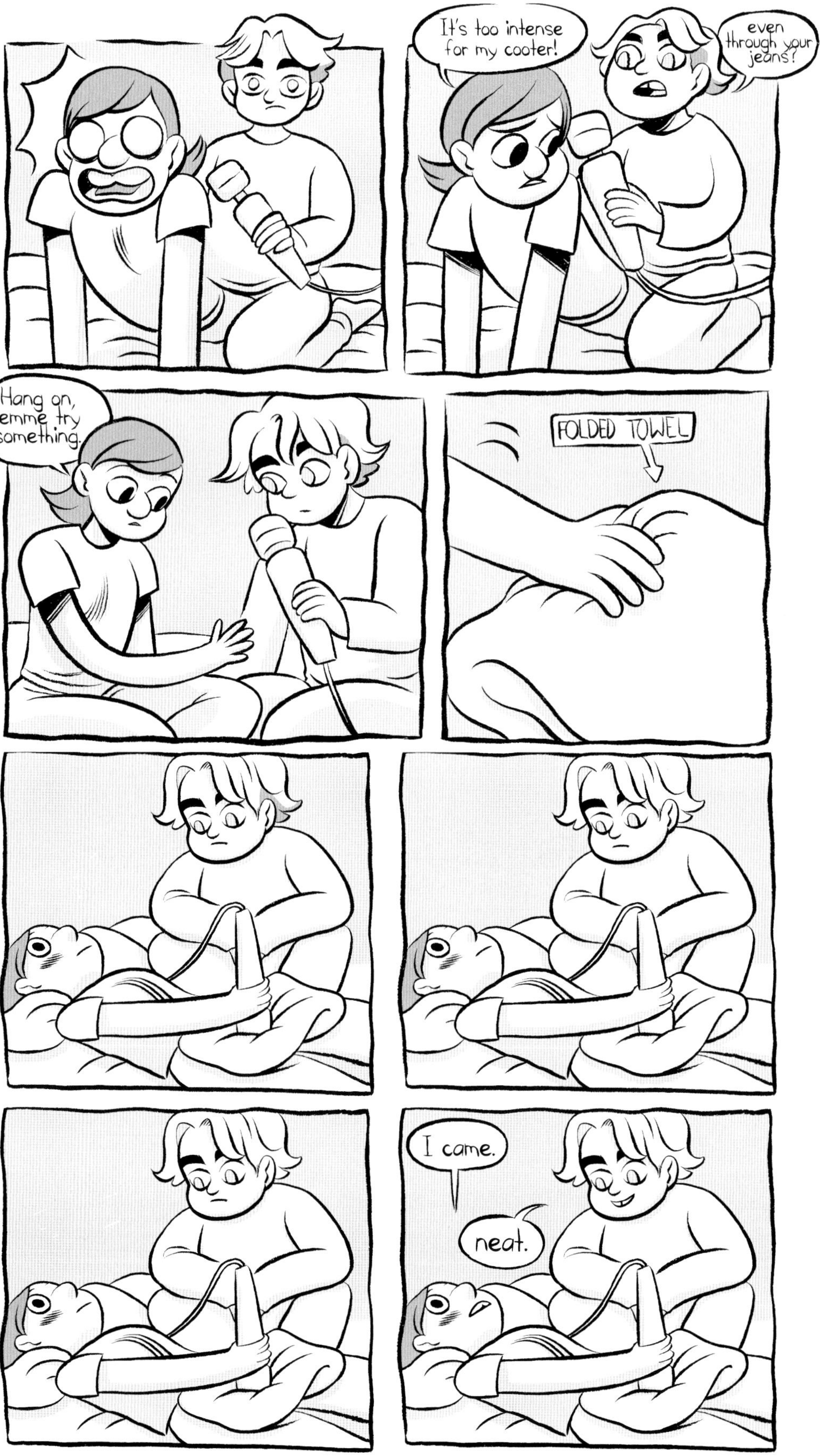
It's too intense for my cooter!
even through your jeans?
Hang on, lemme try something.
FOLDED TOWEL
I came.
neat.

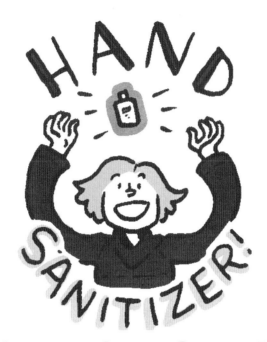

MISTAKES WERE MADE

by Lucy Bellwood

Lucybellwood.com

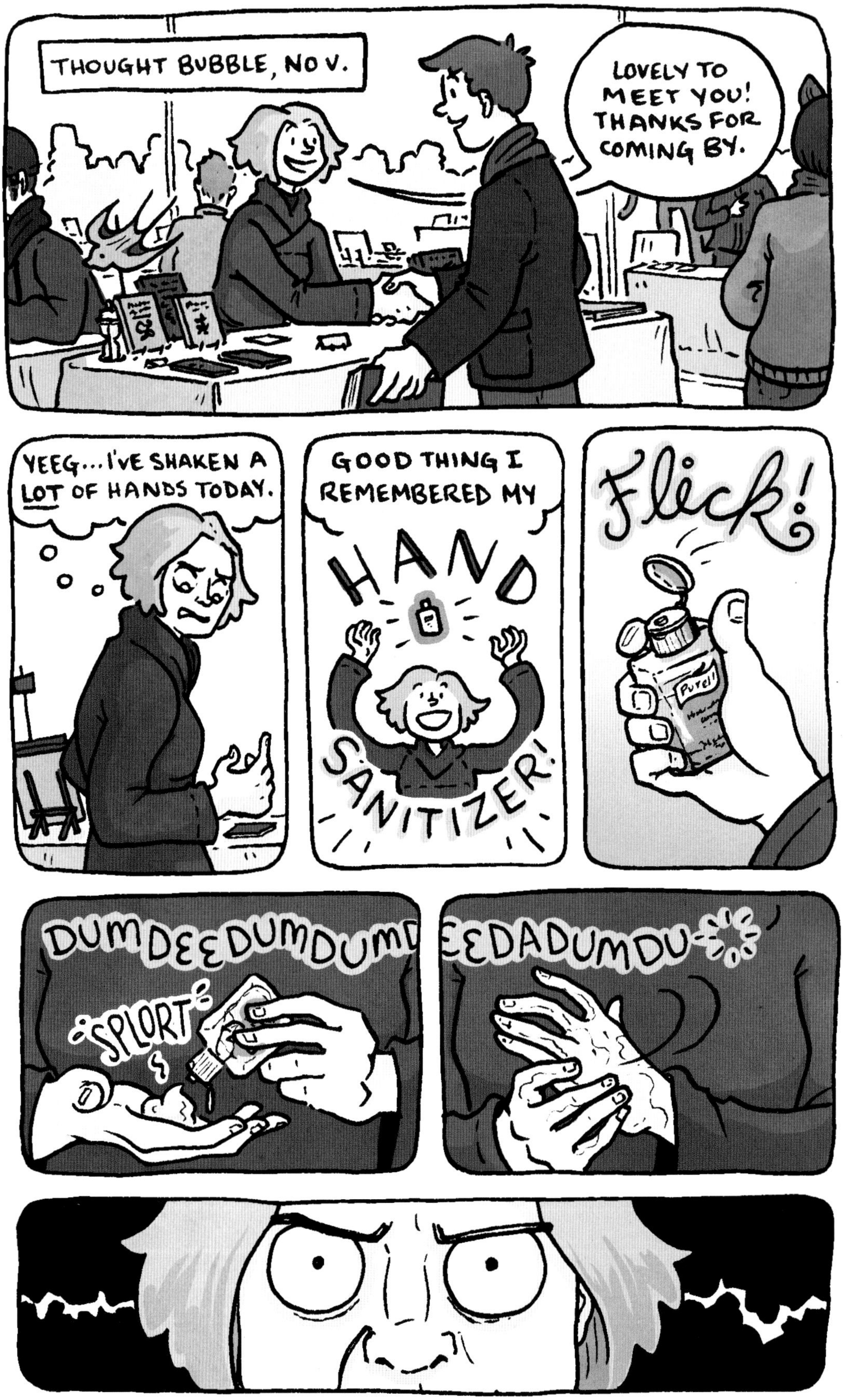

THOUGHT BUBBLE, NOV.
LOVELY TO MEET YOU! THANKS FOR COMING BY.
YEEG... I'VE SHAKEN A LOT OF HANDS TODAY.
GOOD THING I REMEMBERED MY
HAND SANITIZER!
Flick!
Purell
DUMDEEDUMDUMDEEDADUMDU
SPLORT

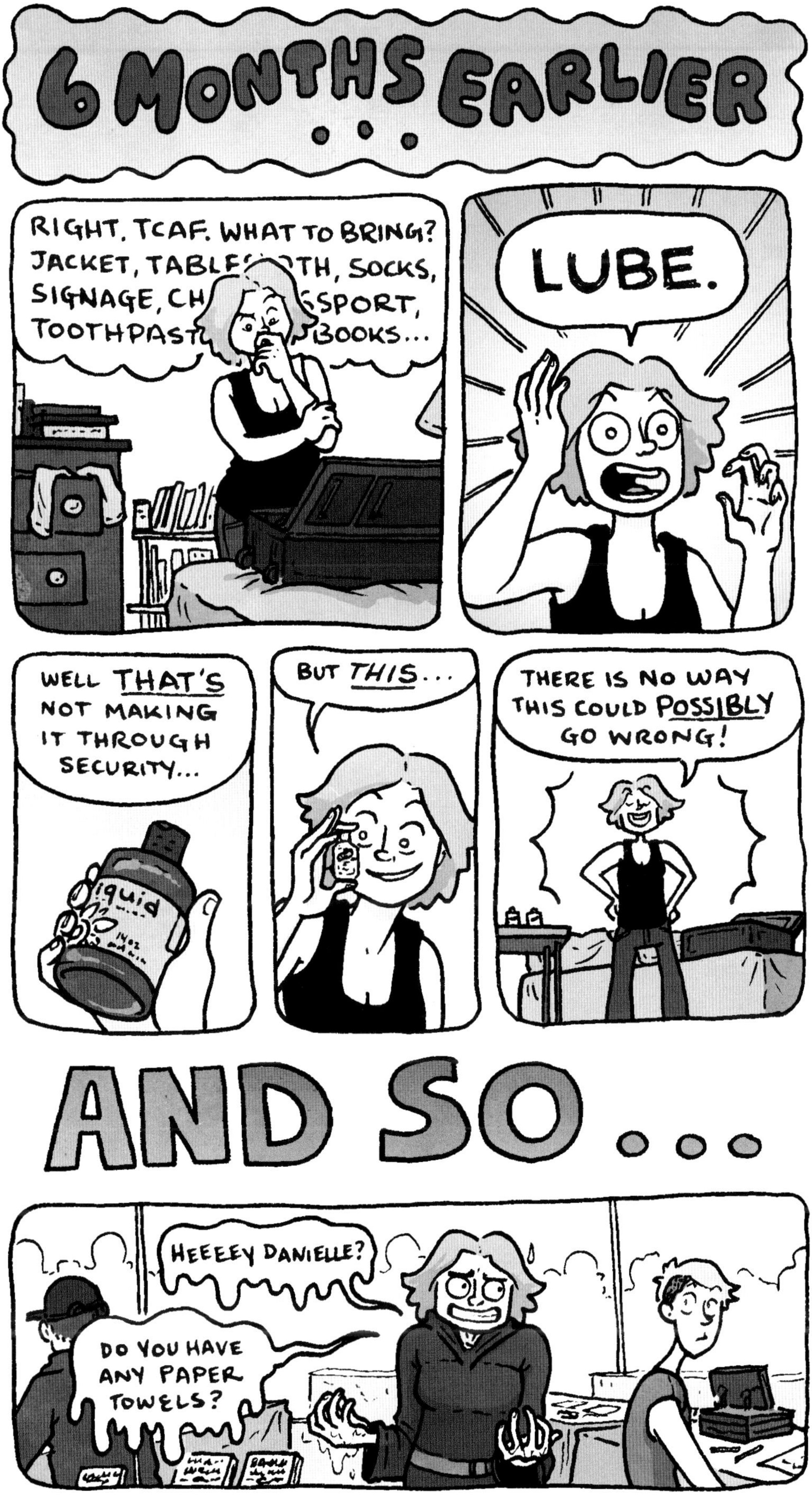
6 MONTHS EARLIER . . .
RIGHT. TCAF. WHAT TO BRING? JACKET, TABLE TH, SOCKS, SIGNAGE, CH SSPORT, TOOTHPAST BOOKS...
LUBE.
WELL THAT'S NOT MAKING IT THROUGH SECURITY...
iquid
BUT THIS...
THERE IS NO WAY THIS COULD POSSIBLY GO WRONG!
AND SO...
HEEEEY DANIELLE?
DO YOU HAVE ANY PAPER TOWELS?

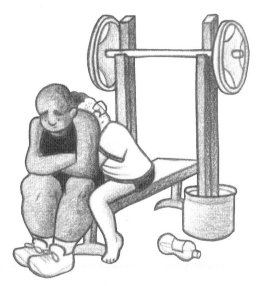

DEFECTIVE
by Melanie Gillman
Melaniegillman.com

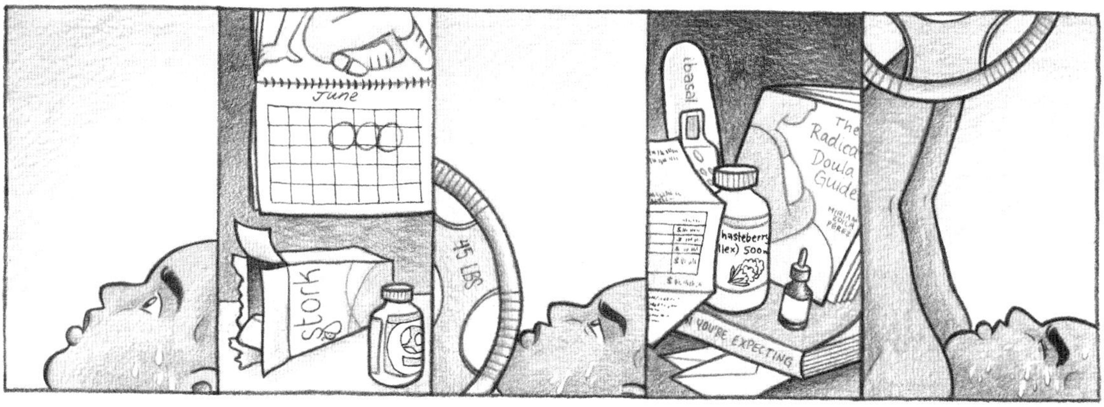
June
stork
45 LBS
basal
YOU'RE EXPECTING

DEFECTIVE

melanie gillman

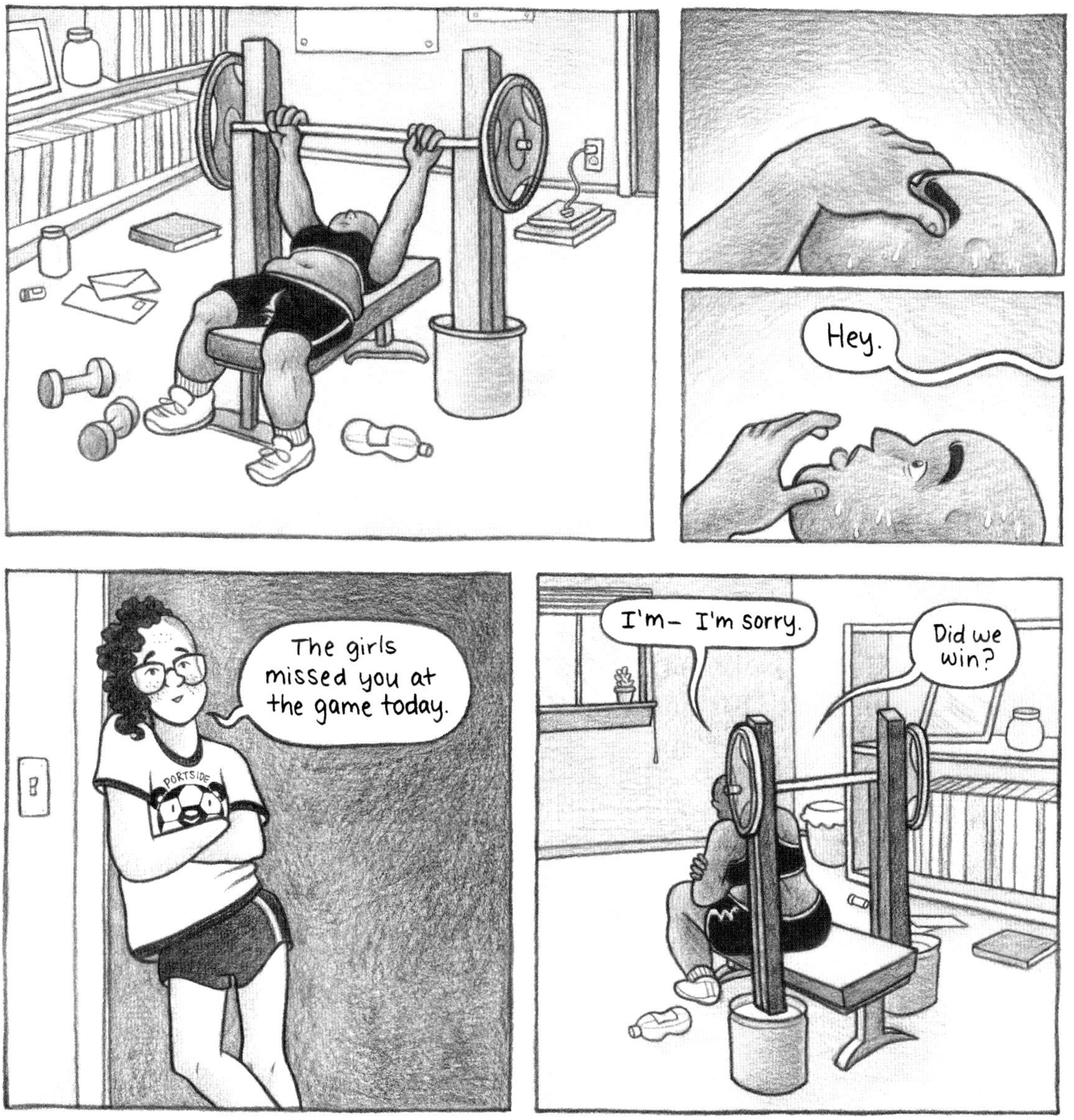
Hey.
The girls missed you at the game today.
PORTSIDE
I'm– I'm sorry.
Did we win?

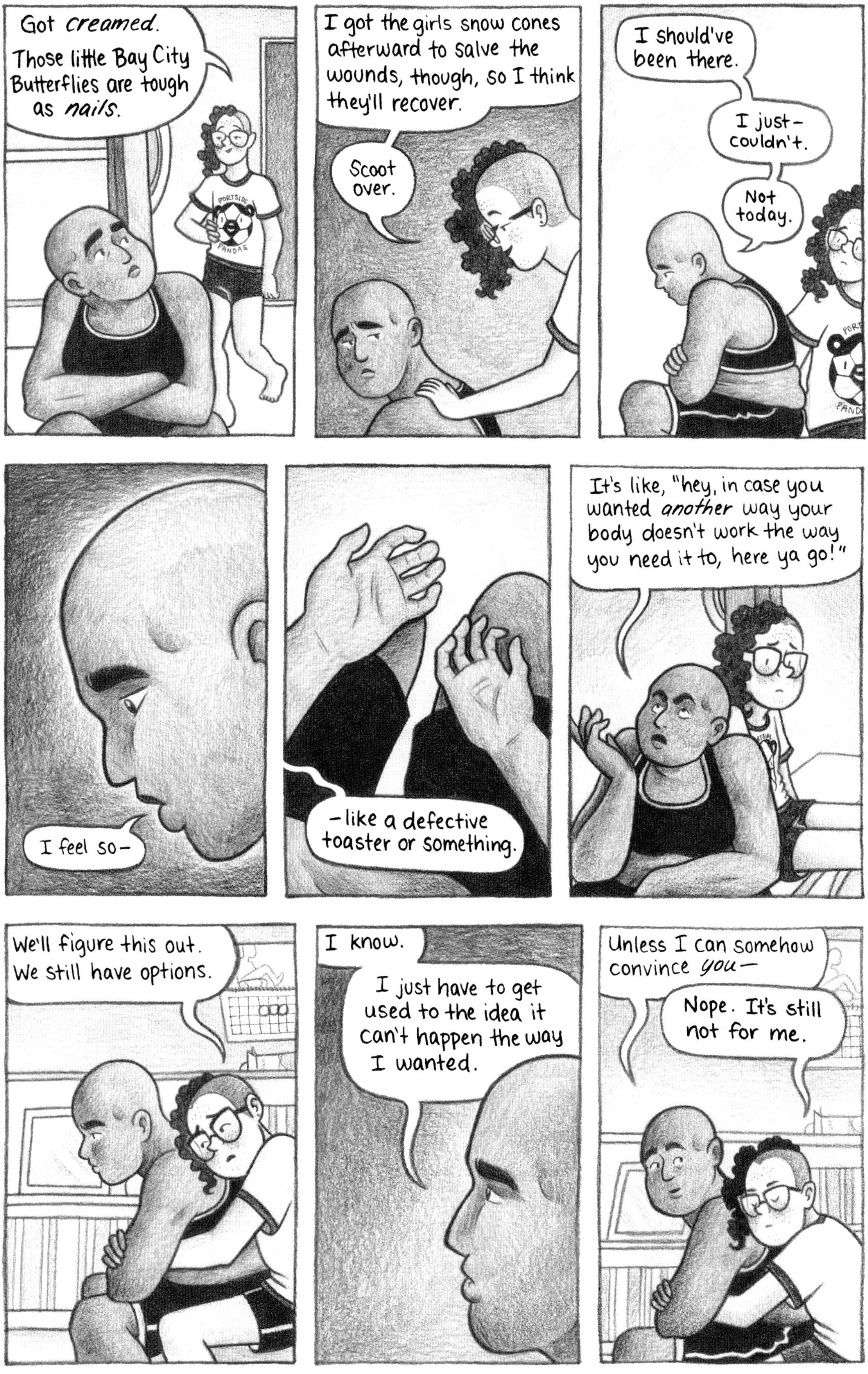
Got *creamed*.
Those little Bay City Butterflies are tough as *nails*.
PORTSIDE PANDAS
I got the girls snow cones afterward to salve the wounds, though, so I think they'll recover.
Scoot over.
I should've been there.
I just— couldn't.
Not today.
I feel so—
—like a defective toaster or something.
It's like, "hey, in case you wanted *another* way your body doesn't work the way you need it to, here ya go!"
We'll figure this out. We still have options.
I know.
I just have to get used to the idea it can't happen the way I wanted.
Unless I can somehow convince *you*—
Nope. It's still not for me.

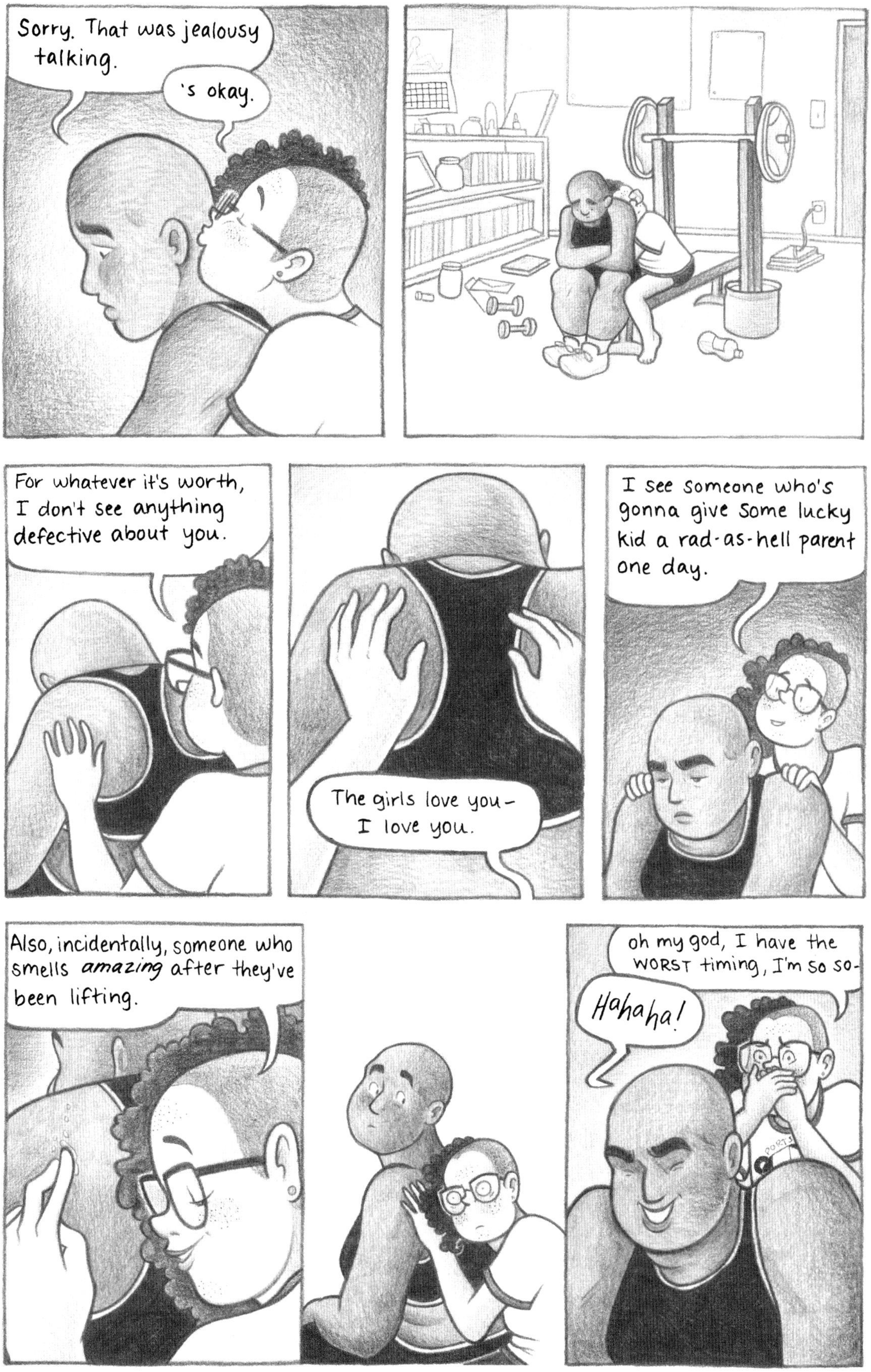
Sorry. That was jealousy talking.
's okay.
For whatever it's worth, I don't see anything defective about you.
The girls love you- I love you.
I see someone who's gonna give some lucky kid a rad-as-hell parent one day.
Also, incidentally, someone who smells *amazing* after they've been lifting.
oh my god, I have the WORST timing, I'm so so-
Hahaha!

It's okay.
You've got quite the alluring mowed-grass-and-grape-snowcone thing going on yourself.
eau de soccer coach

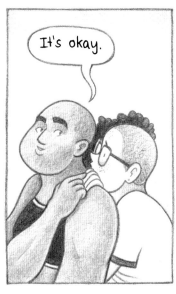

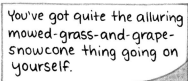

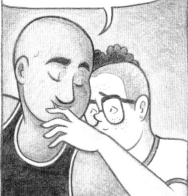

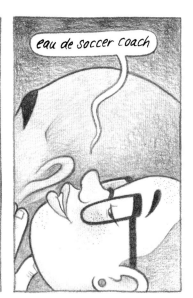

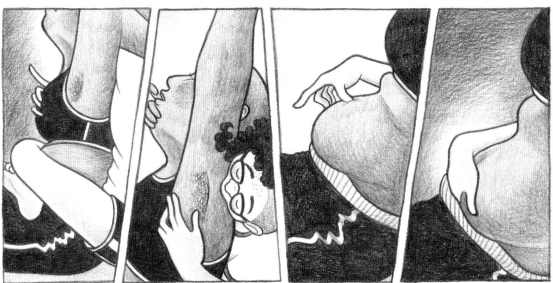

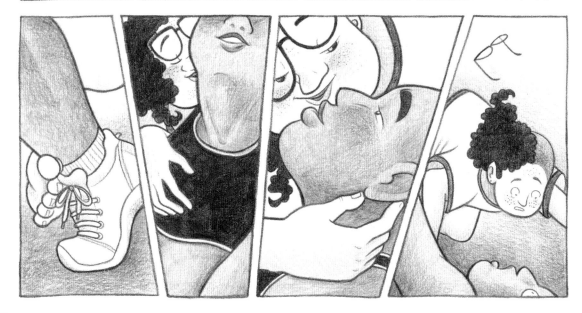

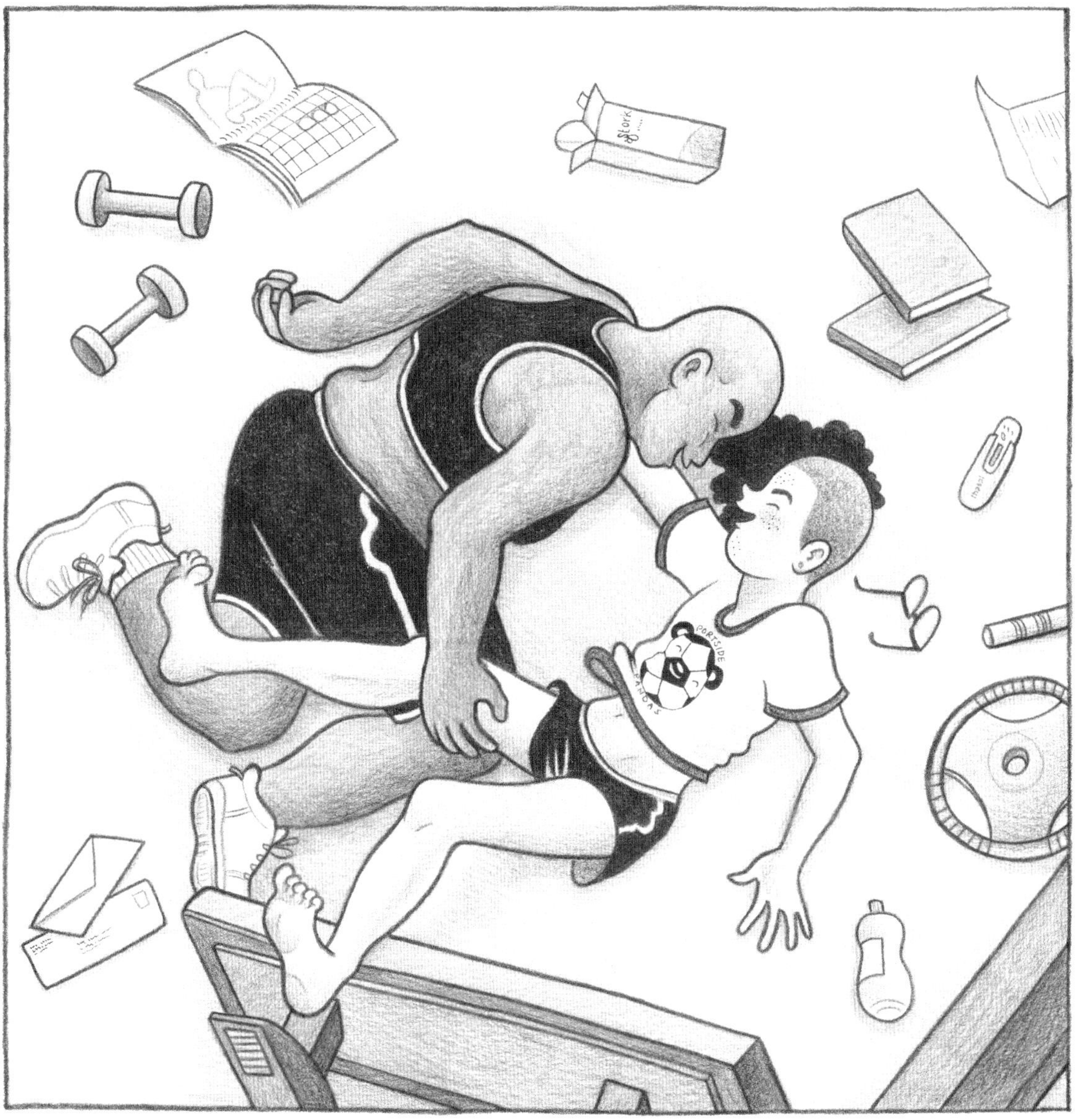

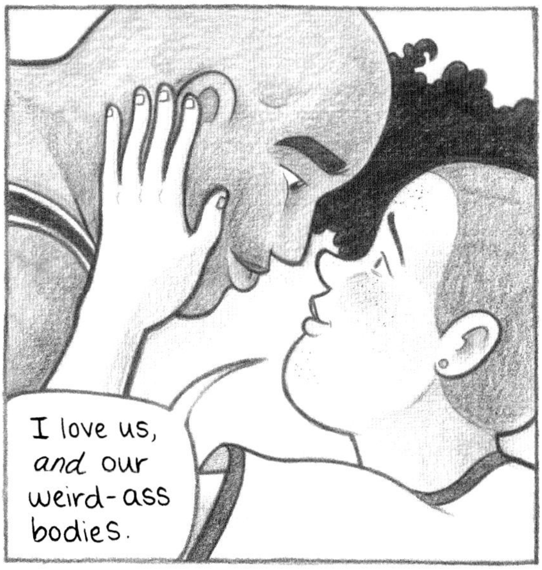
I love us, *and* our weird-ass bodies.

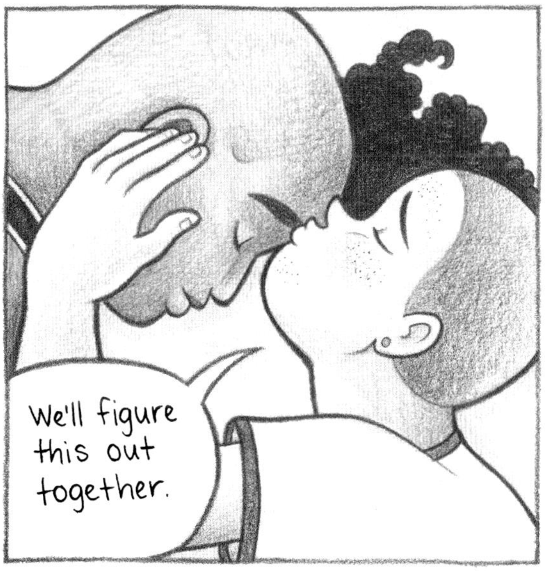
We'll figure this out together.

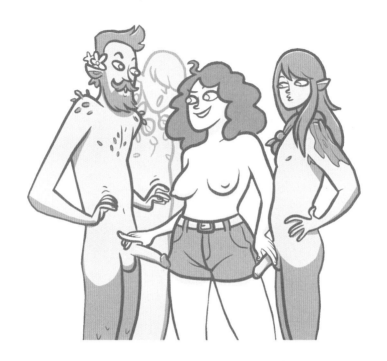

FOREST FRIENDS

by Delidah

FOREST FRIENDS

BY DELIDAH.

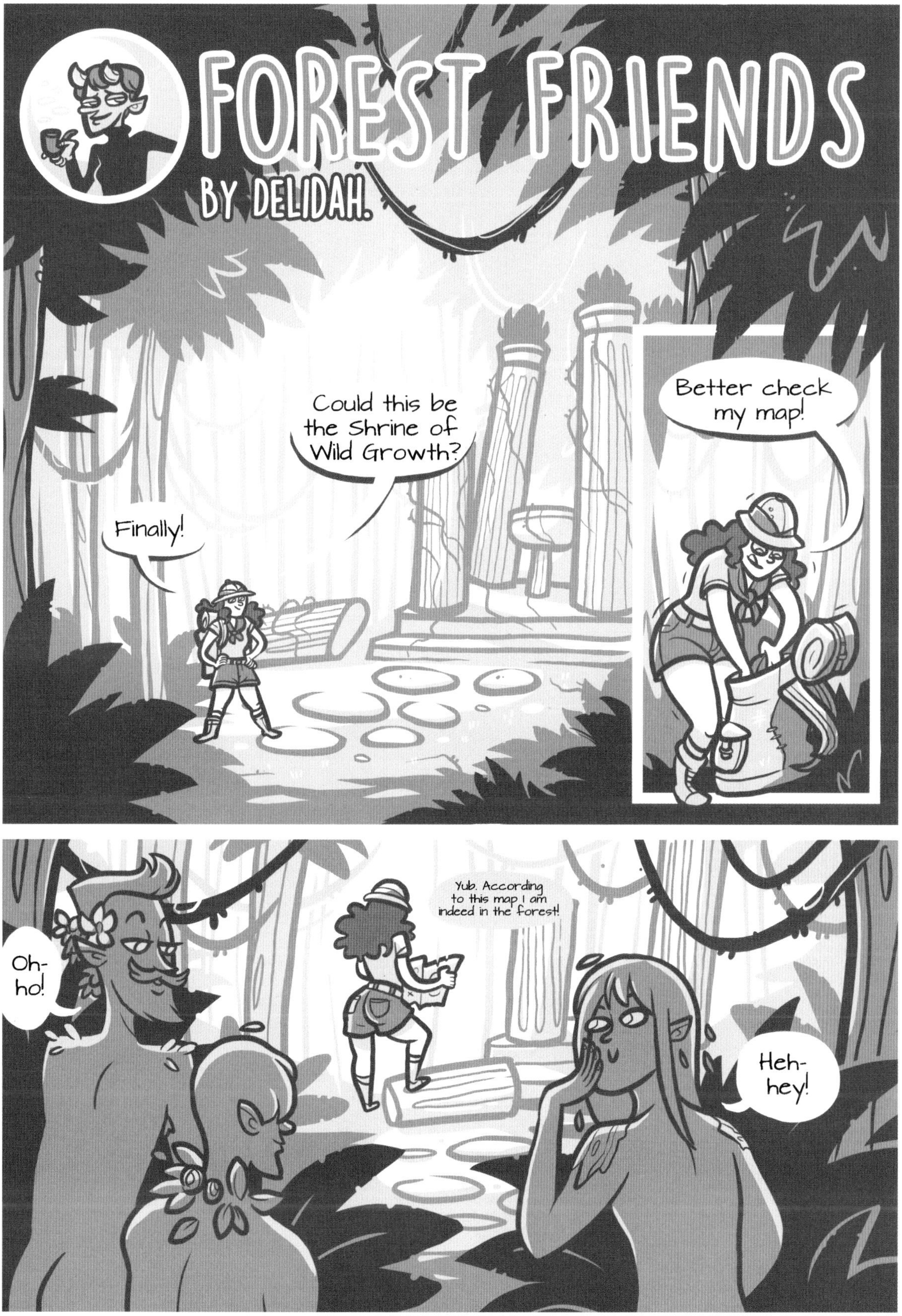
Finally!
Could this be the Shrine of Wild Growth?
Better check my map!
Oh-ho!
Yub. According to this map I am indeed in the forest!
Heh-hey!

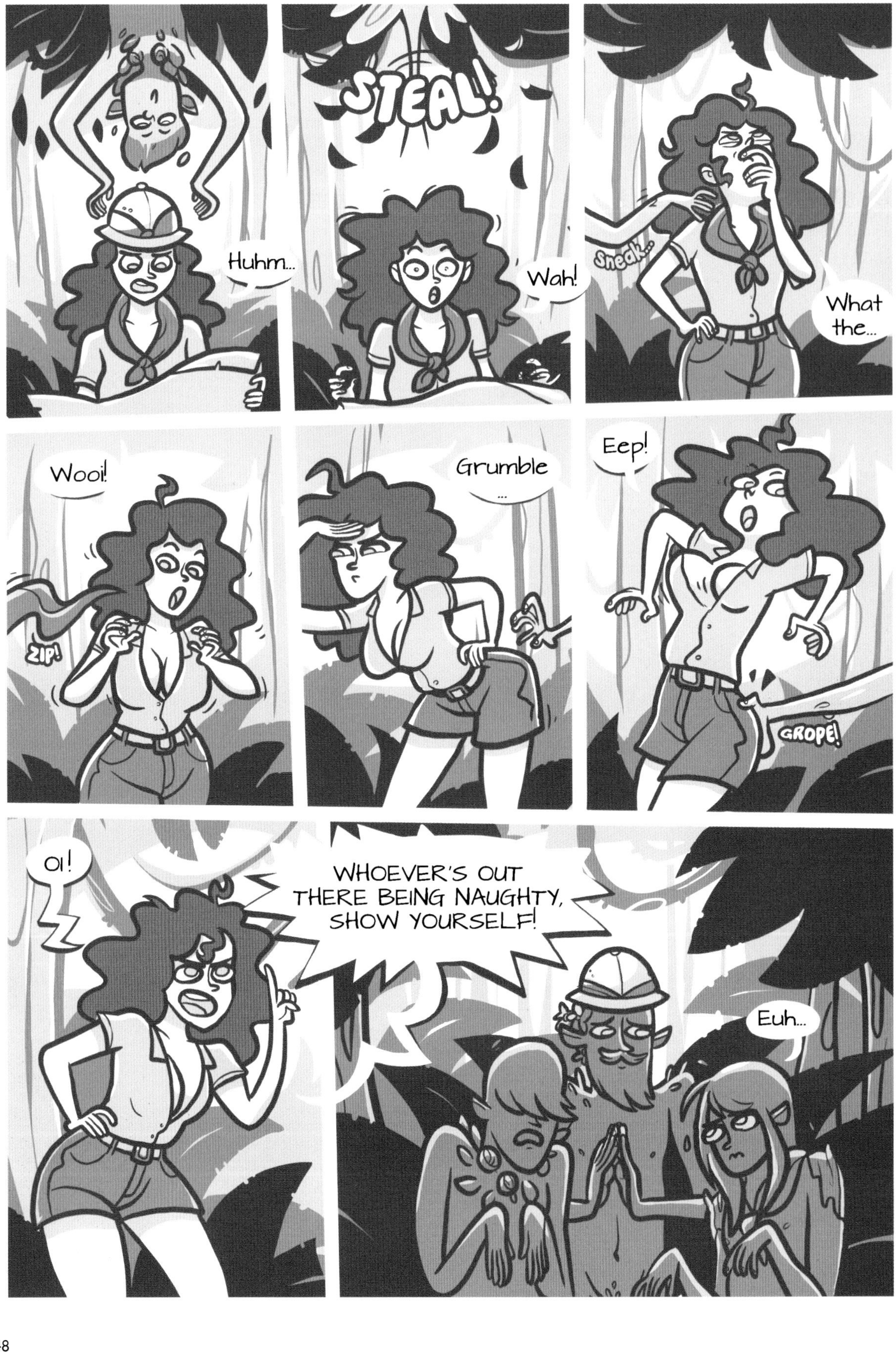
Huhm...
STEAL!
Wah!
Sneak...
What the...
Wooi!
ZIP!
Grumble ...
Eep!
GROPE!
OI!
WHOEVER'S OUT THERE BEING NAUGHTY, SHOW YOURSELF!
Euh...

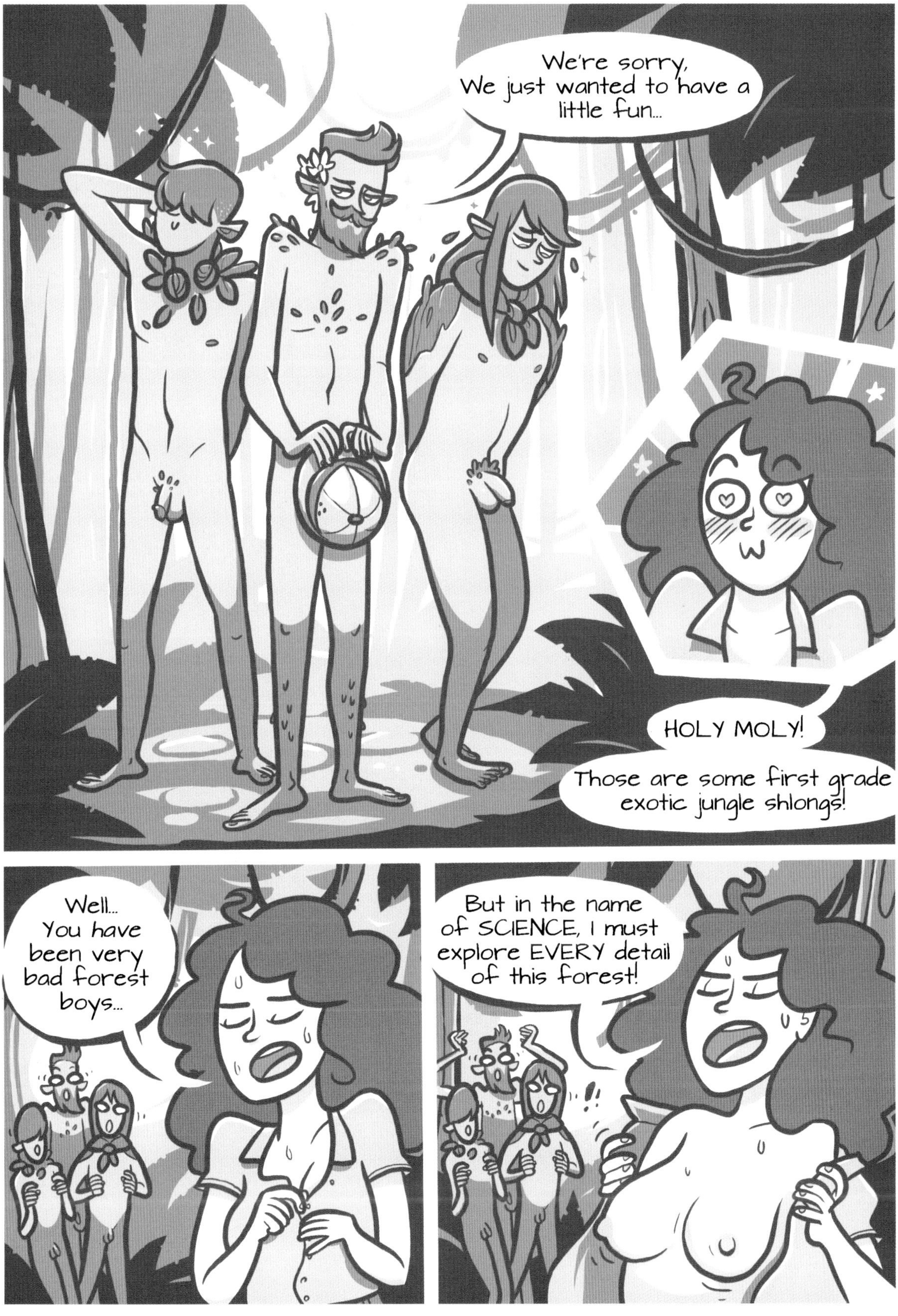
We're sorry,
We just wanted to have a little fun...
HOLY MOLY!
Those are some first grade exotic jungle shlongs!
Well... You have been very bad forest boys...
But in the name of SCIENCE, I must explore EVERY detail of this forest!

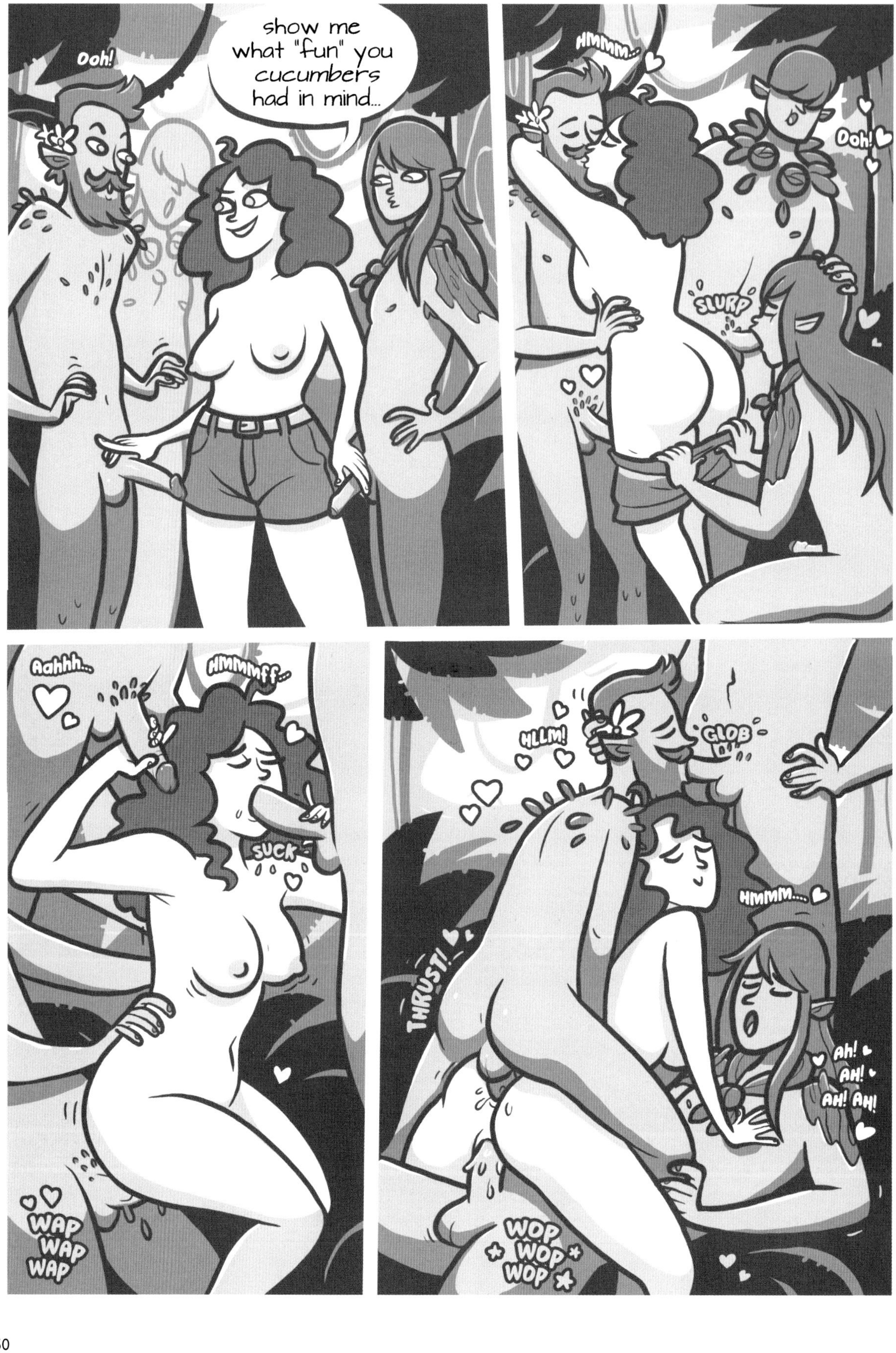
Ooh!
show me what "fun" you cucumbers had in mind...
HMMM...
Ooh!
SLURP
Aahhh...
HMMMff...
SUCK
WAP WAP WAP
HLLM!
GLOB
HMMM....
THRUST!
Ah! AH! AH! AH!
WOP WOP WOP

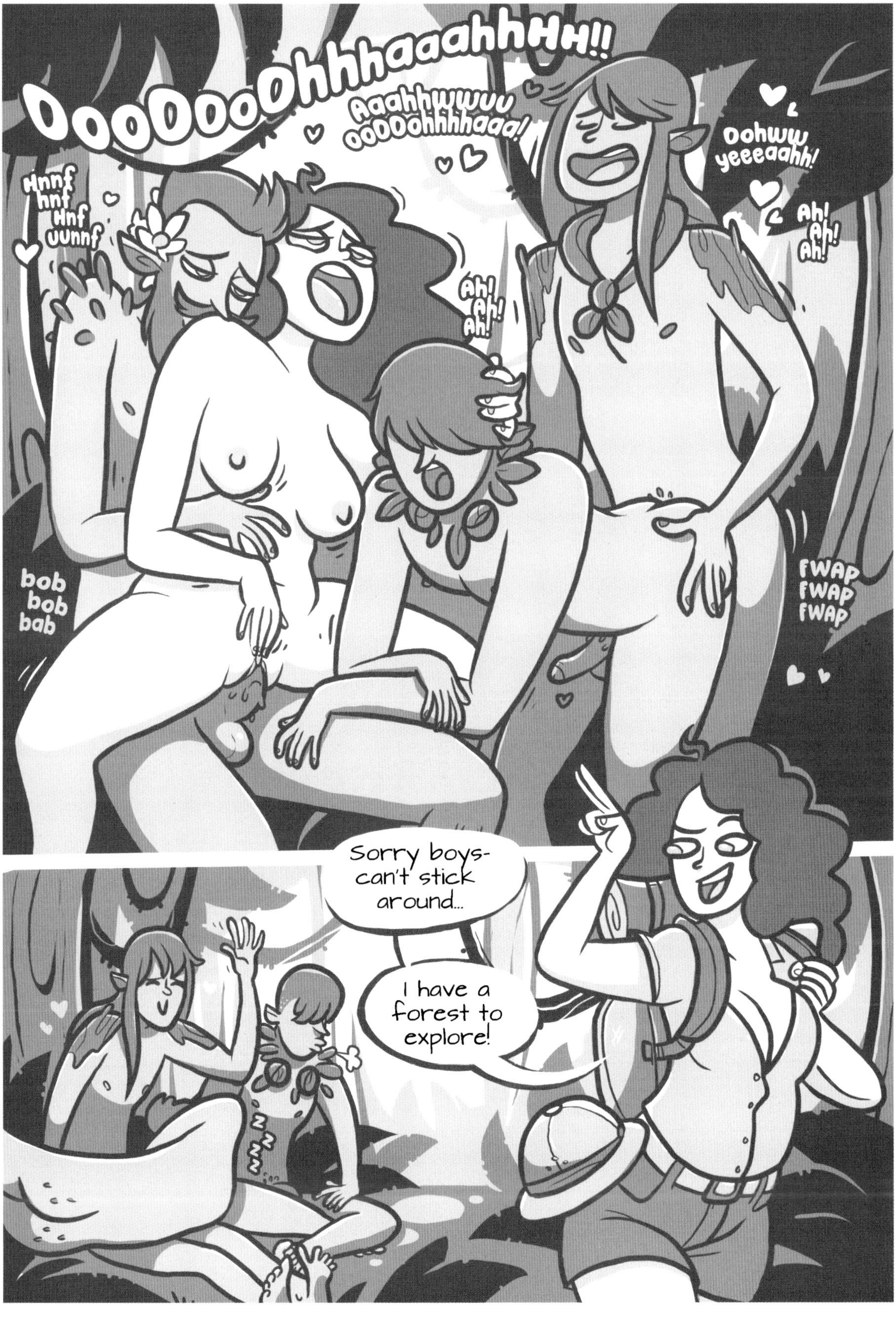
OOODOOOhhhaaahhHH!!
Aaahhwwuu ooDOohhhhaaa!
Oohww yeeeaahh!
Hnnf hnf Hnf uunnf
Ah! Ah! Ah!
Ah! Ah! Ah!
bob bob bab
FWAP FWAP FWAP
Sorry boys-can't stick around...
I have a forest to explore!
Z Z Z

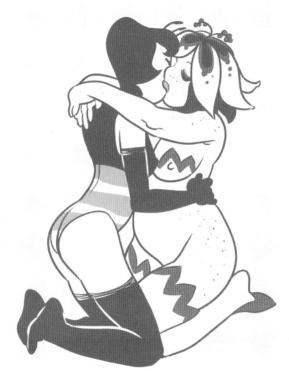

HONEY

by Ghostgreen

Ghostgreen.tumblr.com

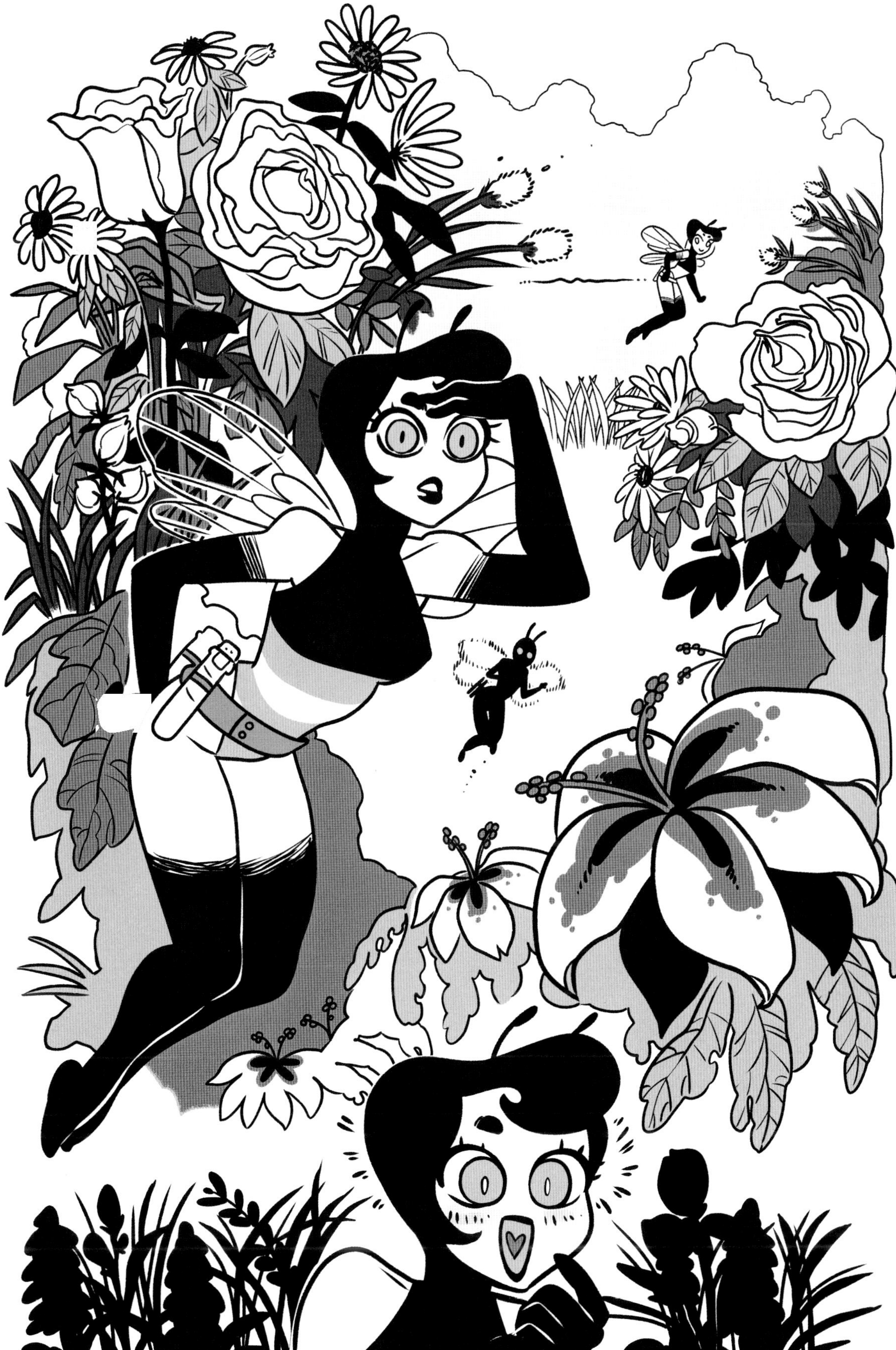

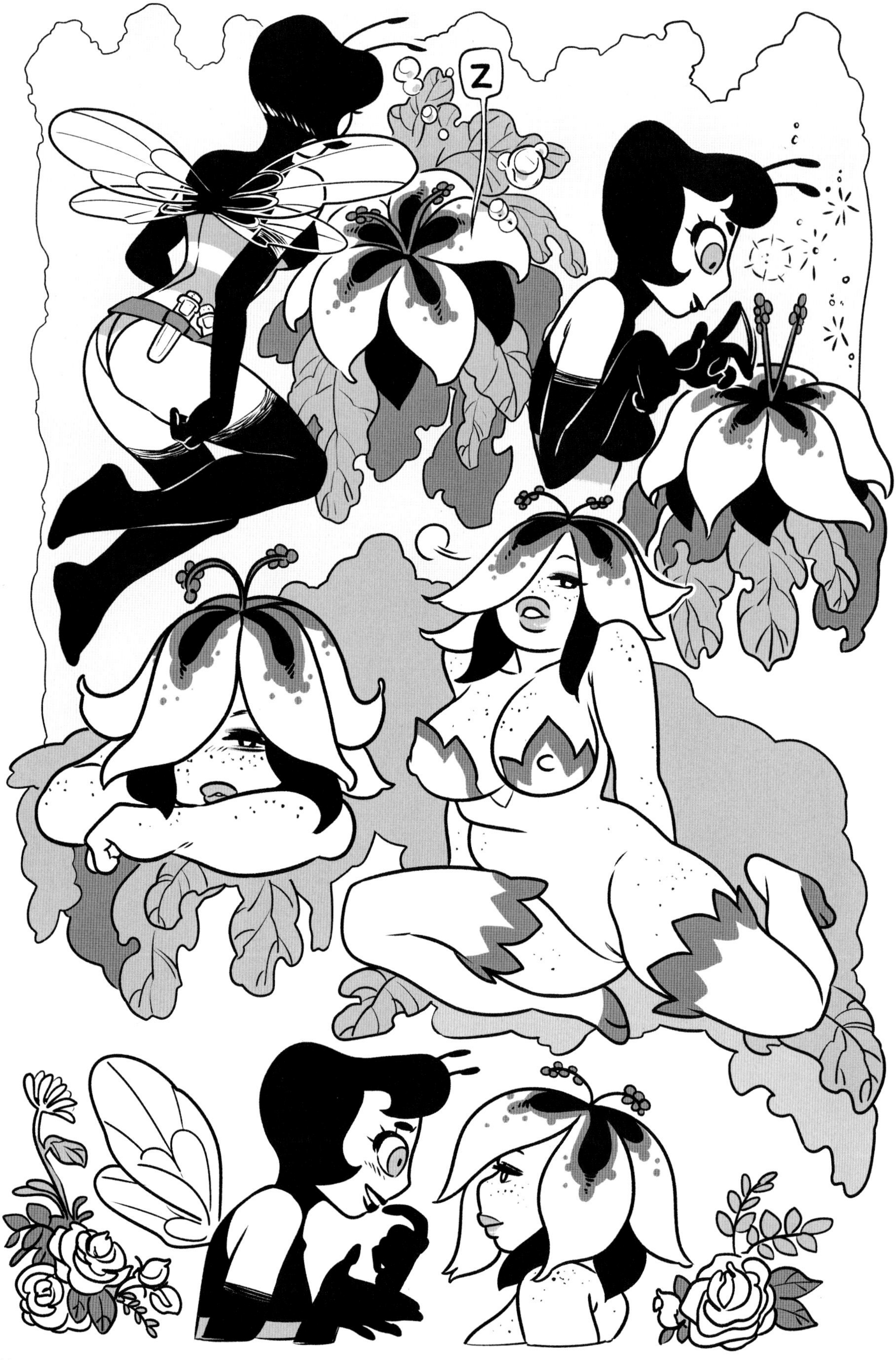
Z

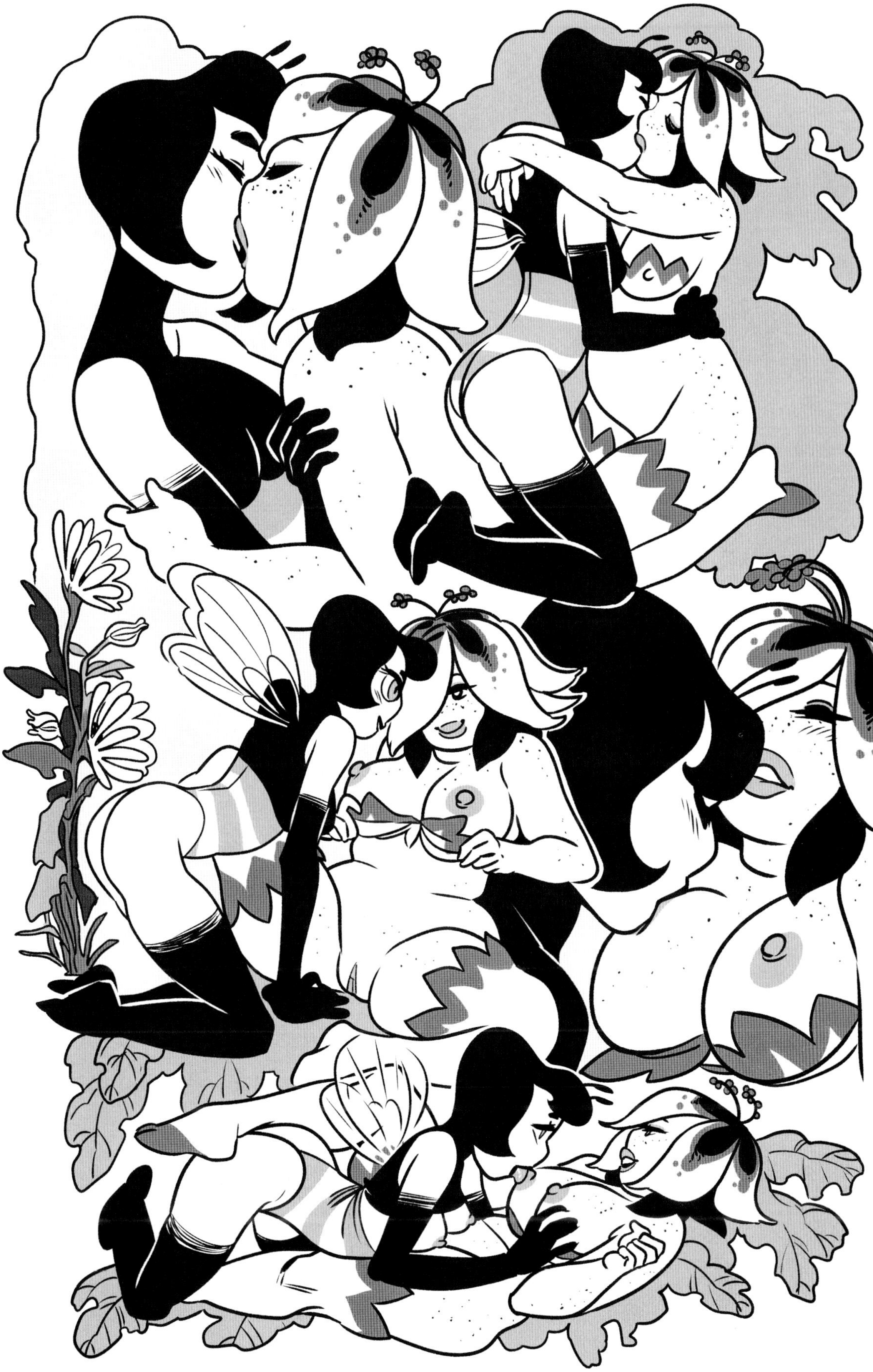

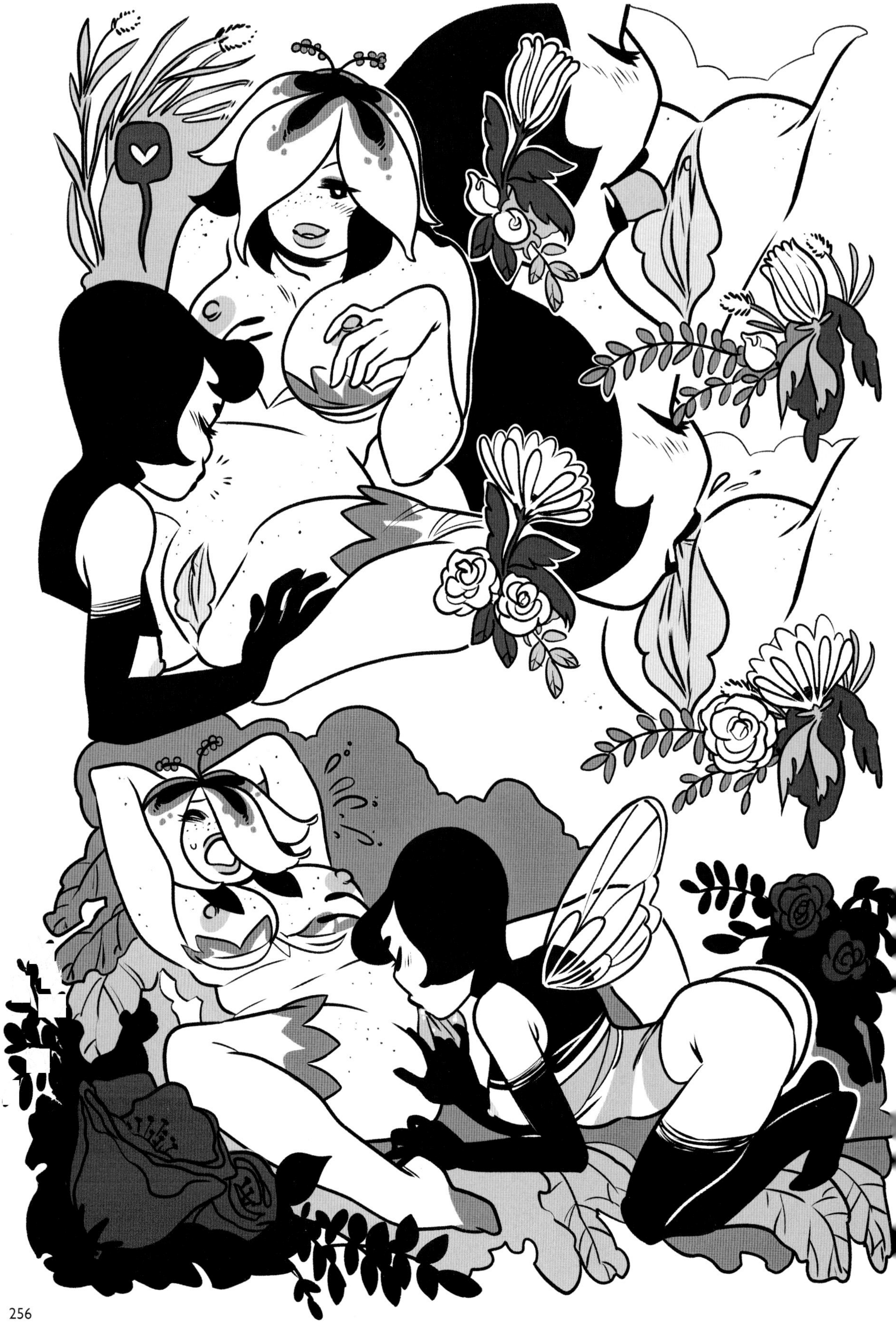

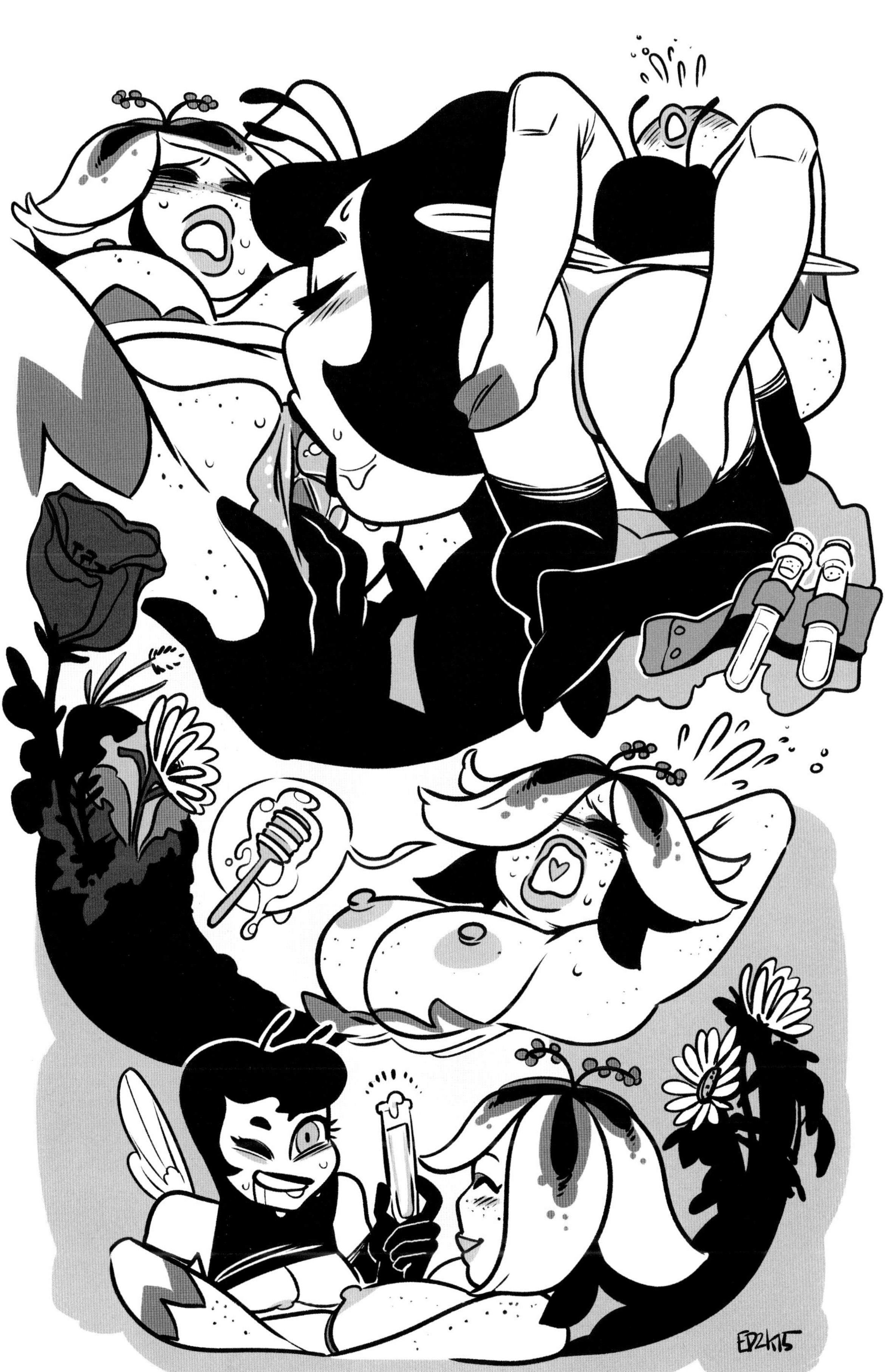
ED2K15

Grindr

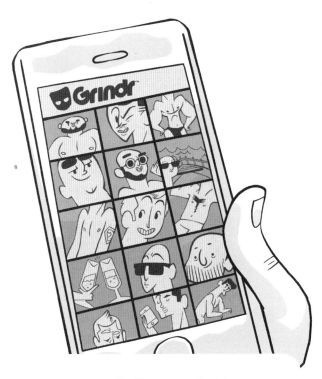

GRINDR

by Reed Black

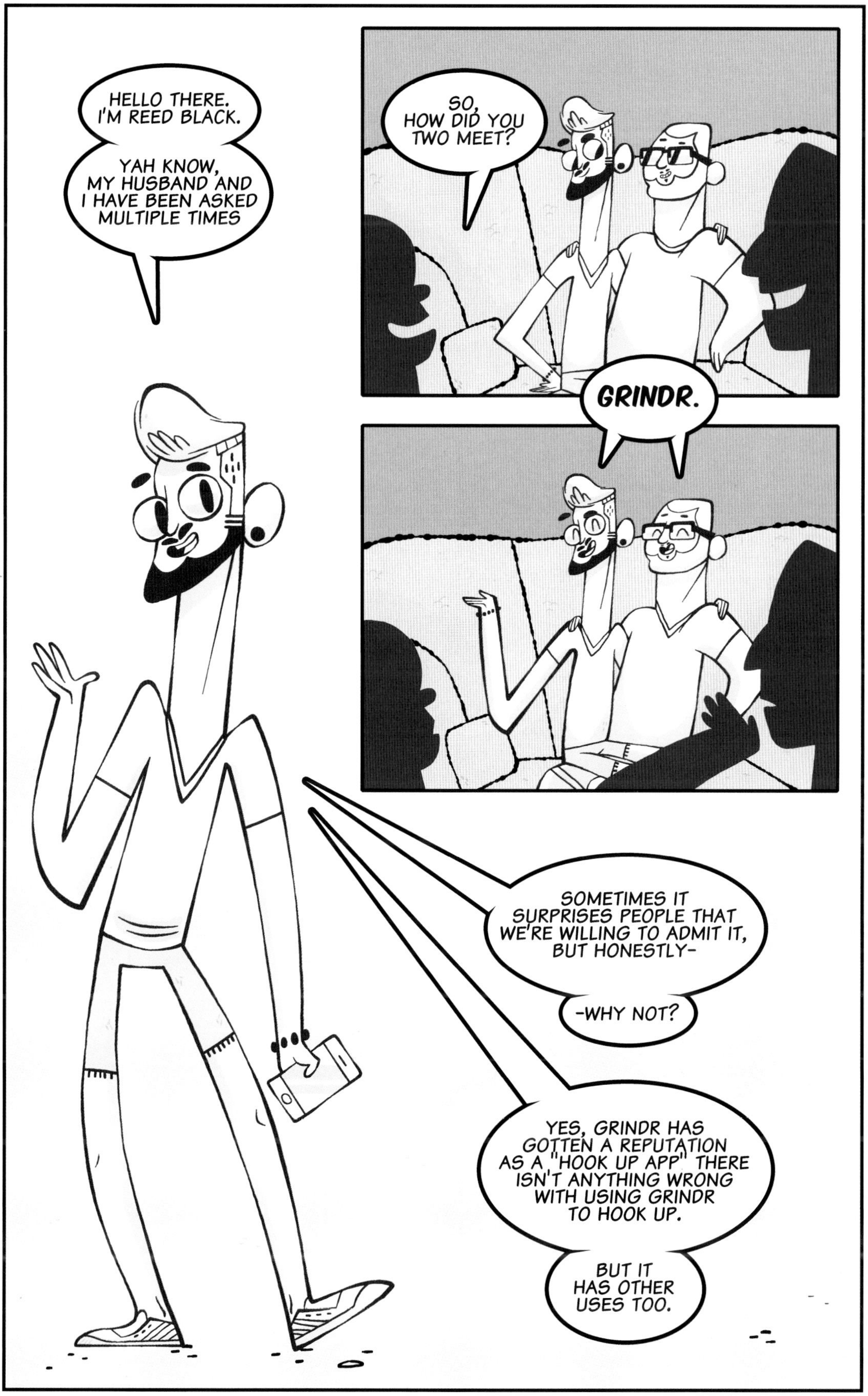
HELLO THERE. I'M REED BLACK.
YAH KNOW, MY HUSBAND AND I HAVE BEEN ASKED MULTIPLE TIMES
SO, HOW DID YOU TWO MEET?
GRINDR.
SOMETIMES IT SURPRISES PEOPLE THAT WE'RE WILLING TO ADMIT IT, BUT HONESTLY-
-WHY NOT?
YES, GRINDR HAS GOTTEN A REPUTATION AS A "HOOK UP APP" THERE ISN'T ANYTHING WRONG WITH USING GRINDR TO HOOK UP.
BUT IT HAS OTHER USES TOO.

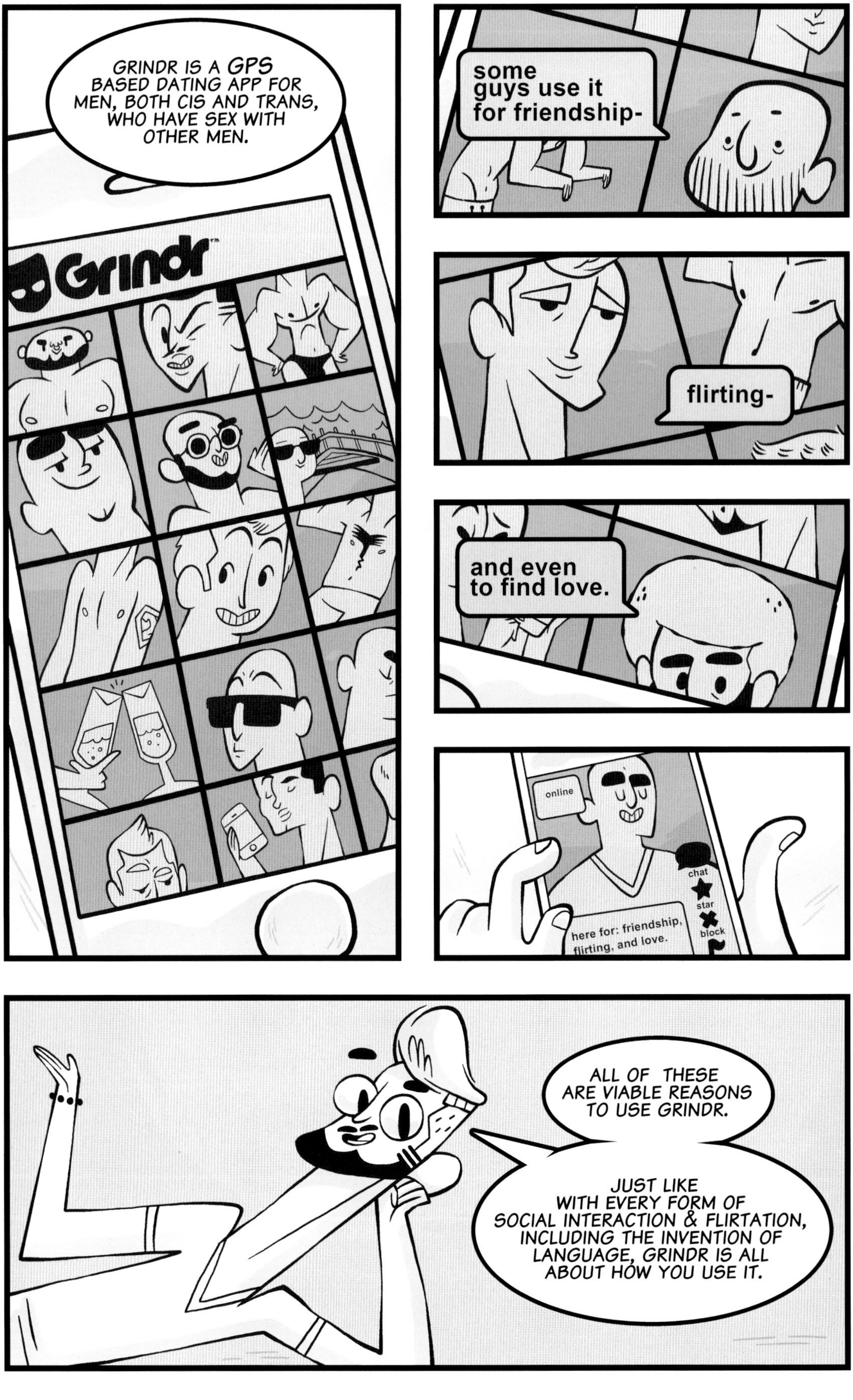
GRINDR IS A GPS BASED DATING APP FOR MEN, BOTH CIS AND TRANS, WHO HAVE SEX WITH OTHER MEN.
Grindr
some guys use it for friendship-
flirting-
and even to find love.
online
chat
star
block
here for: friendship, flirting, and love.
ALL OF THESE ARE VIABLE REASONS TO USE GRINDR.
JUST LIKE WITH EVERY FORM OF SOCIAL INTERACTION & FLIRTATION, INCLUDING THE INVENTION OF LANGUAGE, GRINDR IS ALL ABOUT HOW YOU USE IT.

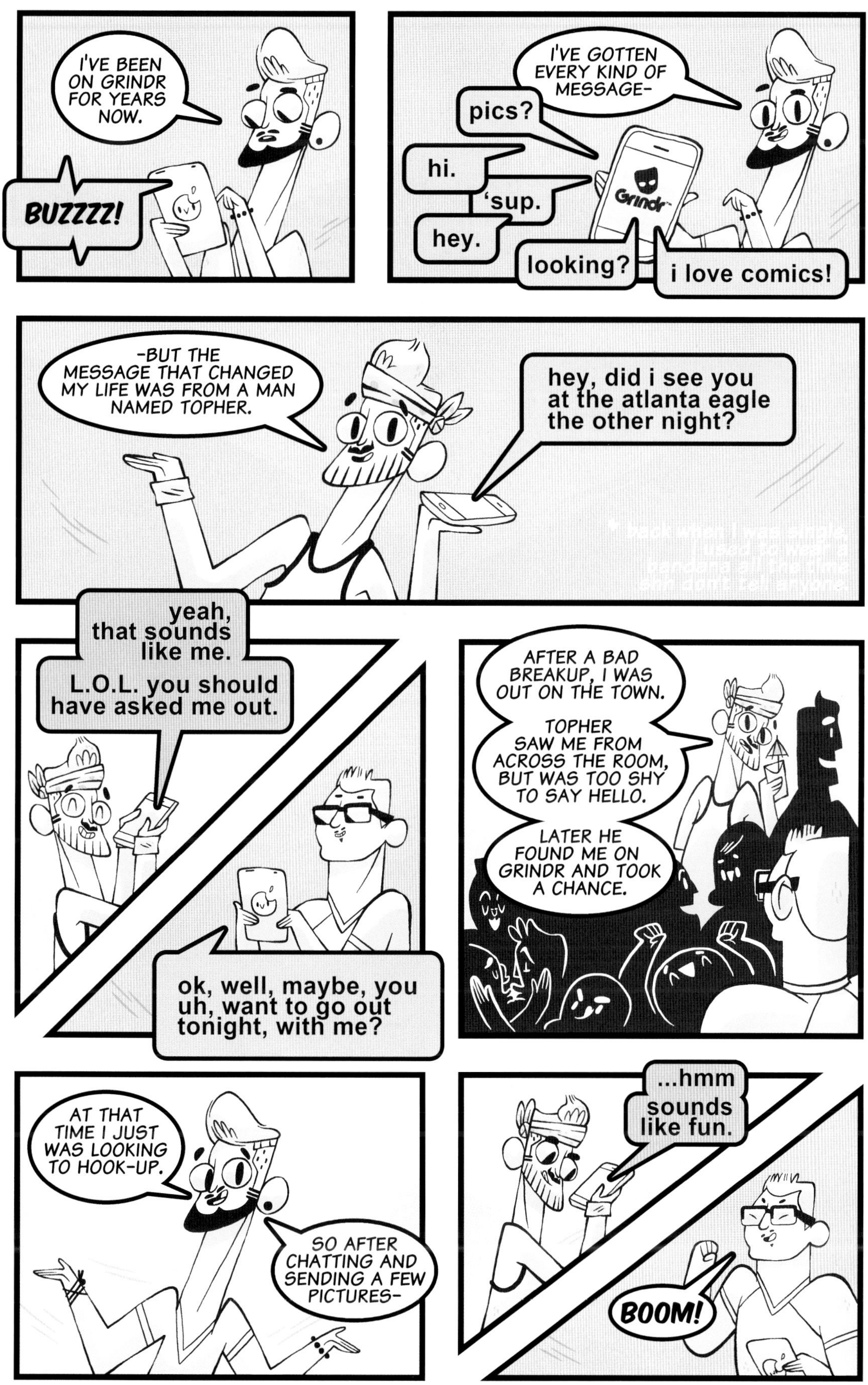
I'VE BEEN ON GRINDR FOR YEARS NOW.
BUZZZZ!
I'VE GOTTEN EVERY KIND OF MESSAGE-
pics?
hi.
'sup.
hey.
Grindr
looking?
i love comics!
-BUT THE MESSAGE THAT CHANGED MY LIFE WAS FROM A MAN NAMED TOPHER.
hey, did i see you at the atlanta eagle the other night?
yeah, that sounds like me.
L.O.L. you should have asked me out.
ok, well, maybe, you uh, want to go out tonight, with me?
AFTER A BAD BREAKUP, I WAS OUT ON THE TOWN.
TOPHER SAW ME FROM ACROSS THE ROOM, BUT WAS TOO SHY TO SAY HELLO.
LATER HE FOUND ME ON GRINDR AND TOOK A CHANCE.
AT THAT TIME I JUST WAS LOOKING TO HOOK-UP.
SO AFTER CHATTING AND SENDING A FEW PICTURES-
...hmm sounds like fun.
BOOM!

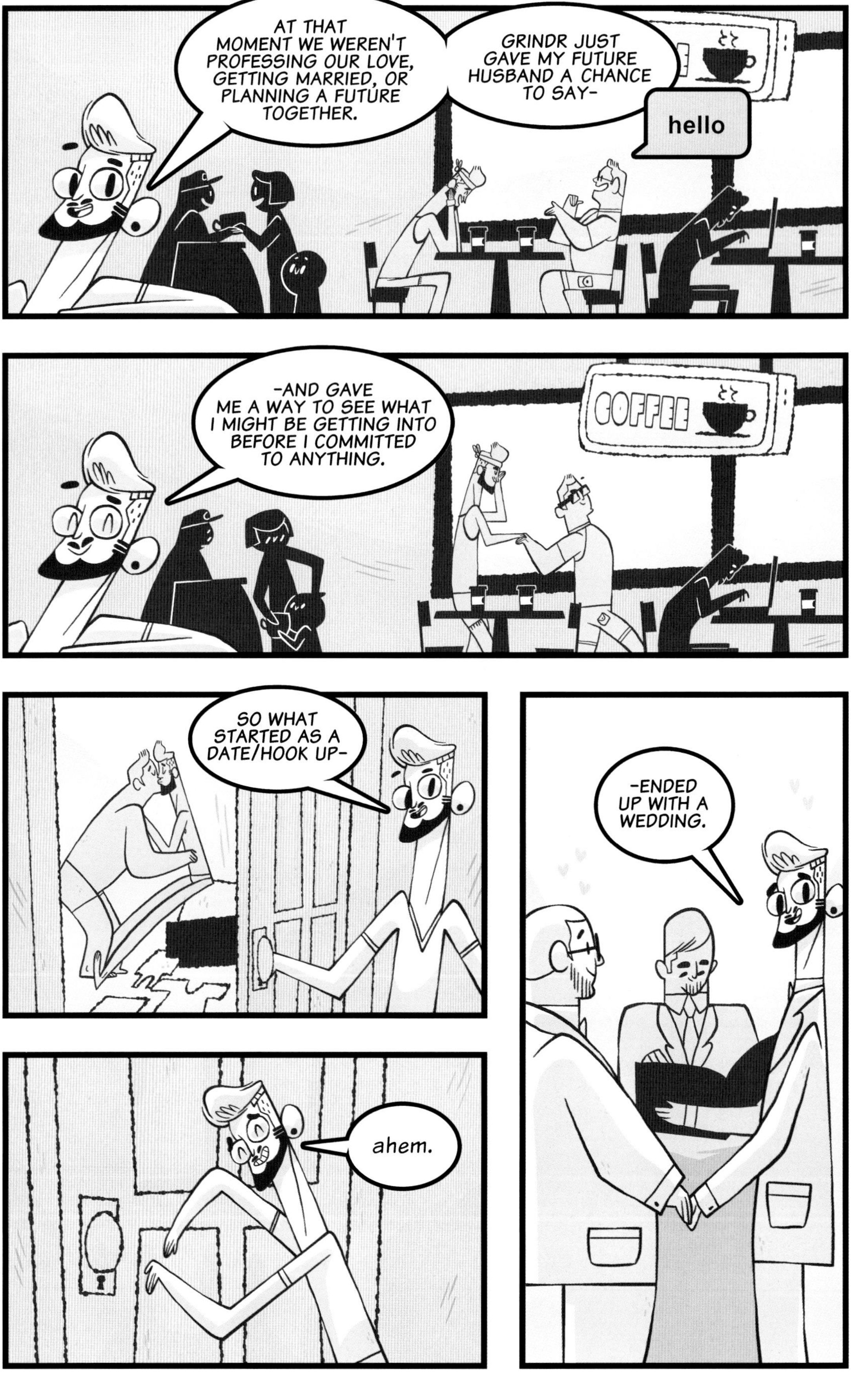
AT THAT MOMENT WE WEREN'T PROFESSING OUR LOVE, GETTING MARRIED, OR PLANNING A FUTURE TOGETHER.
GRINDR JUST GAVE MY FUTURE HUSBAND A CHANCE TO SAY-
hello
-AND GAVE ME A WAY TO SEE WHAT I MIGHT BE GETTING INTO BEFORE I COMMITTED TO ANYTHING.
COFFEE
SO WHAT STARTED AS A DATE/HOOK UP-
ahem.
-ENDED UP WITH A WEDDING.

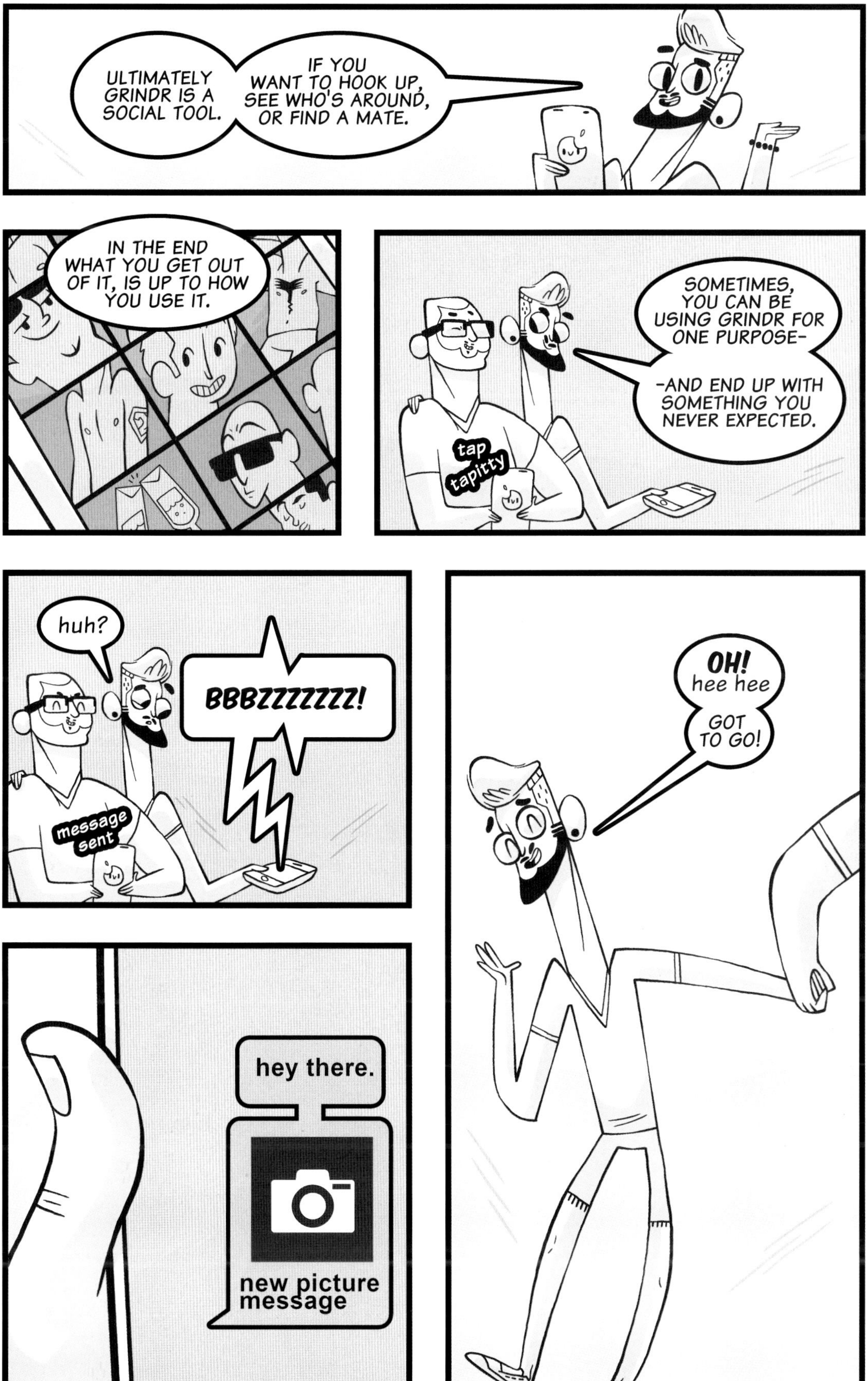
ULTIMATELY GRINDR IS A SOCIAL TOOL.
IF YOU WANT TO HOOK UP, SEE WHO'S AROUND, OR FIND A MATE.
IN THE END WHAT YOU GET OUT OF IT, IS UP TO HOW YOU USE IT.
SOMETIMES, YOU CAN BE USING GRINDR FOR ONE PURPOSE-
-AND END UP WITH SOMETHING YOU NEVER EXPECTED.
tap tapitty
huh?
BBBZZZZZZZ!
message sent
OH! hee hee
GOT TO GO!
hey there.
new picture message

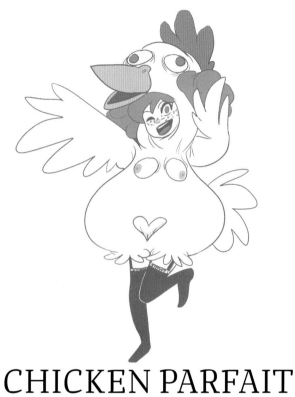

CHICKEN PARFAIT

by Eva Cabrera

Boudikacomics.com

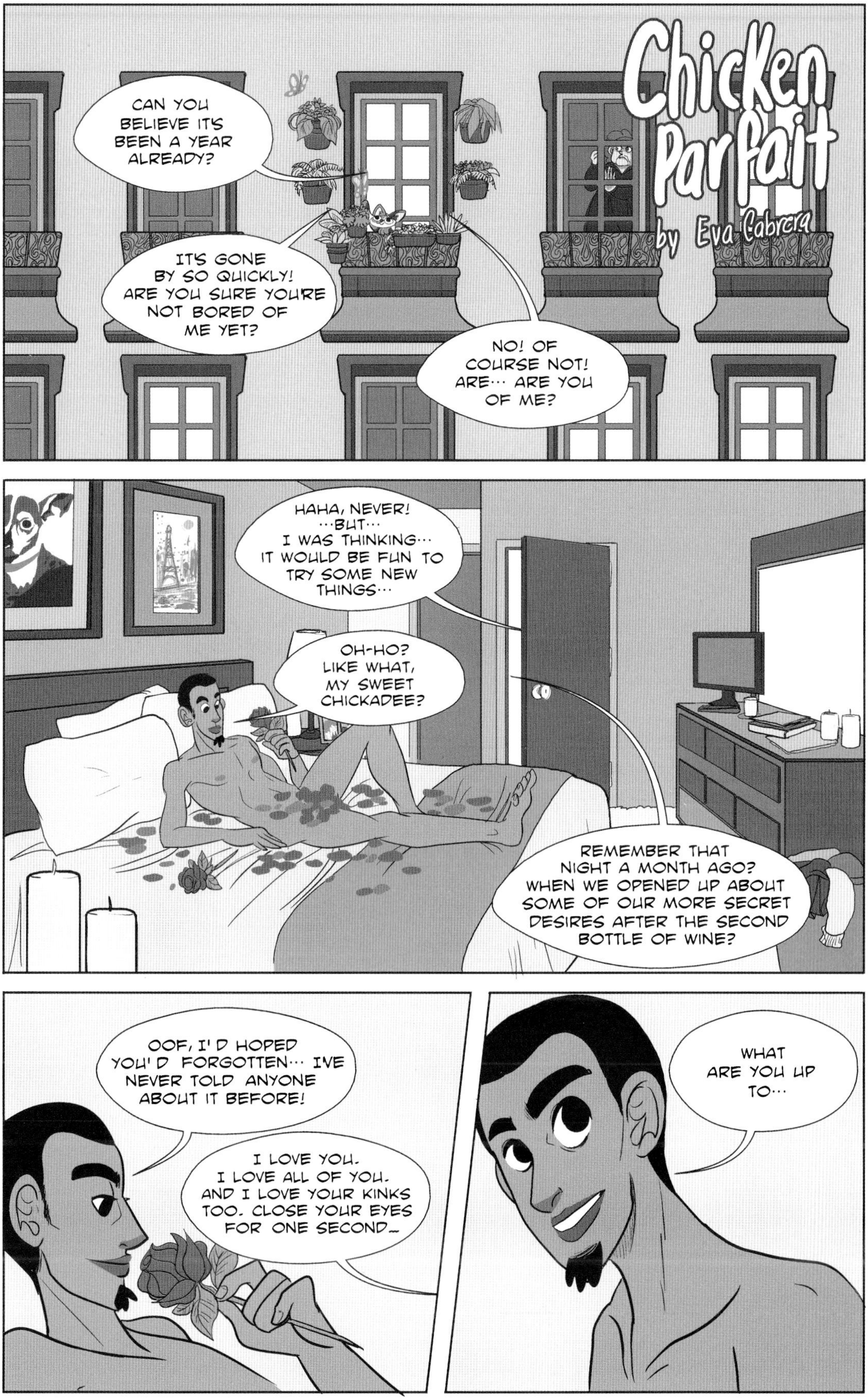
Chicken Parfait
by Eva Cabrera
CAN YOU BELIEVE IT'S BEEN A YEAR ALREADY?
IT'S GONE BY SO QUICKLY! ARE YOU SURE YOU'RE NOT BORED OF ME YET?
NO! OF COURSE NOT! ARE… ARE YOU OF ME?
HAHA, NEVER! …BUT… I WAS THINKING… IT WOULD BE FUN TO TRY SOME NEW THINGS…
OH-HO? LIKE WHAT, MY SWEET CHICKADEE?
REMEMBER THAT NIGHT A MONTH AGO? WHEN WE OPENED UP ABOUT SOME OF OUR MORE SECRET DESIRES AFTER THE SECOND BOTTLE OF WINE?
OOF, I'D HOPED YOU'D FORGOTTEN… I'VE NEVER TOLD ANYONE ABOUT IT BEFORE!
I LOVE YOU. I LOVE ALL OF YOU. AND I LOVE YOUR KINKS TOO. CLOSE YOUR EYES FOR ONE SECOND…
WHAT ARE YOU UP TO…

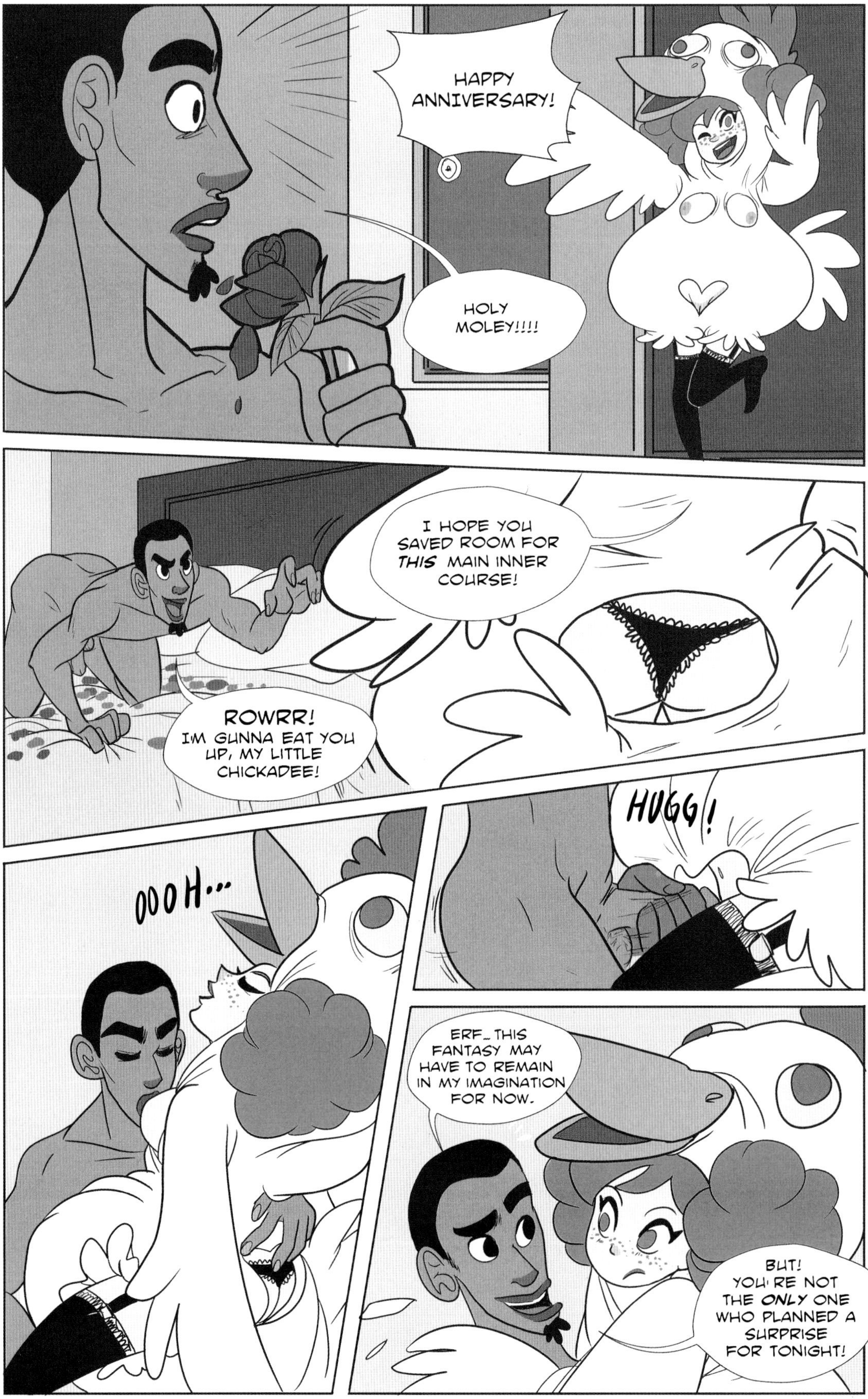
HAPPY ANNIVERSARY!
HOLY MOLEY!!!!
I HOPE YOU SAVED ROOM FOR THIS MAIN INNER COURSE!
ROWRR! I'M GUNNA EAT YOU UP, MY LITTLE CHICKADEE!
HUGG!
OOOH...
ERF_ THIS FANTASY MAY HAVE TO REMAIN IN MY IMAGINATION FOR NOW.
BUT! YOU'RE NOT THE ONLY ONE WHO PLANNED A SURPRISE FOR TONIGHT!

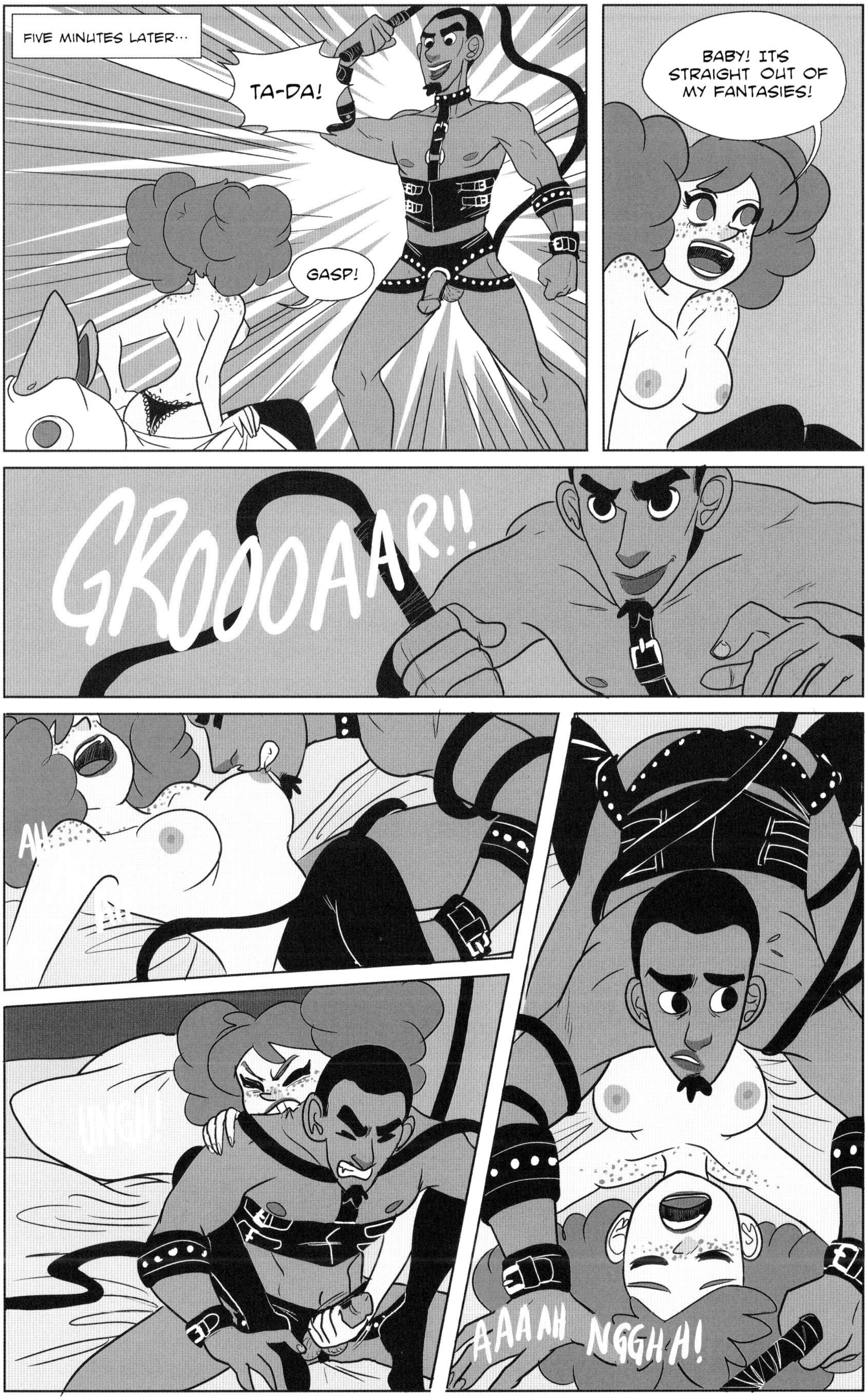
FIVE MINUTES LATER…
TA-DA!
GASP!
BABY! ITS STRAIGHT OUT OF MY FANTASIES!
GROOOAAR!!
AH
UNGH!
AAAAH NGGHAH!

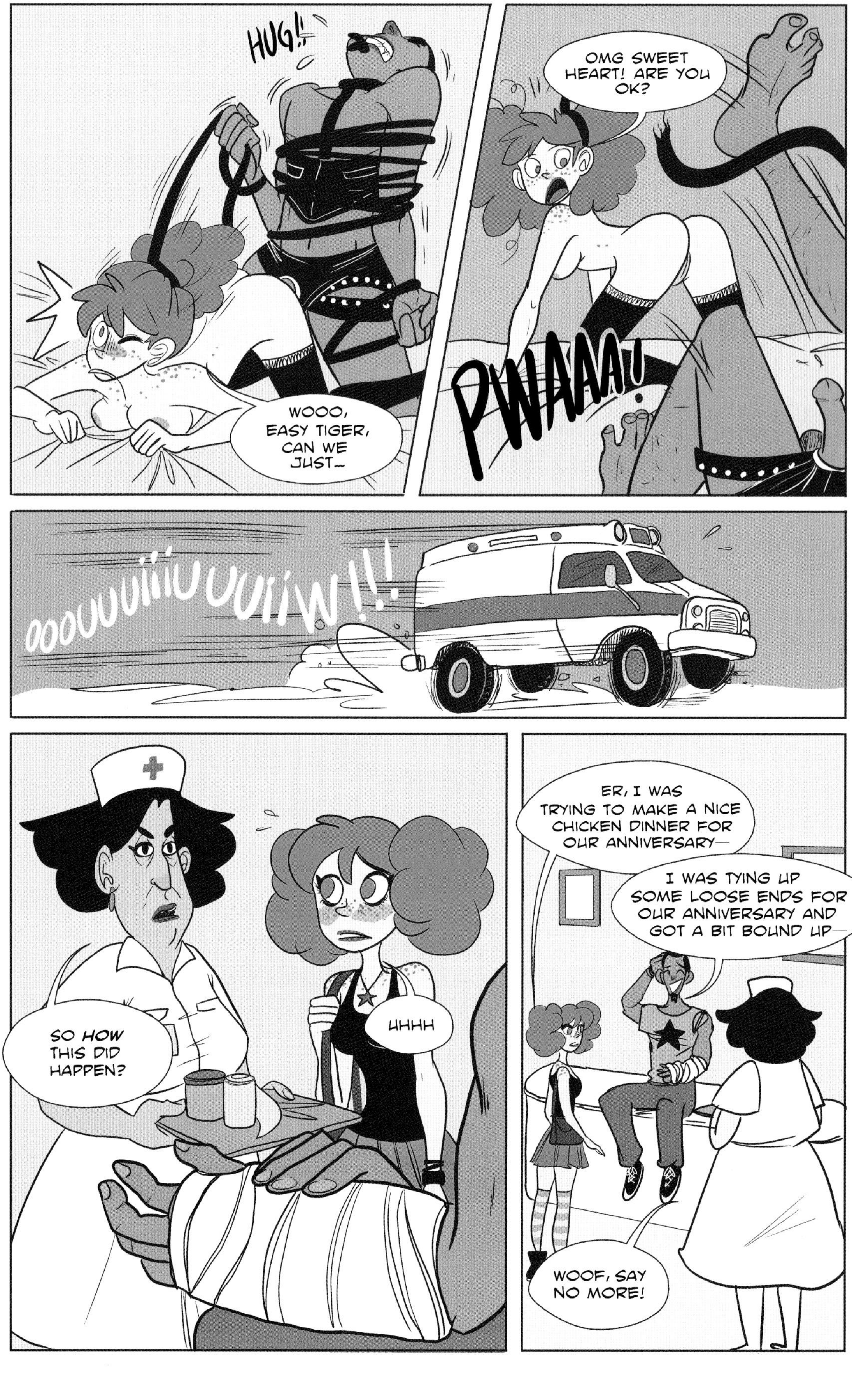
HUG!!
WOOO, EASY TIGER, CAN WE JUST—
OMG SWEET HEART! ARE YOU OK?
PWAAAA!
OOOUUUIIIUUUIIW!!!
SO HOW THIS DID HAPPEN?
UHHH
ER, I WAS TRYING TO MAKE A NICE CHICKEN DINNER FOR OUR ANNIVERSARY—
I WAS TYING UP SOME LOOSE ENDS FOR OUR ANNIVERSARY AND GOT A BIT BOUND UP—
WOOF, SAY NO MORE!

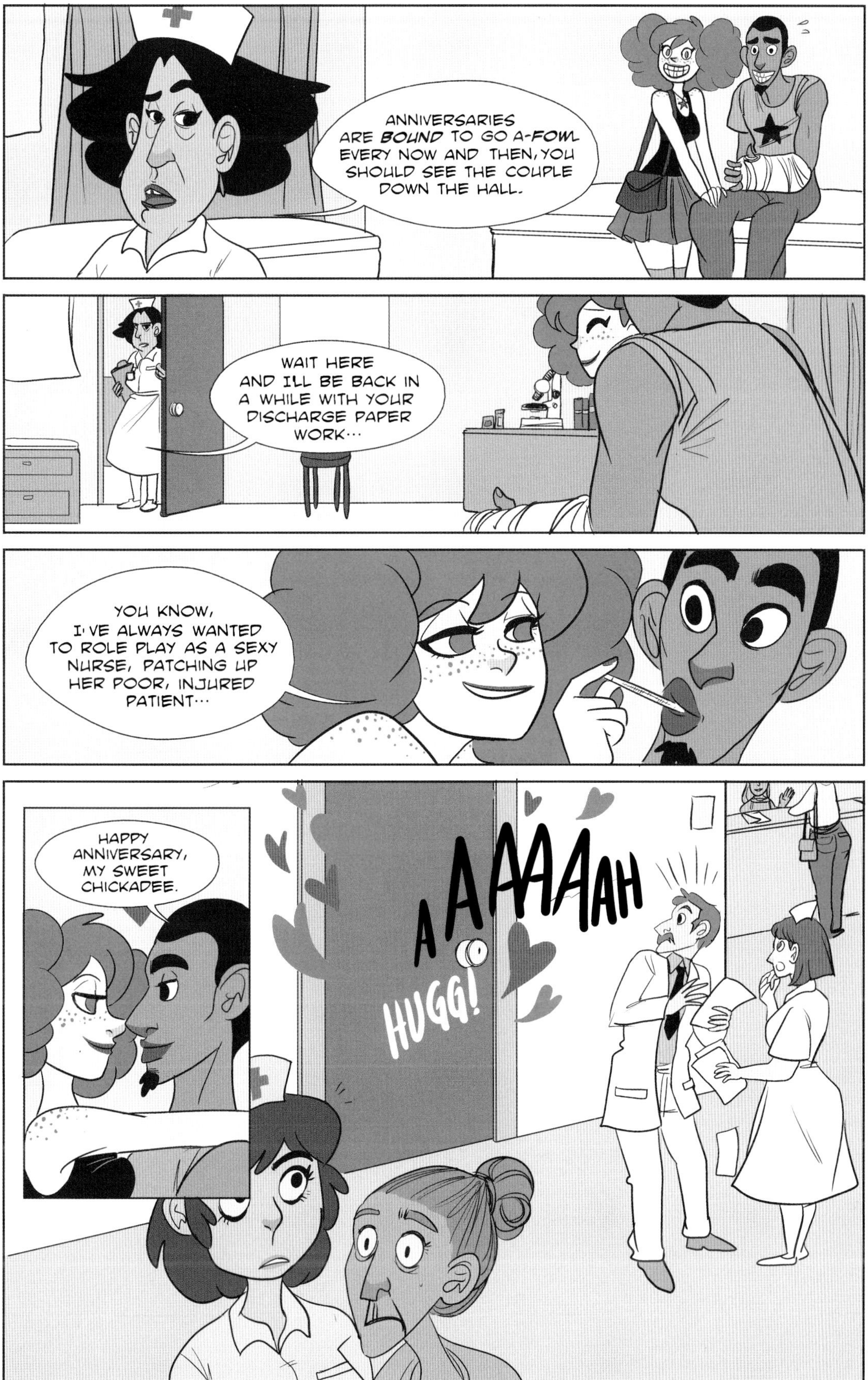
ANNIVERSARIES ARE BOUND TO GO A-FOWL EVERY NOW AND THEN, YOU SHOULD SEE THE COUPLE DOWN THE HALL.
WAIT HERE AND I'LL BE BACK IN A WHILE WITH YOUR DISCHARGE PAPER WORK...
YOU KNOW, I'VE ALWAYS WANTED TO ROLE PLAY AS A SEXY NURSE, PATCHING UP HER POOR, INJURED PATIENT...
HAPPY ANNIVERSARY, MY SWEET CHICKADEE.
AAAAAAH
HUGG!

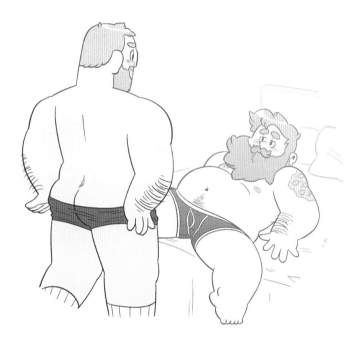

PERFORMANCE ANXIETY

by Drew Green

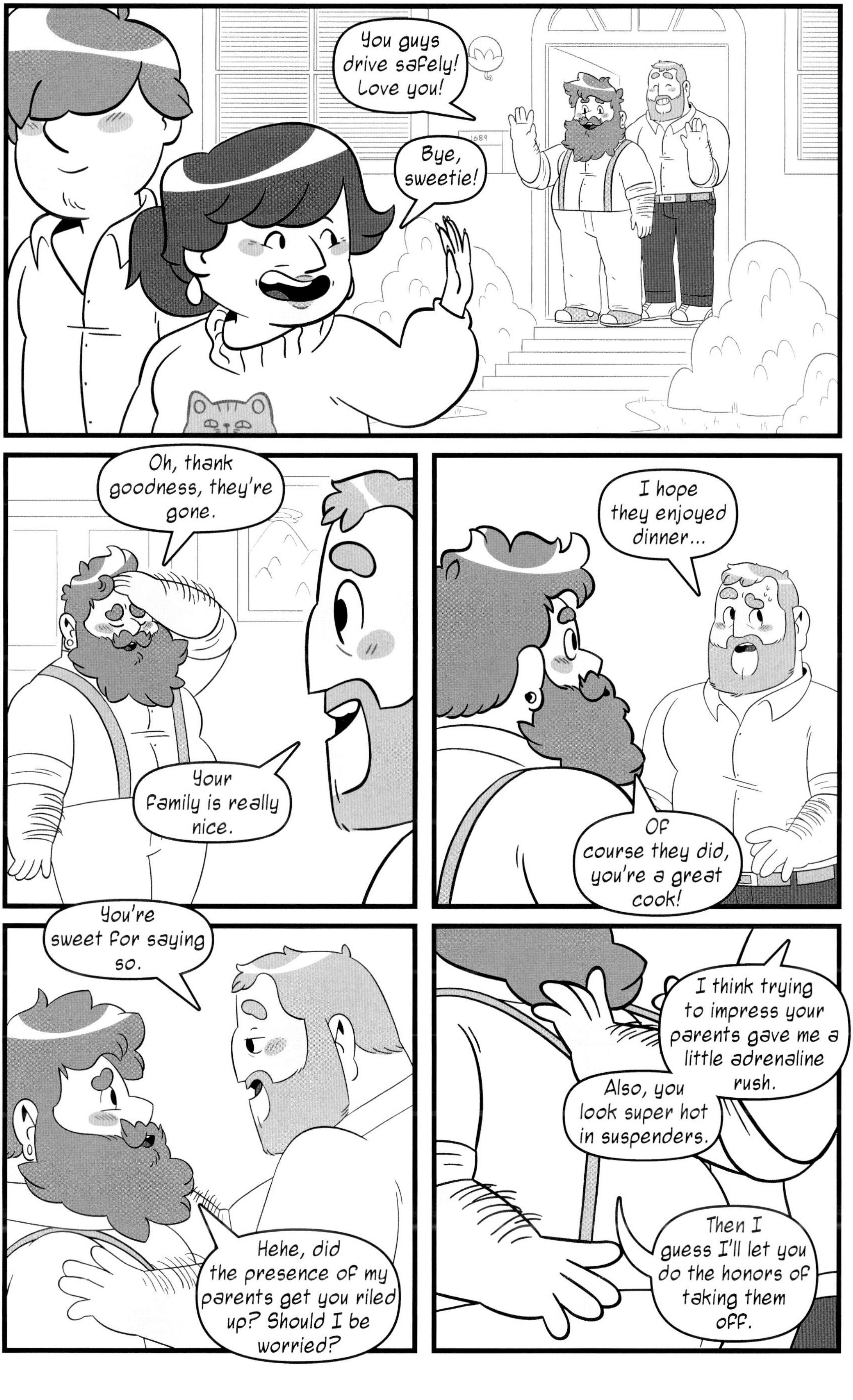

You guys drive safely! Love you!
Bye, sweetie!
1689
Oh, thank goodness, they're gone.
Your family is really nice.
I hope they enjoyed dinner...
Of course they did, you're a great cook!
You're sweet for saying so.
Hehe, did the presence of my parents get you riled up? Should I be worried?
I think trying to impress your parents gave me a little adrenaline rush.
Also, you look super hot in suspenders.
Then I guess I'll let you do the honors of taking them off.

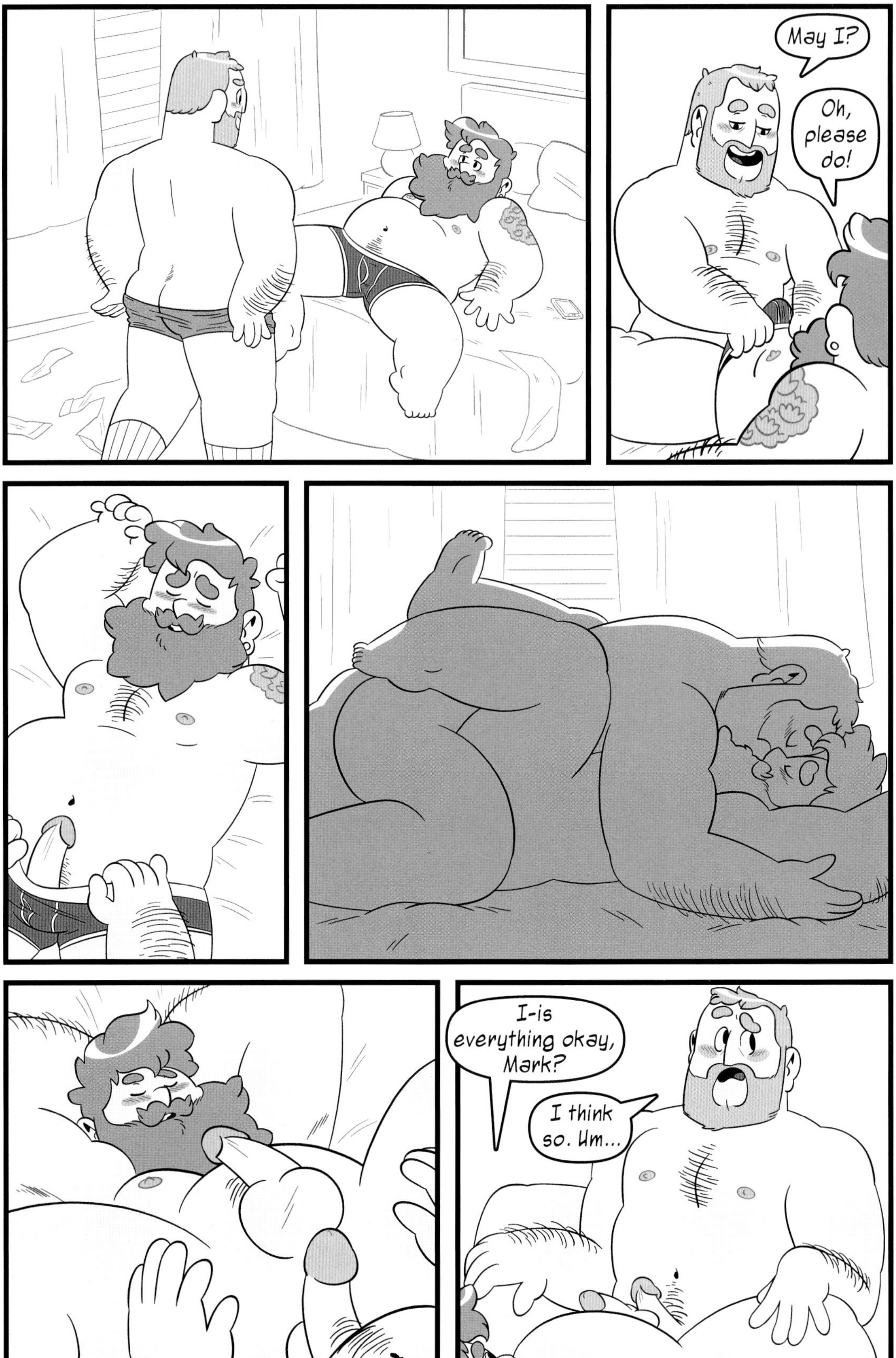
May I?
Oh, please do!
I-is everything okay, Mark?
I think so. Um...

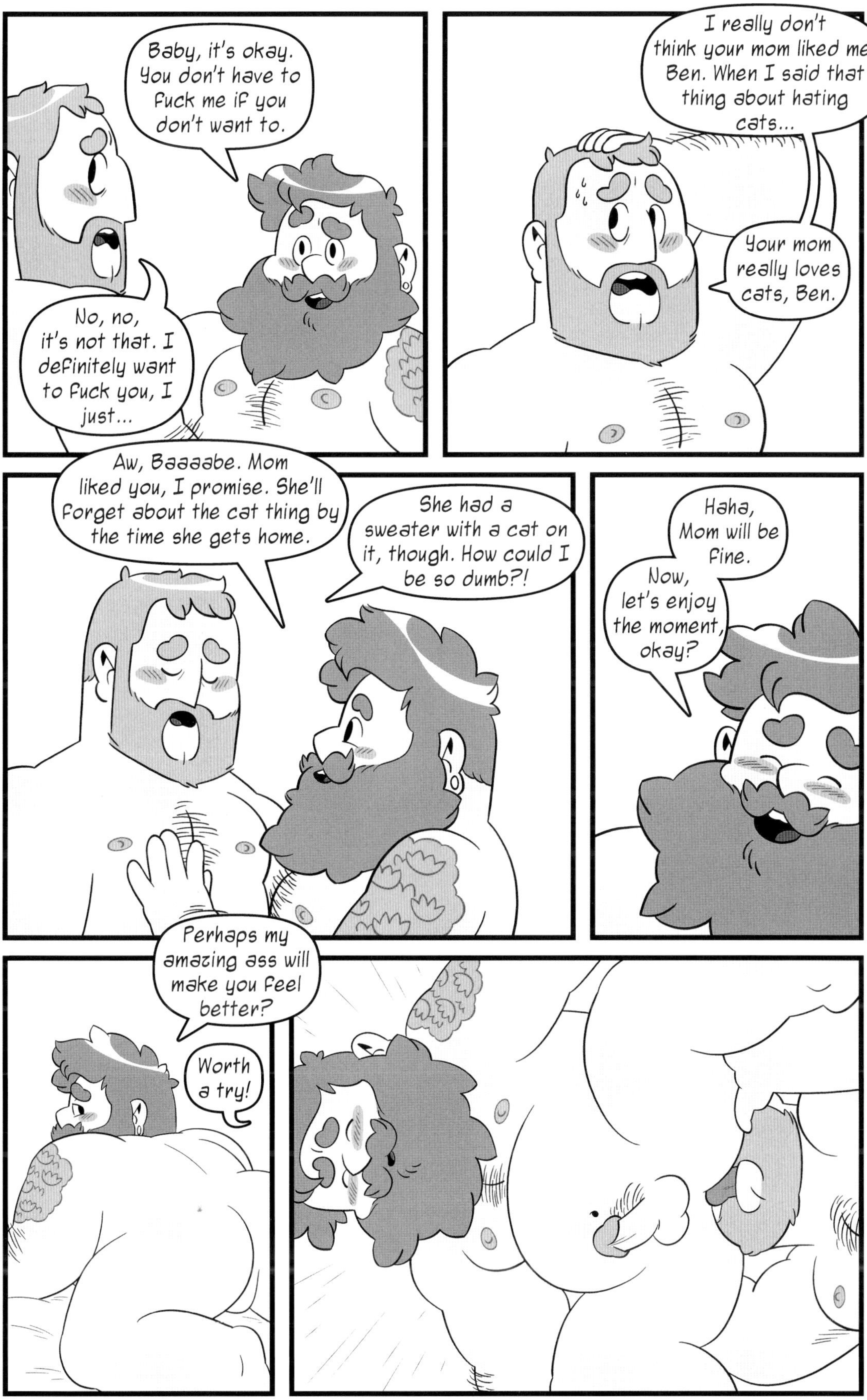
Baby, it's okay. You don't have to fuck me if you don't want to.
No, no, it's not that. I definitely want to fuck you, I just...
I really don't think your mom liked me, Ben. When I said that thing about hating cats...
Your mom really loves cats, Ben.
Aw, Baaaabe. Mom liked you, I promise. She'll forget about the cat thing by the time she gets home.
She had a sweater with a cat on it, though. How could I be so dumb?!
Haha, Mom will be fine.
Now, let's enjoy the moment, okay?
Perhaps my amazing ass will make you feel better?
Worth a try!

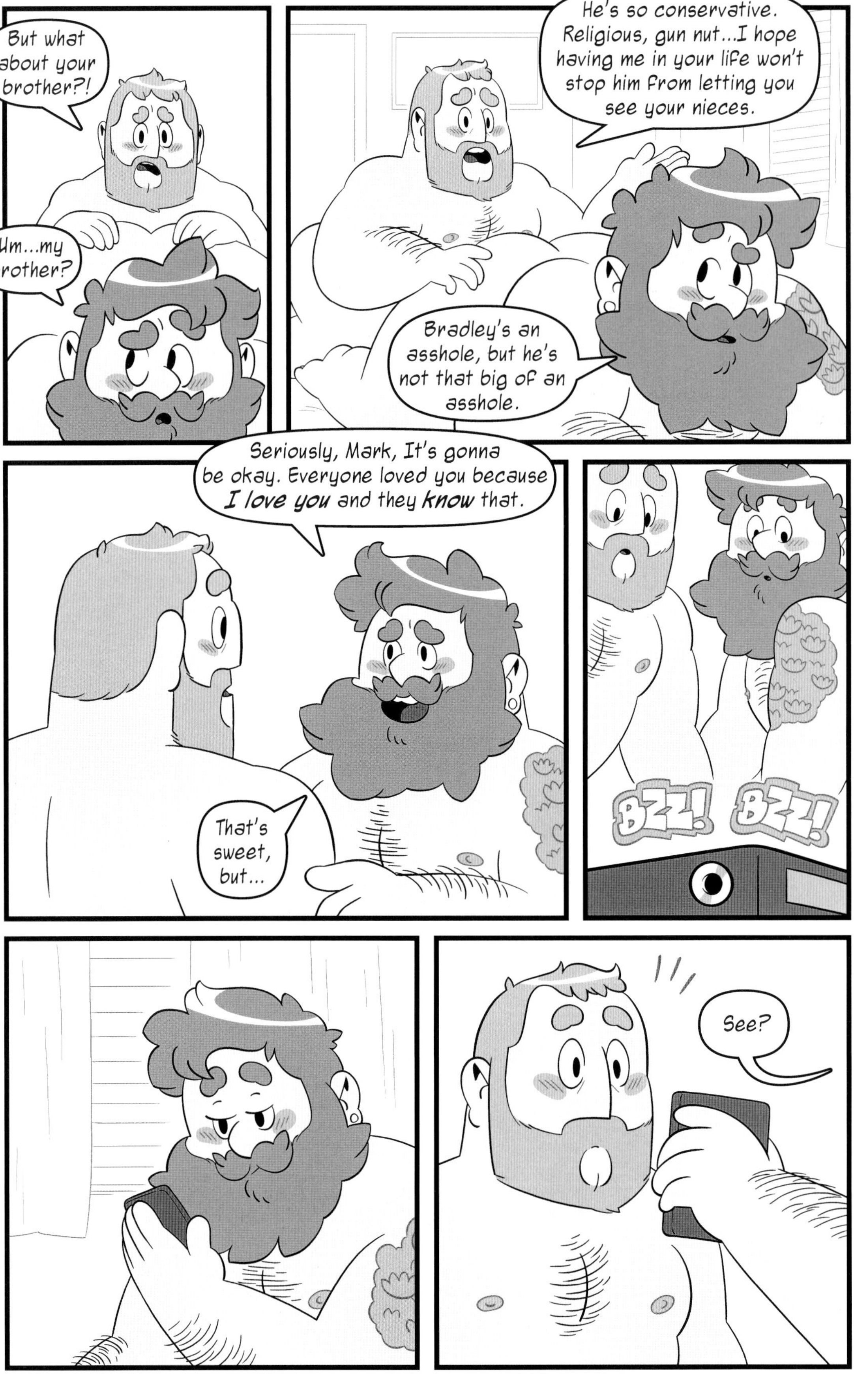
But what about your brother?!
Um...my brother?
He's so conservative. Religious, gun nut...I hope having me in your life won't stop him from letting you see your nieces.
Bradley's an asshole, but he's not that big of an asshole.
Seriously, Mark, It's gonna be okay. Everyone loved you because *I love you* and they *know* that.
That's sweet, but...
BZZ! BZZ!
See?

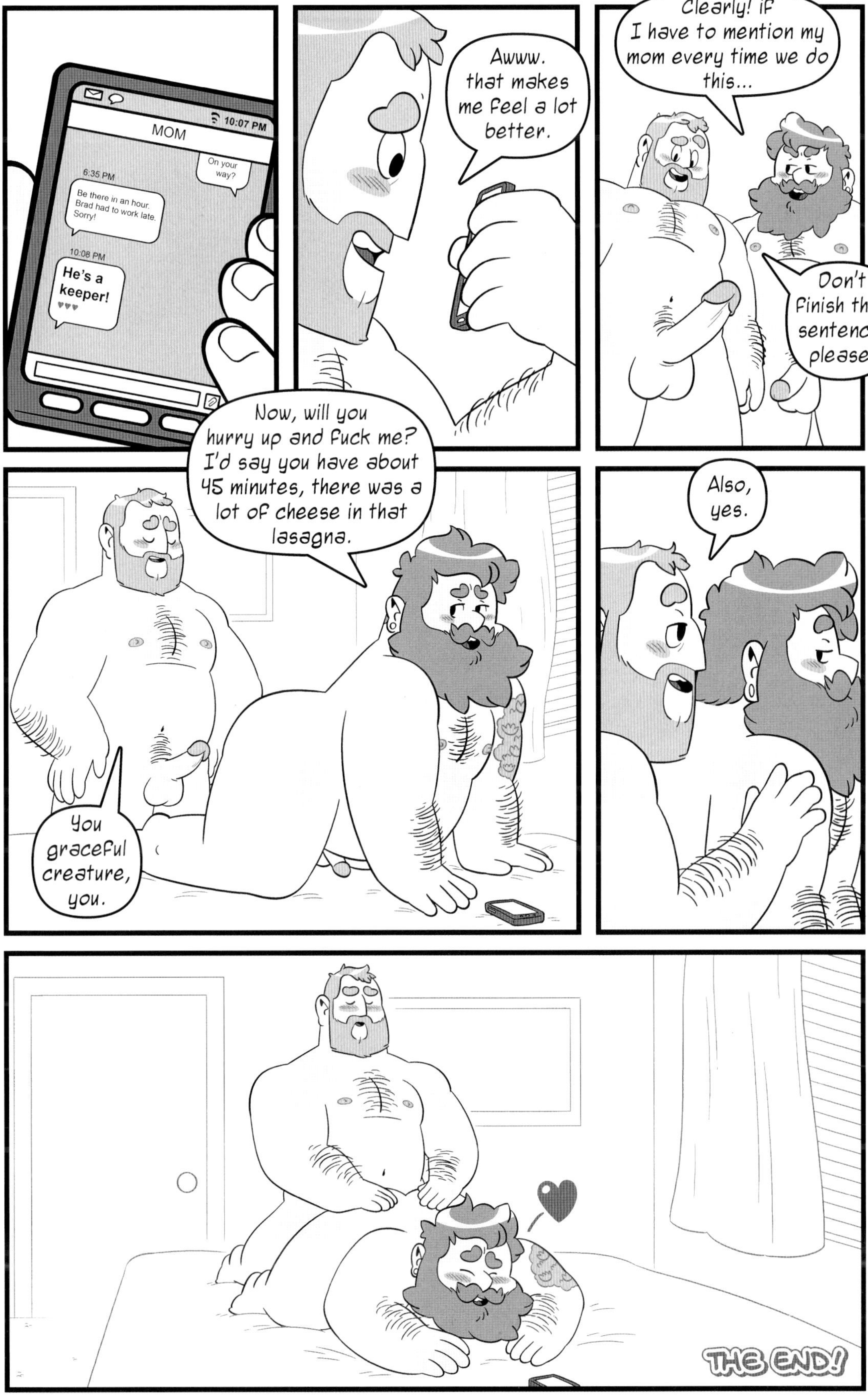
MOM
10:07 PM
On your way?
6:35 PM
Be there in an hour. Brad had to work late. Sorry!
10:08 PM
He's a keeper!
Awww. that makes me feel a lot better.
Clearly! if I have to mention my mom every time we do this...
Don't finish that sentence, please.
Now, will you hurry up and fuck me? I'd say you have about 45 minutes, there was a lot of cheese in that lasagna.
You graceful creature, you.
Also, yes.
THE END!

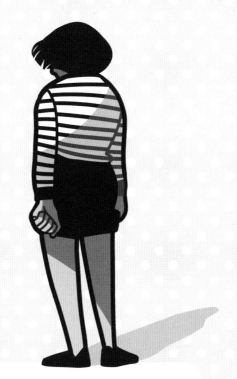

ACE

by Kiku H

Geniusbee.tumblr.com

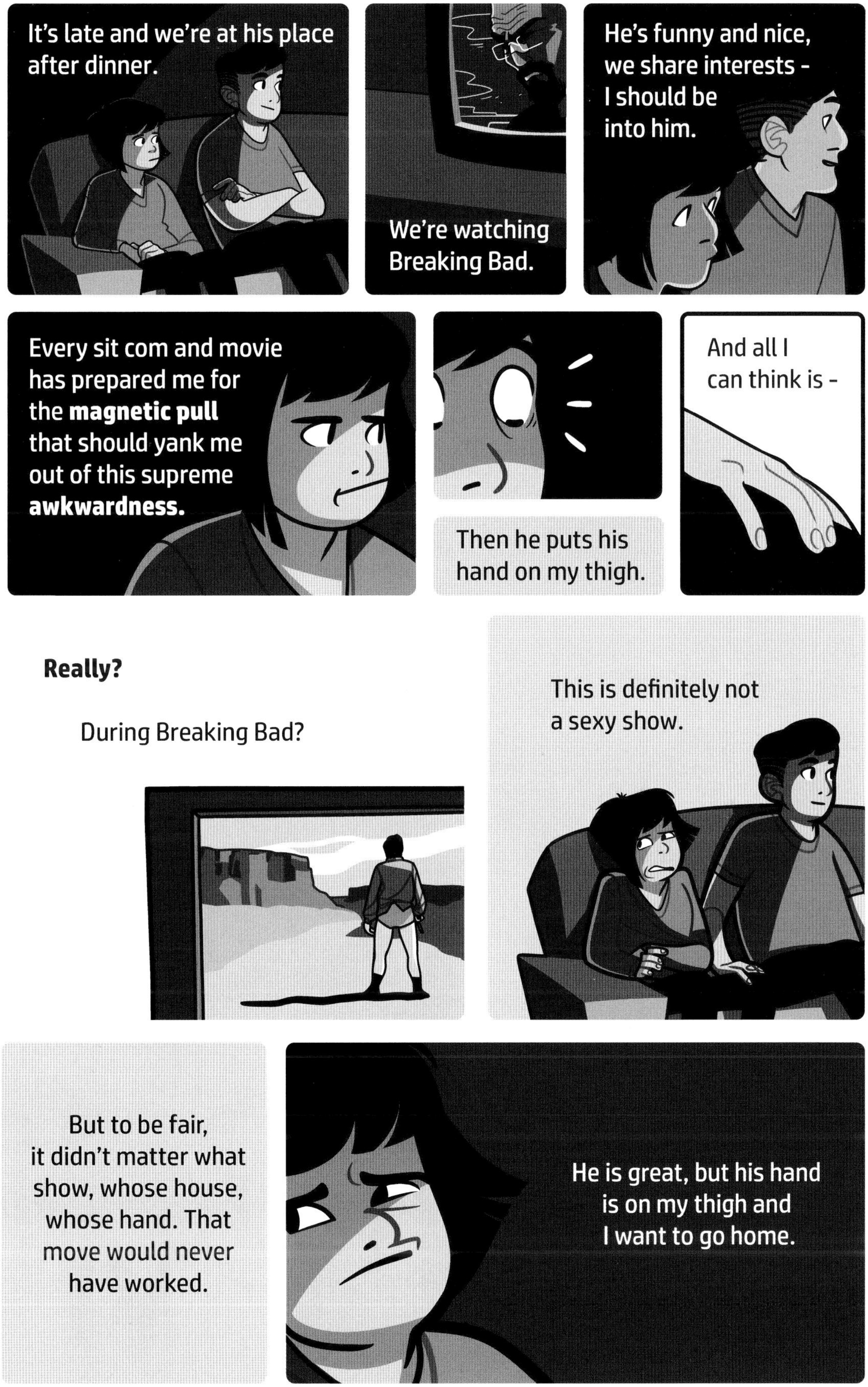
It's late and we're at his place after dinner.
We're watching Breaking Bad.
He's funny and nice, we share interests - I should be into him.
Every sit com and movie has prepared me for the **magnetic pull** that should yank me out of this supreme **awkwardness.**
Then he puts his hand on my thigh.
And all I can think is -
Really?
During Breaking Bad?
This is definitely not a sexy show.
But to be fair, it didn't matter what show, whose house, whose hand. That move would never have worked.
He is great, but his hand is on my thigh and I want to go home.

ASEXUALITY!

(People identify as Ace for short)!

I spent most of my life unaware that this word existed. Sex was not something I thought about much, but when I did it was with a sense of distant inevitability. Sex was normal, maybe even vital. Reading about asexuality finally gave a name to my experiences, but it wasn't a relief. It terrified me.

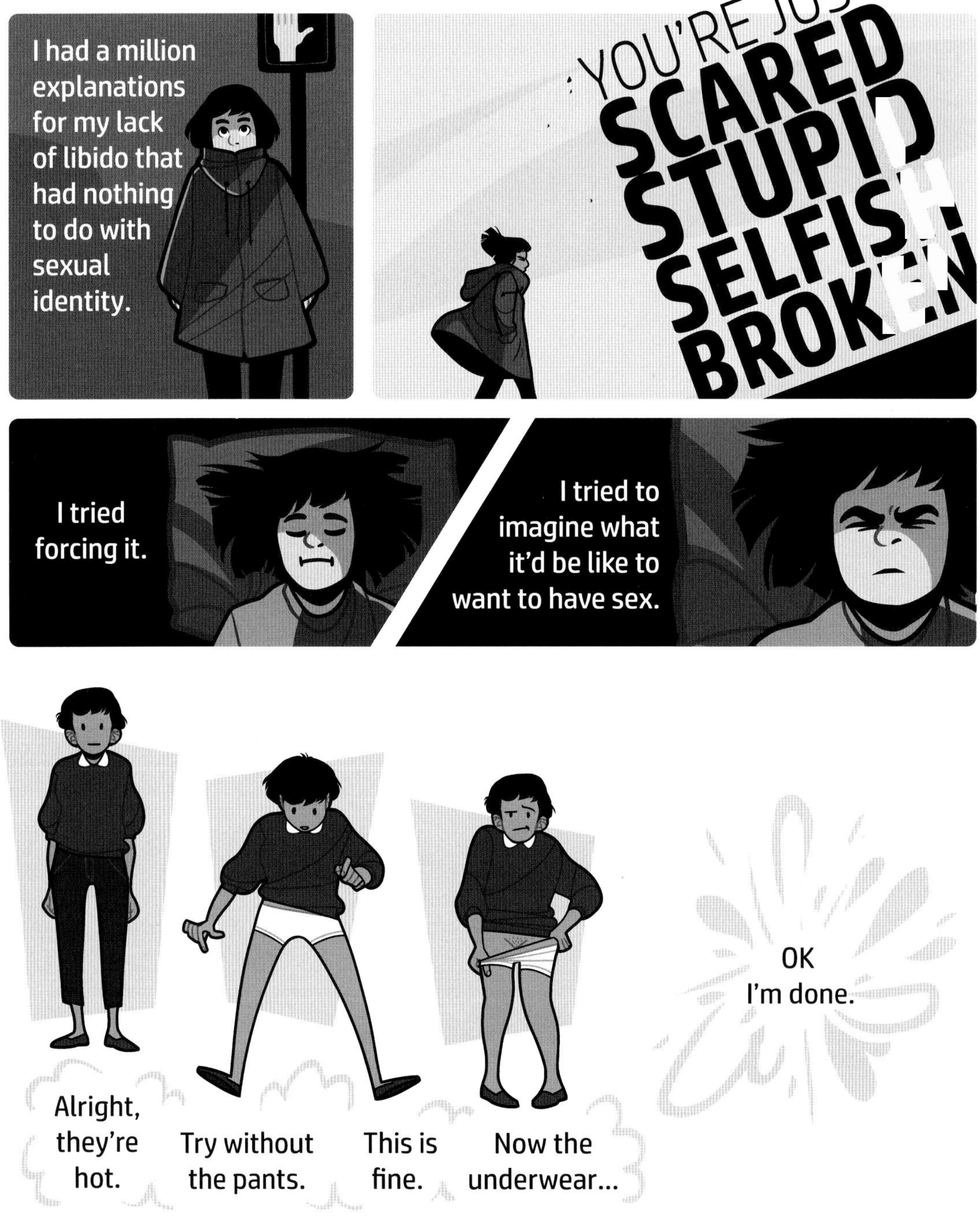

I had a million explanations for my lack of libido that had nothing to do with sexual identity.
YOU'RE JUST
SCARED
STUPID
SELFISH
BROKEN
I tried forcing it.
I tried to imagine what it'd be like to want to have sex.
Alright, they're hot.
Try without the pants.
This is fine.
Now the underwear...
OK
I'm done.

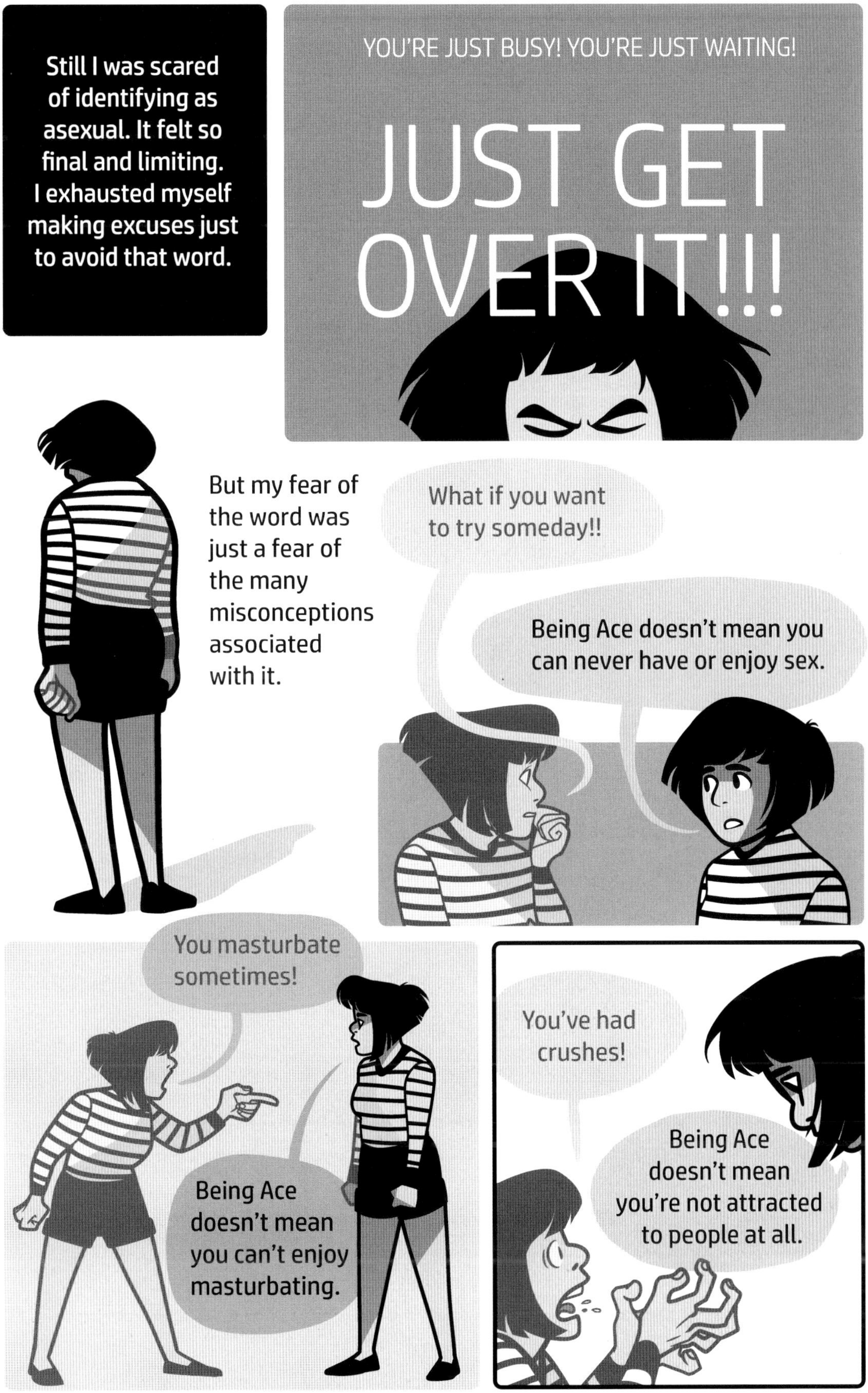
Still I was scared of identifying as asexual. It felt so final and limiting. I exhausted myself making excuses just to avoid that word.
YOU'RE JUST BUSY! YOU'RE JUST WAITING!
JUST GET OVER IT!!!
But my fear of the word was just a fear of the many misconceptions associated with it.
What if you want to try someday!!
Being Ace doesn't mean you can never have or enjoy sex.
You masturbate sometimes!
Being Ace doesn't mean you can't enjoy masturbating.
You've had crushes!
Being Ace doesn't mean you're not attracted to people at all.

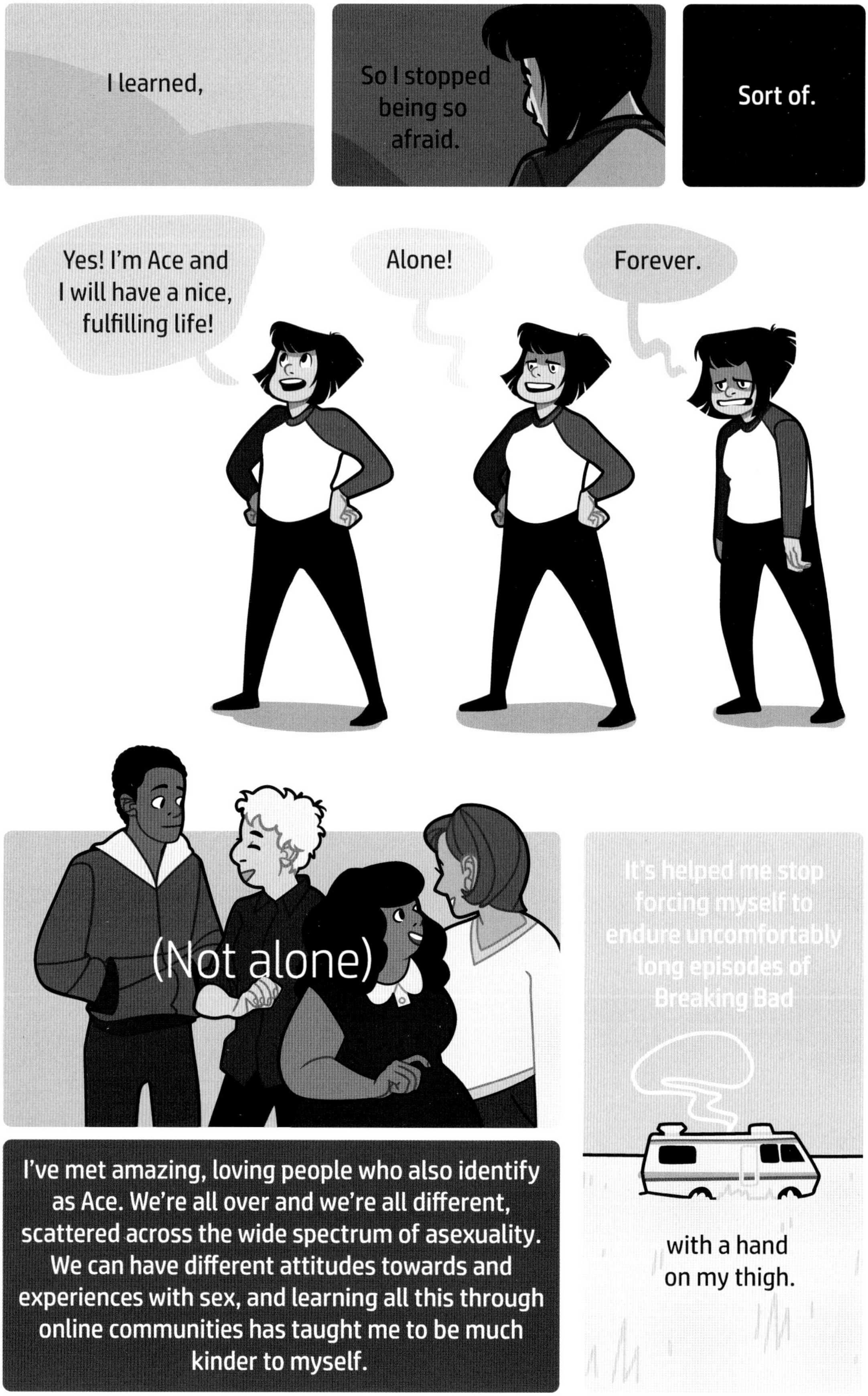
I learned,
So I stopped being so afraid.
Sort of.
Yes! I'm Ace and I will have a nice, fulfilling life!
Alone!
Forever.
(Not alone)
I've met amazing, loving people who also identify as Ace. We're all over and we're all different, scattered across the wide spectrum of asexuality. We can have different attitudes towards and experiences with sex, and learning all this through online communities has taught me to be much kinder to myself.
It's helped me stop forcing myself to endure uncomfortably long episodes of Breaking Bad
with a hand on my thigh.

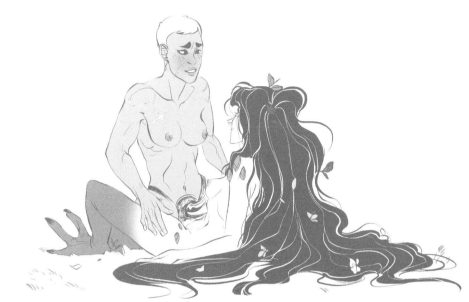

BEWARE THE WOOD WITCH

by Claudia Aguirre

Boudikacomics.com

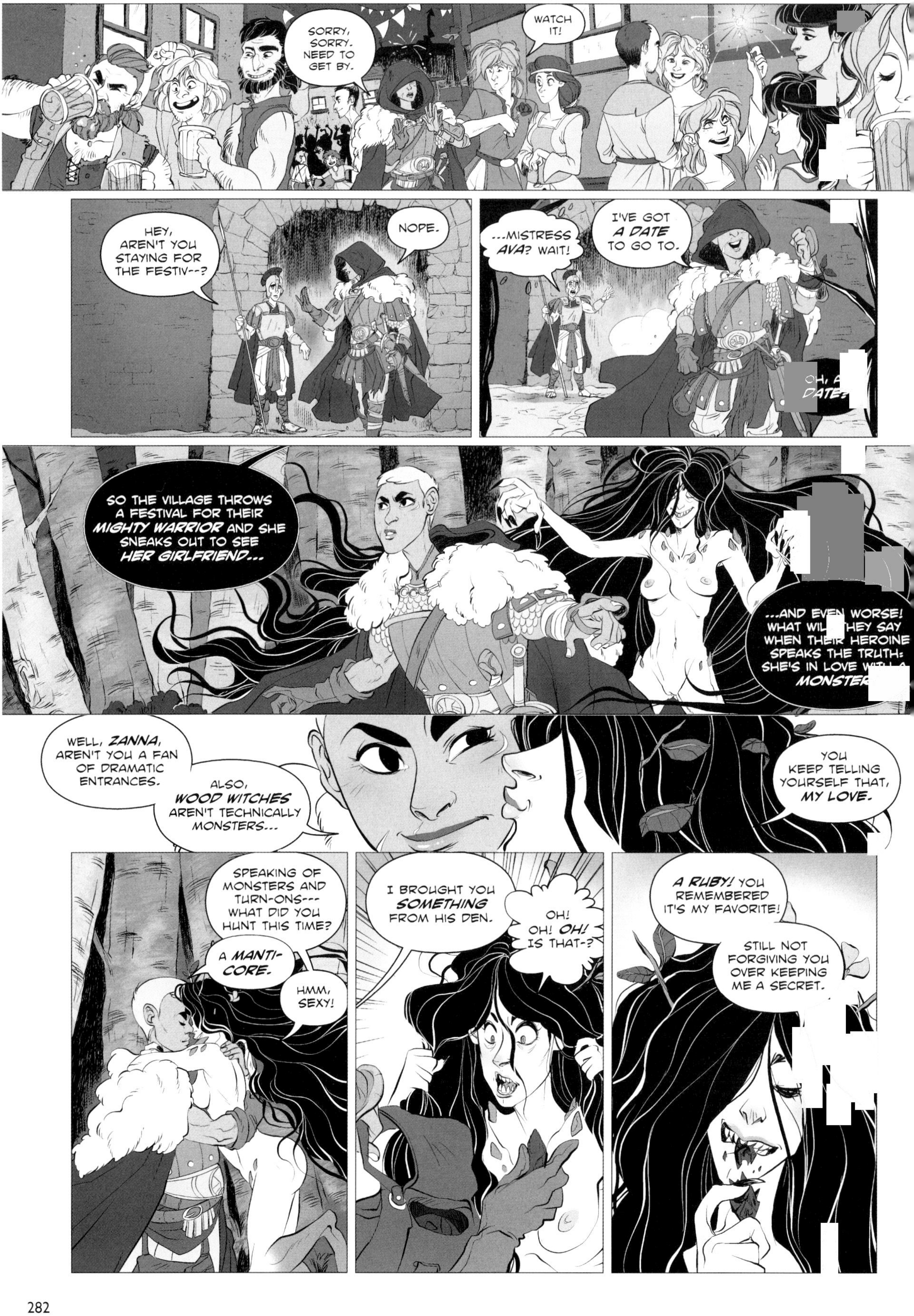
SORRY, SORRY. NEED TO GET BY.
WATCH IT!
HEY, AREN'T YOU STAYING FOR THE FESTIV--?
NOPE.
...MISTRESS AVA? WAIT!
I'VE GOT A DATE TO GO TO.
OH, A DATE?
SO THE VILLAGE THROWS A FESTIVAL FOR THEIR MIGHTY WARRIOR AND SHE SNEAKS OUT TO SEE HER GIRLFRIEND...
...AND EVEN WORSE! WHAT WILL THEY SAY WHEN THE[illegible] HEROINE SPEAKS THE TRUTH: SHE'S IN LOVE WITH A MONSTER
WELL, ZANNA, AREN'T YOU A FAN OF DRAMATIC ENTRANCES.
ALSO, WOOD WITCHES AREN'T TECHNICALLY MONSTERS...
YOU KEEP TELLING YOURSELF THAT, MY LOVE.
SPEAKING OF MONSTERS AND TURN-ONS--- WHAT DID YOU HUNT THIS TIME?
A MANTI-CORE.
HMM, SEXY!
I BROUGHT YOU SOMETHING FROM HIS DEN.
OH! OH! OH! IS THAT-?
A RUBY! YOU REMEMBERED IT'S MY FAVORITE!
STILL NOT FORGIVING YOU OVER KEEPING ME A SECRET.

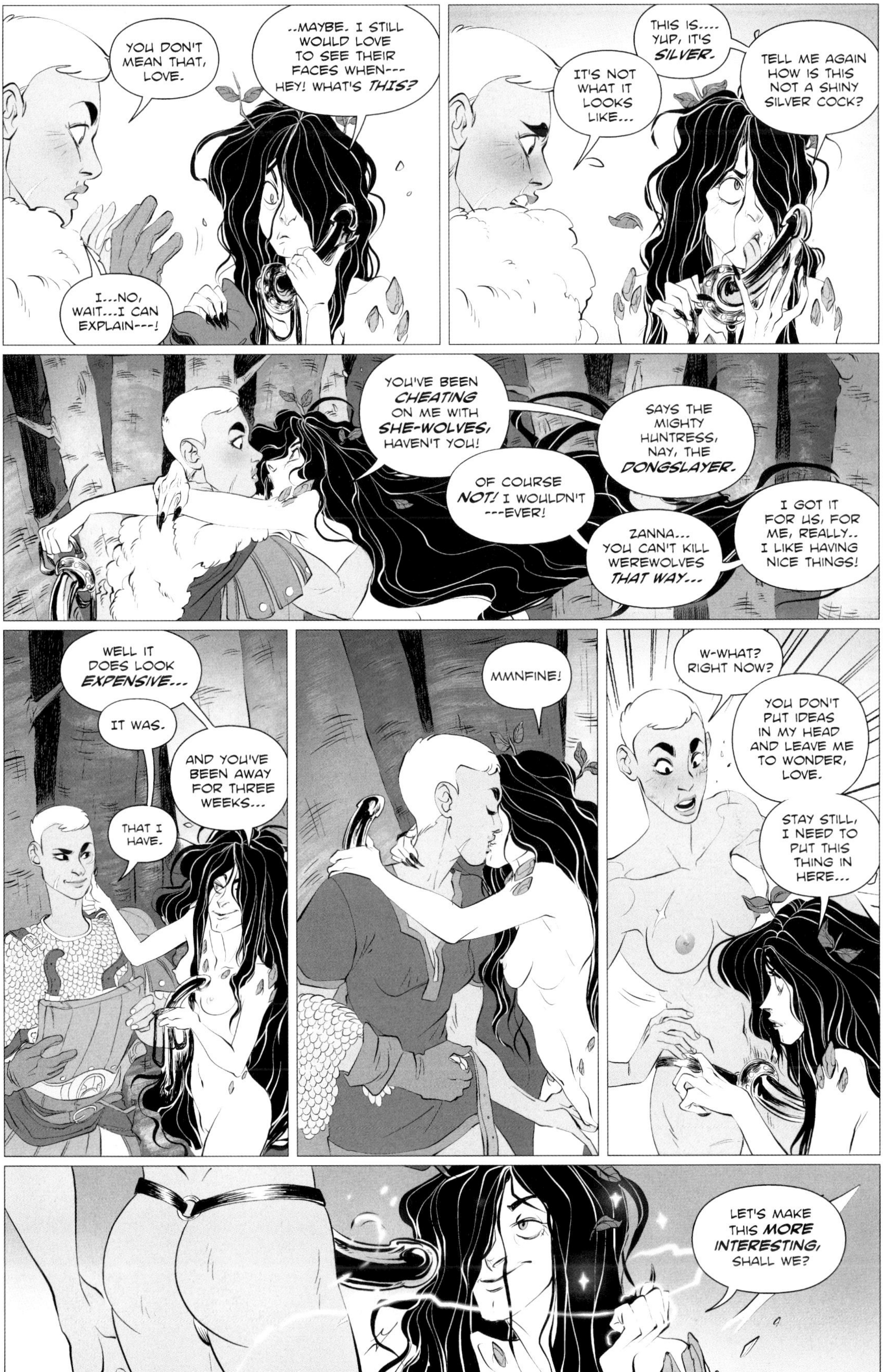
YOU DON'T MEAN THAT, LOVE.
..MAYBE. I STILL WOULD LOVE TO SEE THEIR FACES WHEN--- HEY! WHAT'S THIS?
I...NO, WAIT...I CAN EXPLAIN---!
THIS IS.... YUP, IT'S SILVER.
IT'S NOT WHAT IT LOOKS LIKE...
TELL ME AGAIN HOW IS THIS NOT A SHINY SILVER COCK?
YOU'VE BEEN CHEATING ON ME WITH SHE-WOLVES, HAVEN'T YOU!
OF COURSE NOT! I WOULDN'T ---EVER!
SAYS THE MIGHTY HUNTRESS, NAY, THE DONGSLAYER.
ZANNA... YOU CAN'T KILL WEREWOLVES THAT WAY...
I GOT IT FOR US, FOR ME, REALLY.. I LIKE HAVING NICE THINGS!
WELL IT DOES LOOK EXPENSIVE...
IT WAS.
AND YOU'VE BEEN AWAY FOR THREE WEEKS...
THAT I HAVE.
MMNFINE!
W-WHAT? RIGHT NOW?
YOU DON'T PUT IDEAS IN MY HEAD AND LEAVE ME TO WONDER, LOVE.
STAY STILL, I NEED TO PUT THIS THING IN HERE...
LET'S MAKE THIS MORE INTERESTING, SHALL WE?

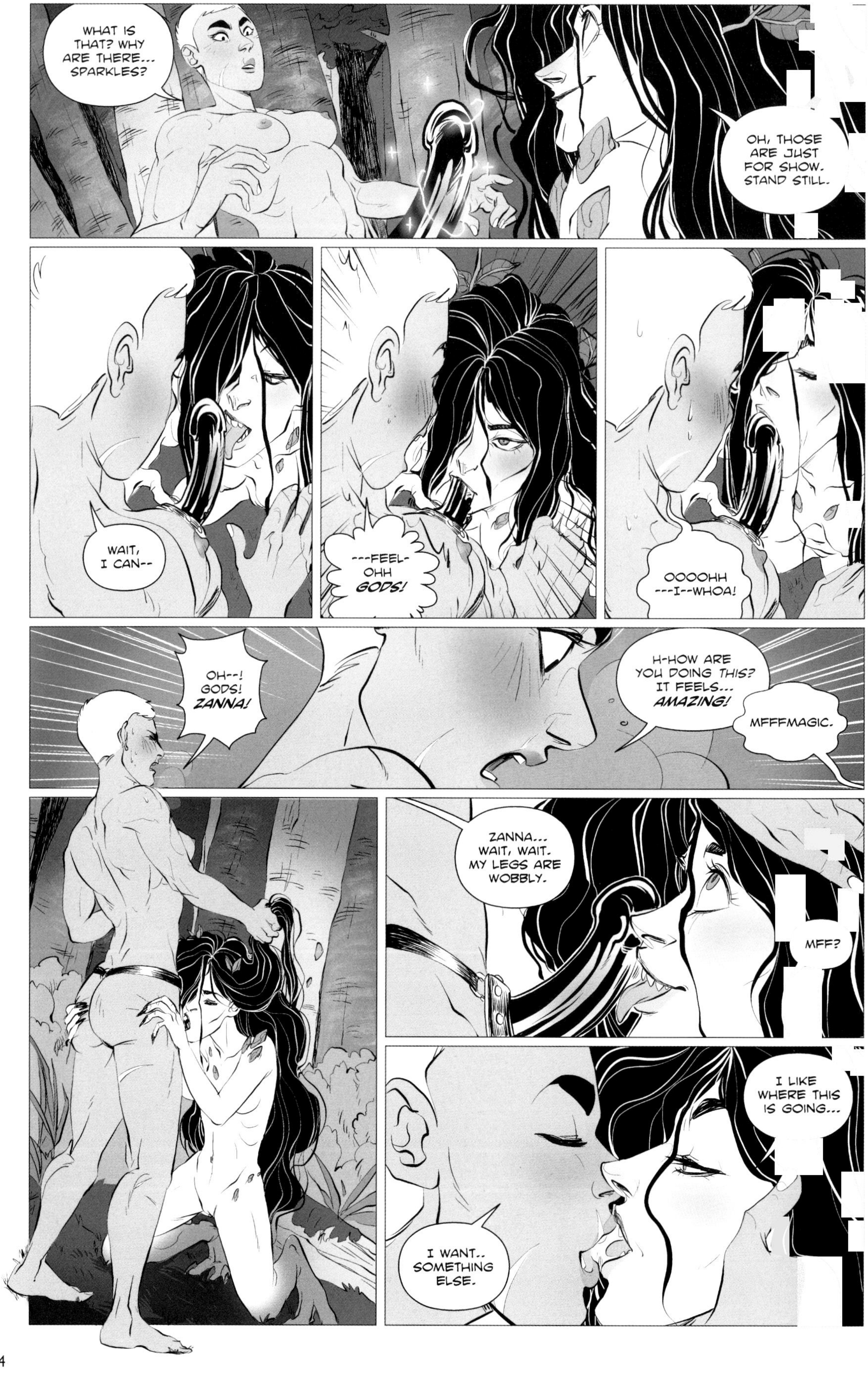
WHAT IS THAT? WHY ARE THERE... SPARKLES?
OH, THOSE ARE JUST FOR SHOW. STAND STILL.
WAIT, I CAN--
---FEEL- OHH GODS!
OOOOHH ---I--WHOA!
OH--! GODS! ZANNA!
H-HOW ARE YOU DOING THIS? IT FEELS... AMAZING!
MFFFMAGIC.
ZANNA... WAIT, WAIT. MY LEGS ARE WOBBLY.
MFF?
I LIKE WHERE THIS IS GOING...
I WANT.. SOMETHING ELSE.

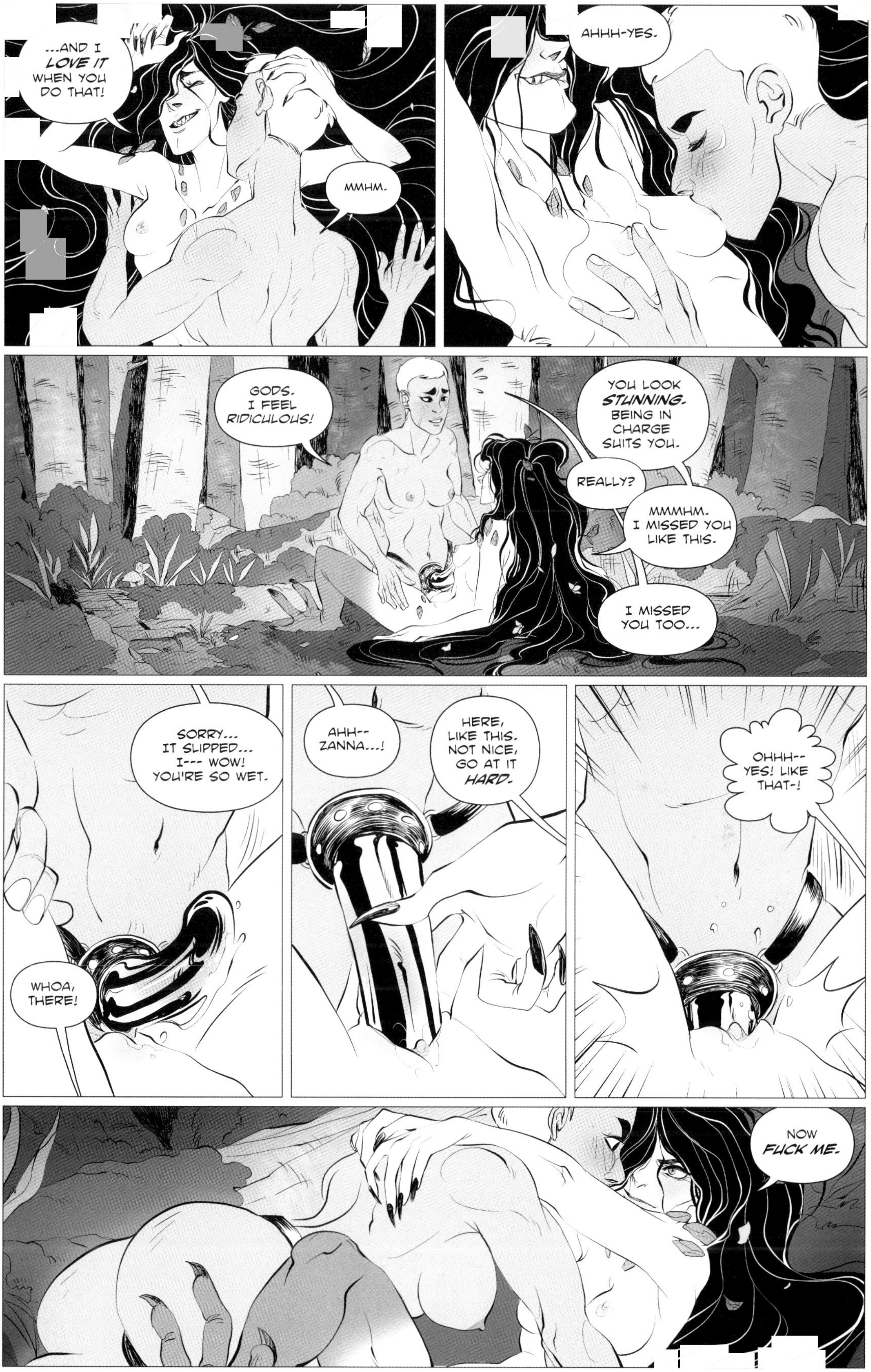
...AND I LOVE IT WHEN YOU DO THAT!
MMHM.
AHHH-YES.
GODS. I FEEL RIDICULOUS!
YOU LOOK STUNNING. BEING IN CHARGE SUITS YOU.
REALLY?
MMMHM. I MISSED YOU LIKE THIS.
I MISSED YOU TOO...
SORRY... IT SLIPPED... I--- WOW! YOU'RE SO WET.
WHOA, THERE!
AHH-- ZANNA...!
HERE, LIKE THIS. NOT NICE, GO AT IT HARD.
OHHH-- YES! LIKE THAT-!
NOW FUCK ME.

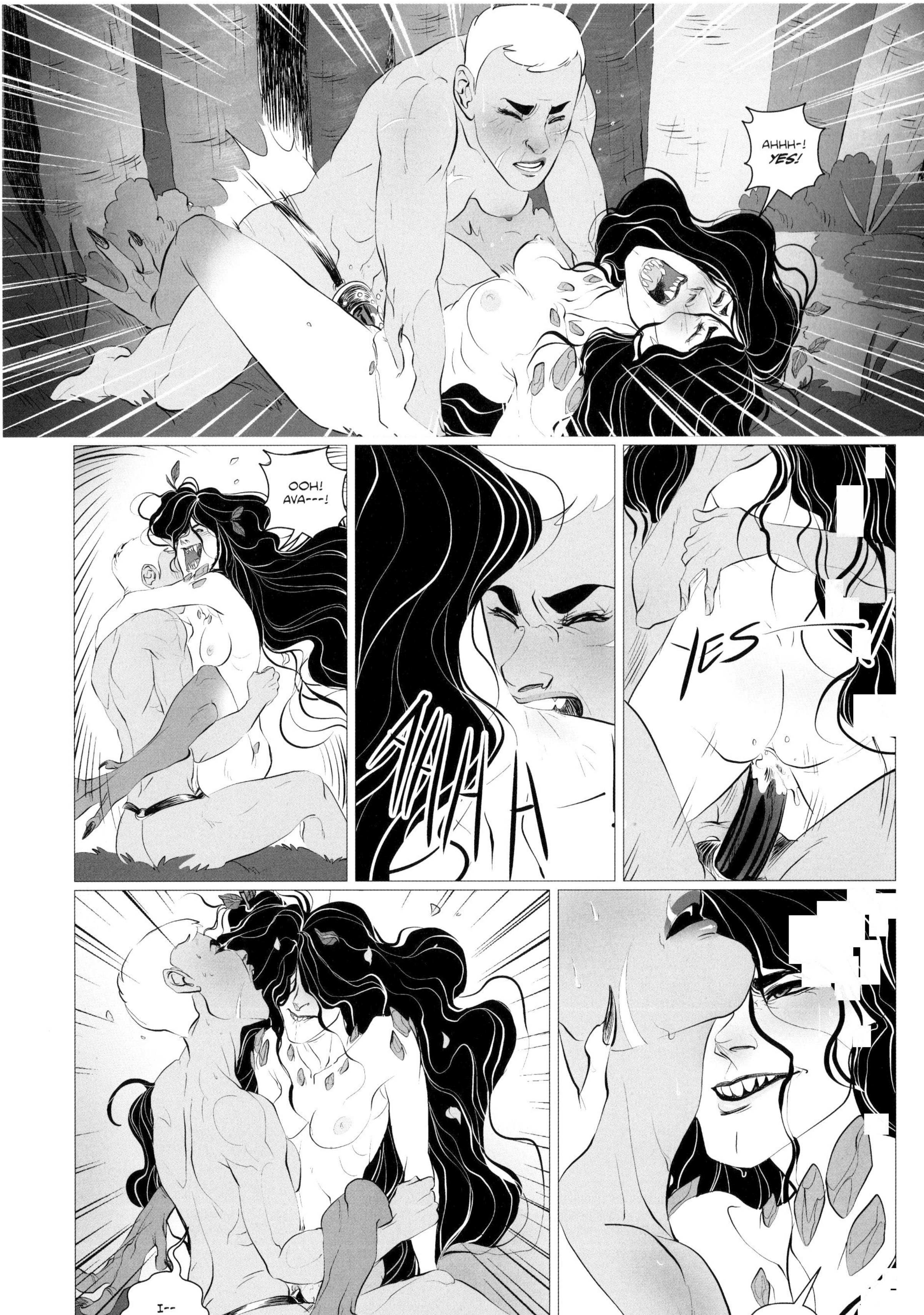
AHHH-! YES!
OOH! AVA---!
YES
I-- I'M..
DO IT.

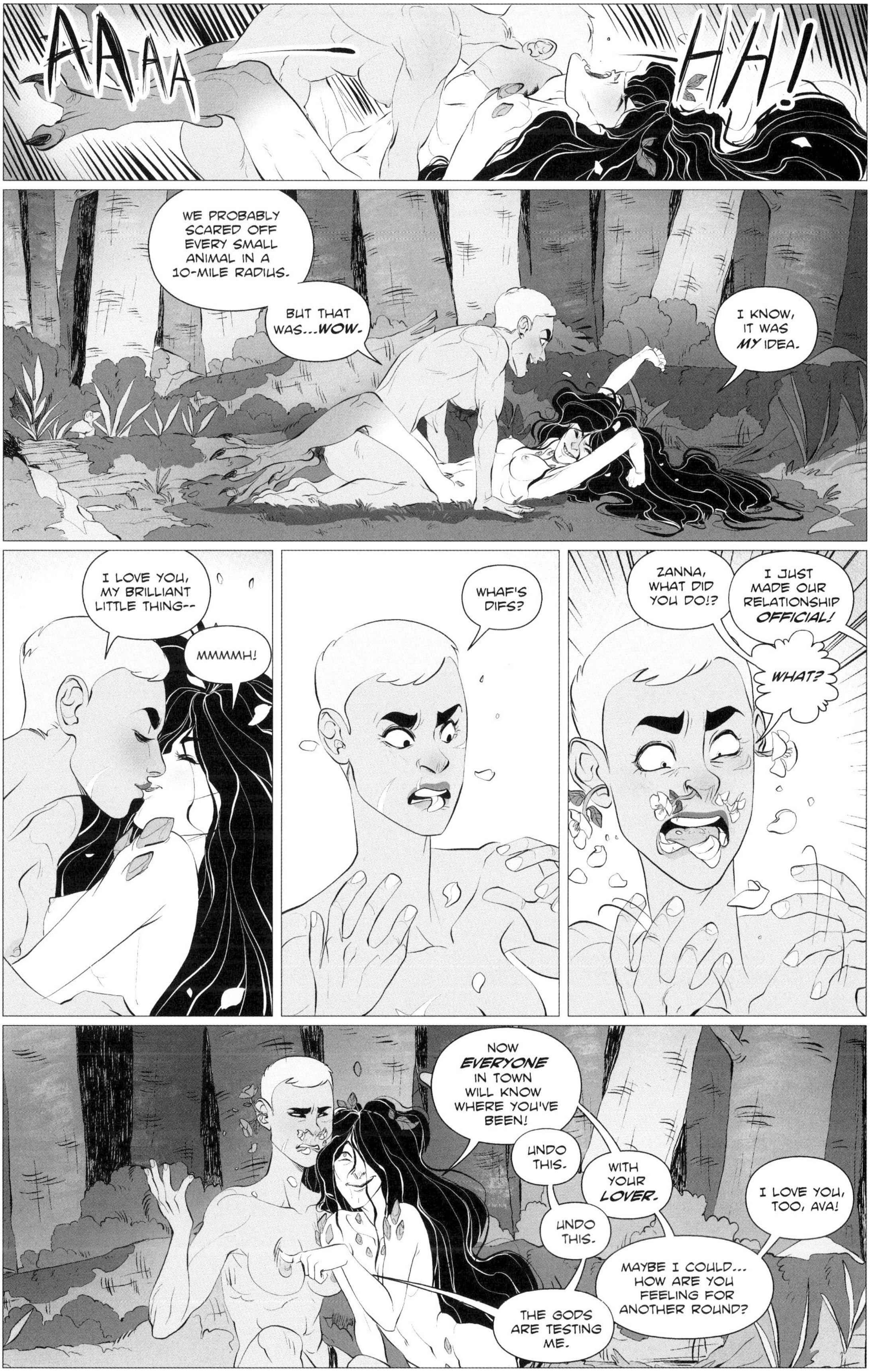
AAAAA—HH!
WE PROBABLY SCARED OFF EVERY SMALL ANIMAL IN A 10-MILE RADIUS.
BUT THAT WAS...WOW.
I KNOW, IT WAS MY IDEA.
I LOVE YOU, MY BRILLIANT LITTLE THING--
MMMMH!
WHAF'S DIFS?
ZANNA, WHAT DID YOU DO!?
I JUST MADE OUR RELATIONSHIP OFFICIAL!
WHAT?
NOW EVERYONE IN TOWN WILL KNOW WHERE YOU'VE BEEN!
UNDO THIS.
WITH YOUR LOVER.
UNDO THIS.
I LOVE YOU, TOO, AVA!
MAYBE I COULD... HOW ARE YOU FEELING FOR ANOTHER ROUND?
THE GODS ARE TESTING ME.

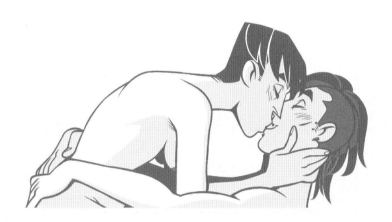

WHAT'S THE BUZZ
by Benjamin

6wholesilabus.tumblr.com

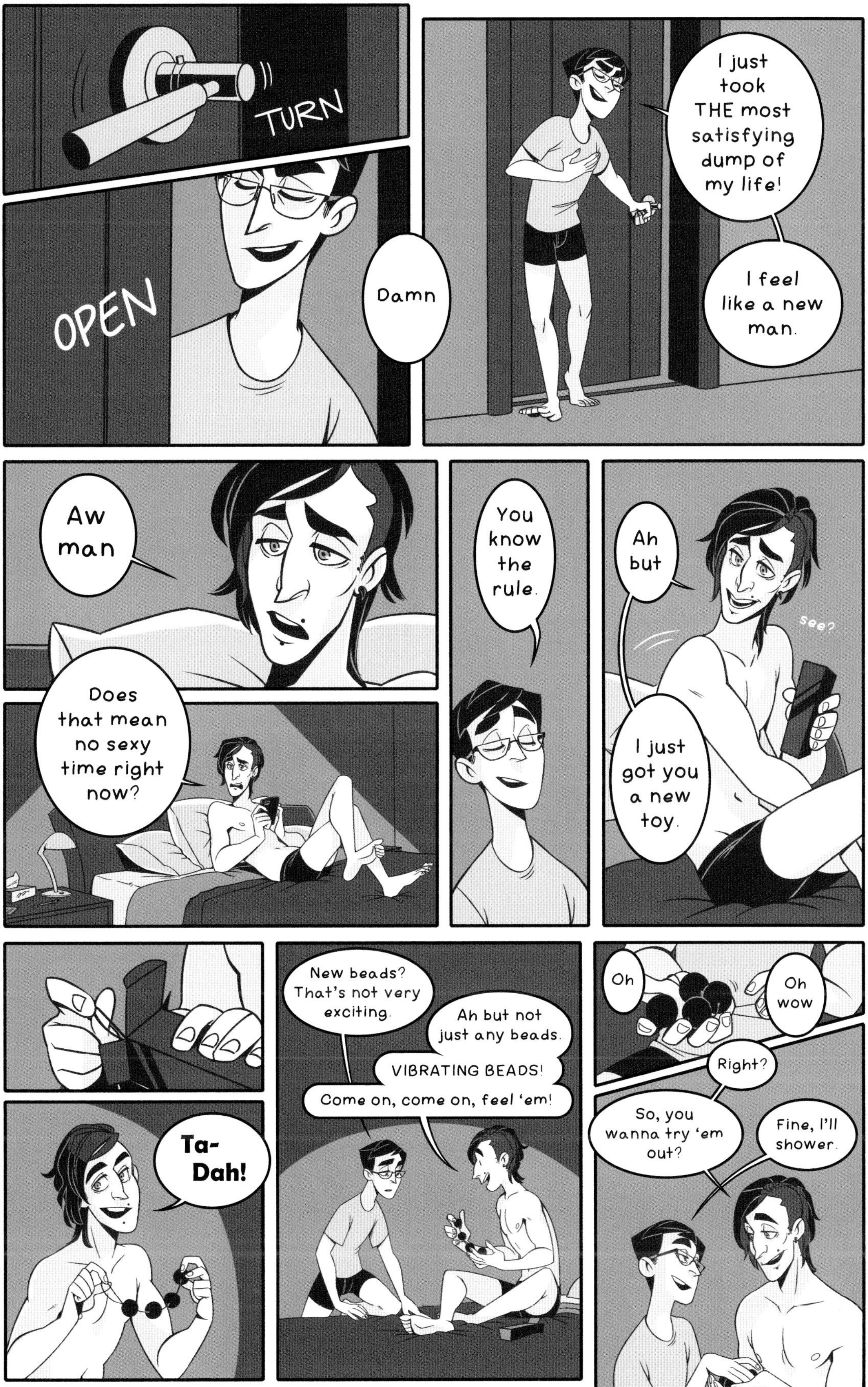
TURN
OPEN
Damn
I just took THE most satisfying dump of my life!
I feel like a new man.
Aw man
Does that mean no sexy time right now?
You know the rule.
Ah but
see?
I just got you a new toy.
Ta-Dah!
New beads? That's not very exciting.
Ah but not just any beads.
VIBRATING BEADS!
Come on, come on, feel 'em!
Oh
Oh wow
Right?
So, you wanna try 'em out?
Fine, I'll shower.

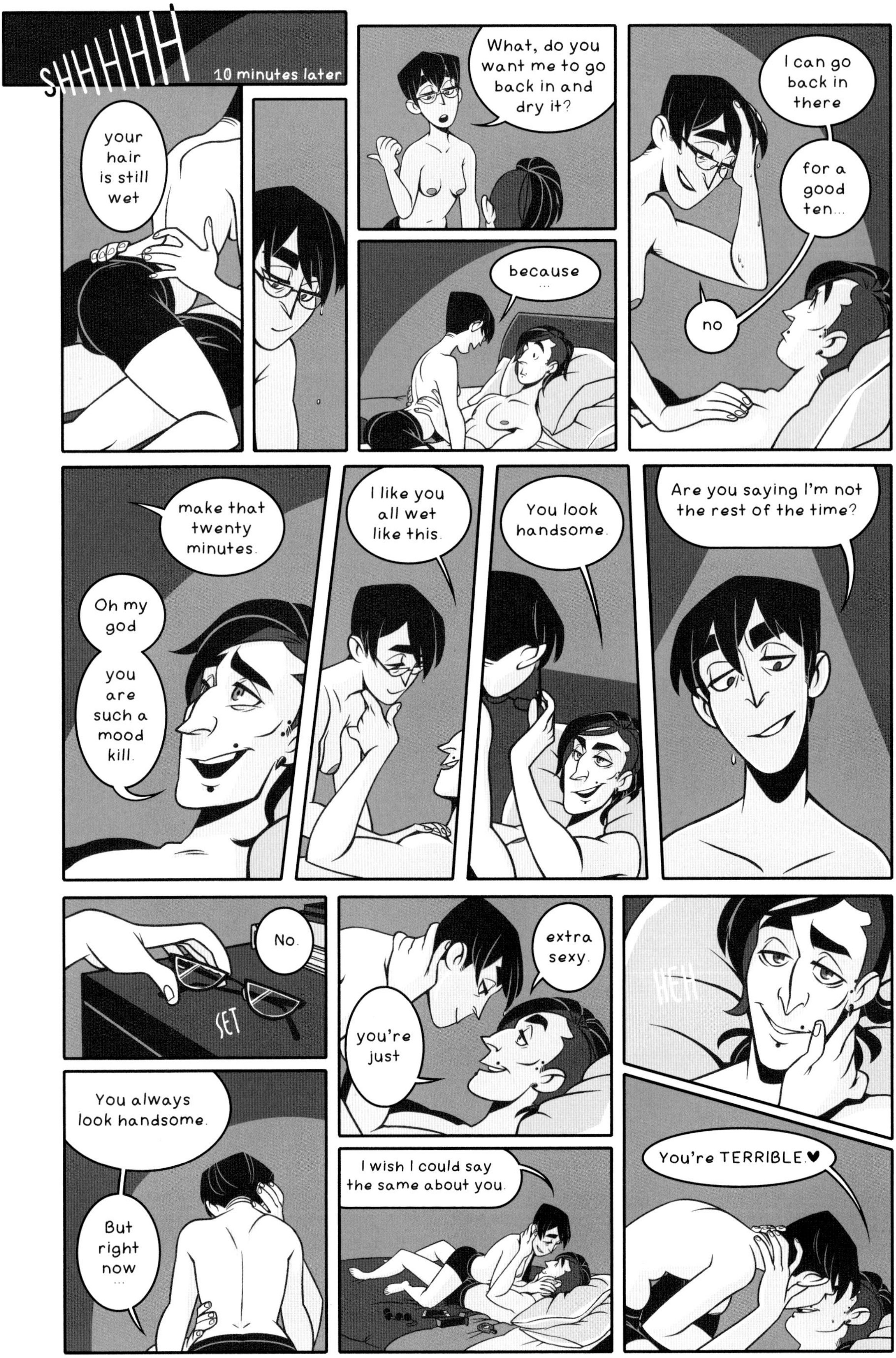
SHHHHHH
10 minutes later
your hair is still wet
What, do you want me to go back in and dry it?
because ...
I can go back in there
for a good ten...
no
make that twenty minutes.
Oh my god
you are such a mood kill.
I like you all wet like this.
You look handsome.
Are you saying I'm not the rest of the time?
No.
SET
You always look handsome.
But right now ...
extra sexy.
you're just
I wish I could say the same about you.
HEH
You're TERRIBLE.♥

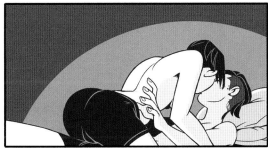

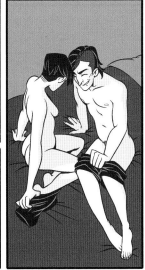

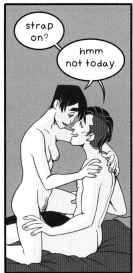

strap on?

hmm not today.

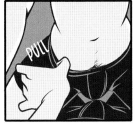

PULL

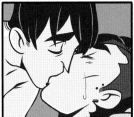

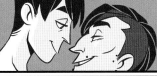

Well, let me know if you change your mind

you know I'm always down.

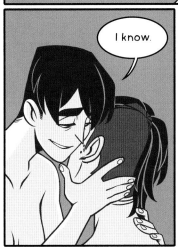

I know.

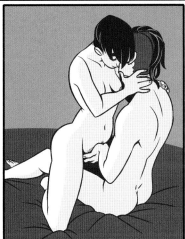

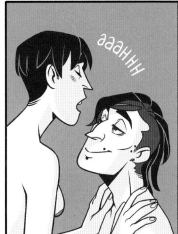

aaaHHH

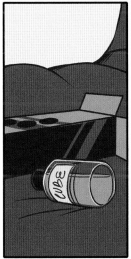

CUBE

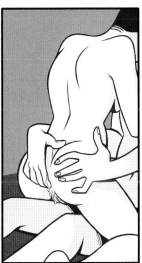

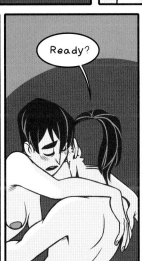

Ready?

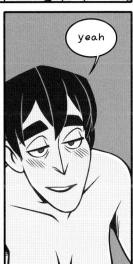

yeah

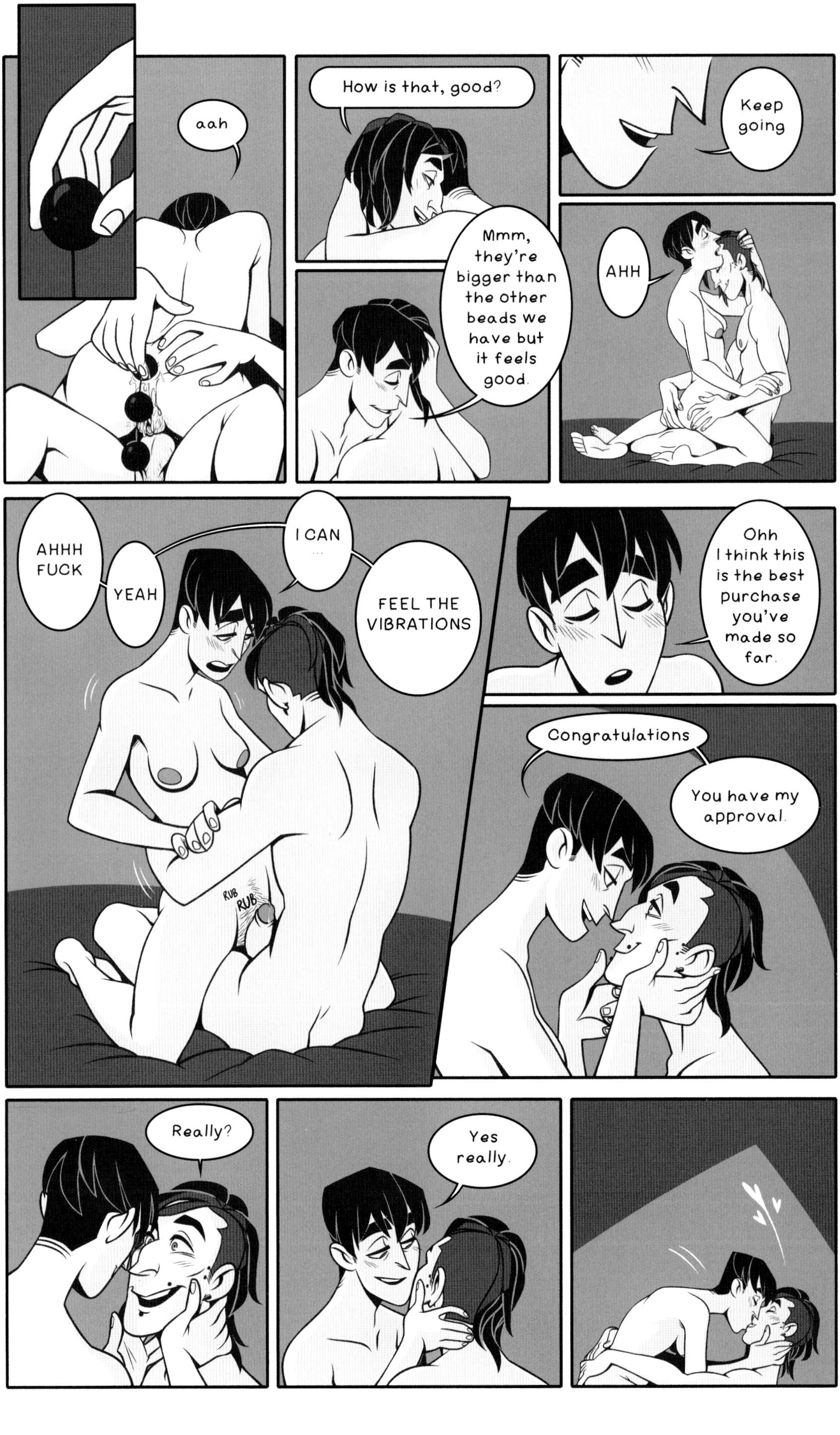
aah
How is that, good?
Keep going
Mmm, they're bigger than the other beads we have but it feels good.
AHH
AHHH FUCK
YEAH
I CAN
FEEL THE VIBRATIONS
RUB
RUB
Ohh I think this is the best purchase you've made so far.
Congratulations
You have my approval.
Really?
Yes really.

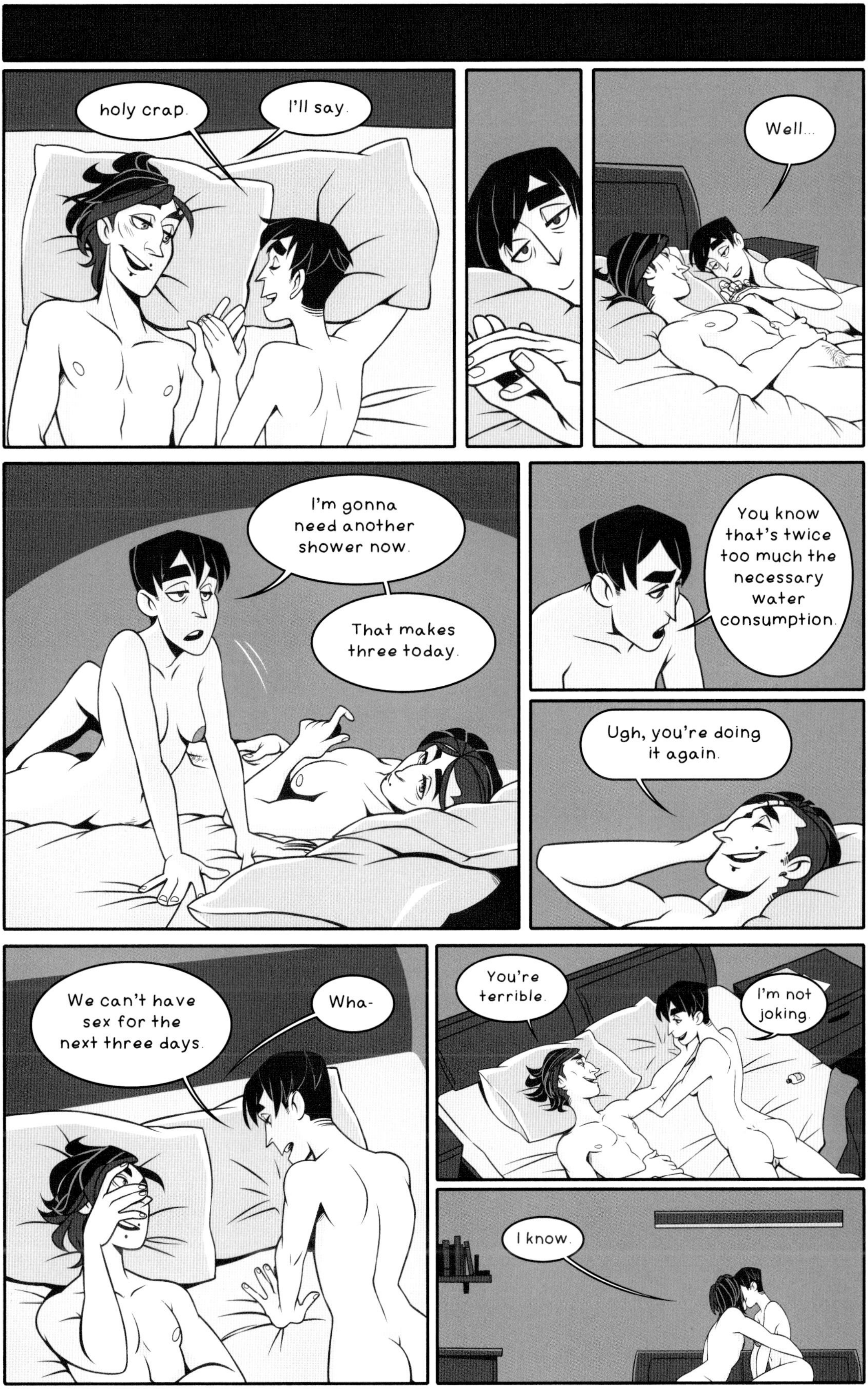
holy crap.
I'll say.
Well...
I'm gonna need another shower now.
That makes three today.
You know that's twice too much the necessary water consumption.
Ugh, you're doing it again.
We can't have sex for the next three days.
Wha-
You're terrible.
I'm not joking.
I know.

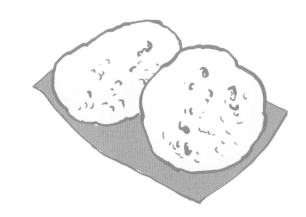

MENSTRUAL SPONGE

by Dwam

Sang-noir.net

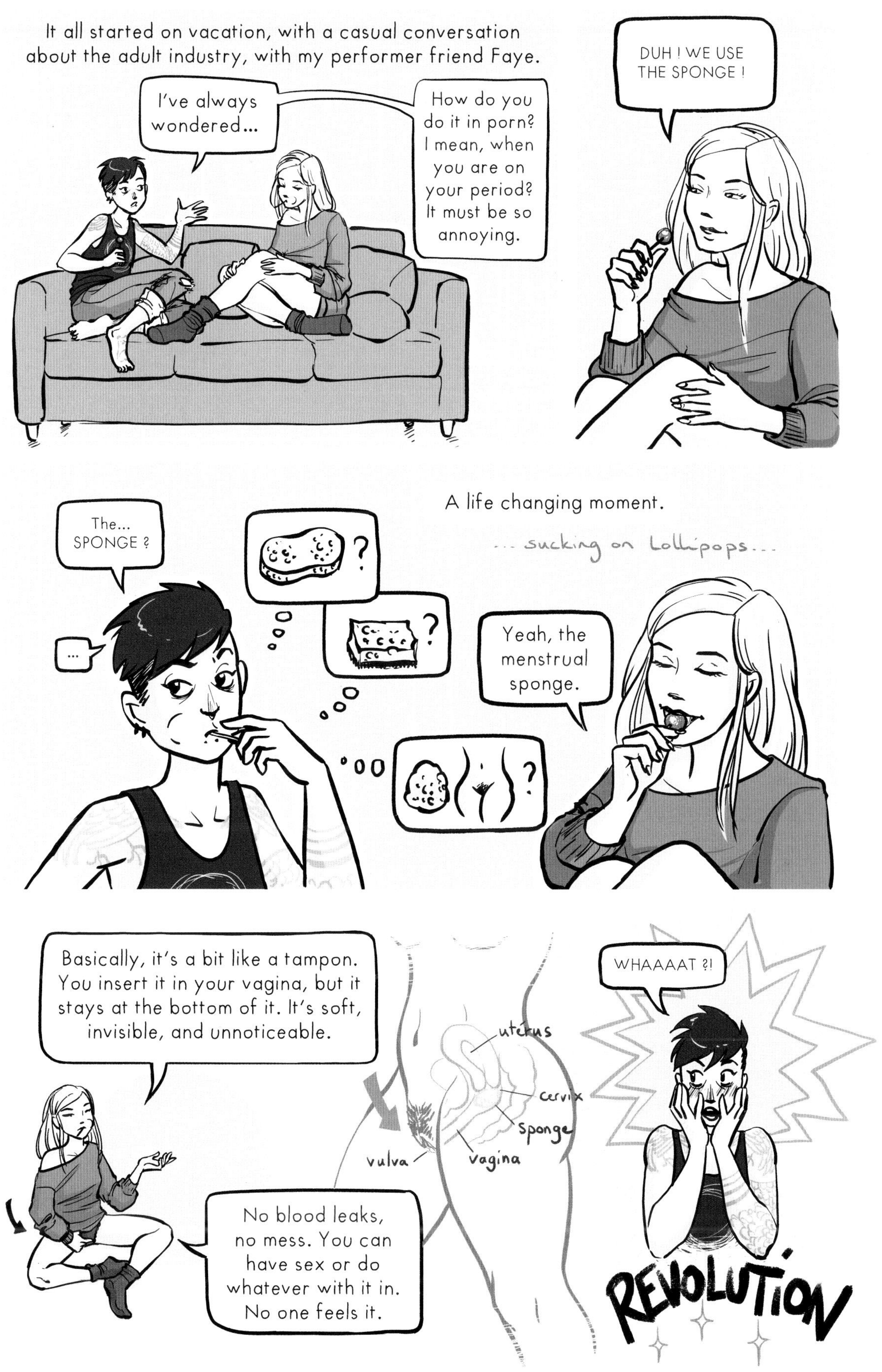

It all started on vacation, with a casual conversation about the adult industry, with my performer friend Faye.
I've always wondered...
How do you do it in porn? I mean, when you are on your period? It must be so annoying.
DUH ! WE USE THE SPONGE !
The... SPONGE ?
...
A life changing moment.
... sucking on Lollipops...
Yeah, the menstrual sponge.
Basically, it's a bit like a tampon. You insert it in your vagina, but it stays at the bottom of it. It's soft, invisible, and unnoticeable.
utérus
cervix
sponge
vulva
vagina
No blood leaks, no mess. You can have sex or do whatever with it in. No one feels it.
WHAAAAT ?!
REVOLUTION

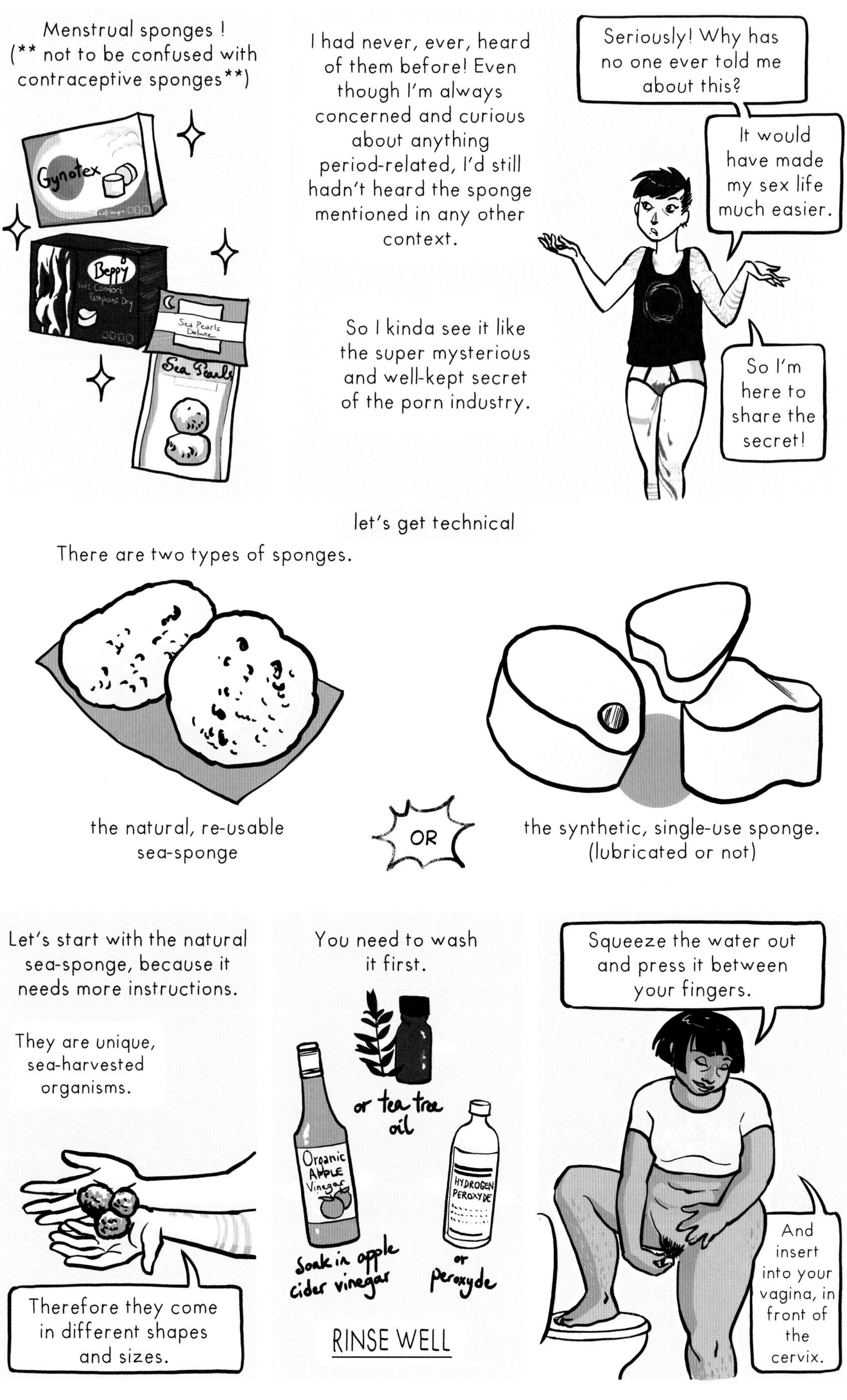

Menstrual sponges ! (** not to be confused with contraceptive sponges**)
Gynotex
Beppy
Soft Comfort Tampons Dry
Sea Pearls Deluxe
Sea Pearls
I had never, ever, heard of them before! Even though I'm always concerned and curious about anything period-related, I'd still hadn't heard the sponge mentioned in any other context.
So I kinda see it like the super mysterious and well-kept secret of the porn industry.
Seriously! Why has no one ever told me about this?
It would have made my sex life much easier.
So I'm here to share the secret!
let's get technical
There are two types of sponges.
the natural, re-usable sea-sponge
OR
the synthetic, single-use sponge. (lubricated or not)
Let's start with the natural sea-sponge, because it needs more instructions.
They are unique, sea-harvested organisms.
Therefore they come in different shapes and sizes.
You need to wash it first.
or tea tree oil
Organic APPLE Vinegar
HYDROGEN PEROXYDE
Soak in apple cider vinegar
or Peroxyde
RINSE WELL
Squeeze the water out and press it between your fingers.
And insert into your vagina, in front of the cervix.

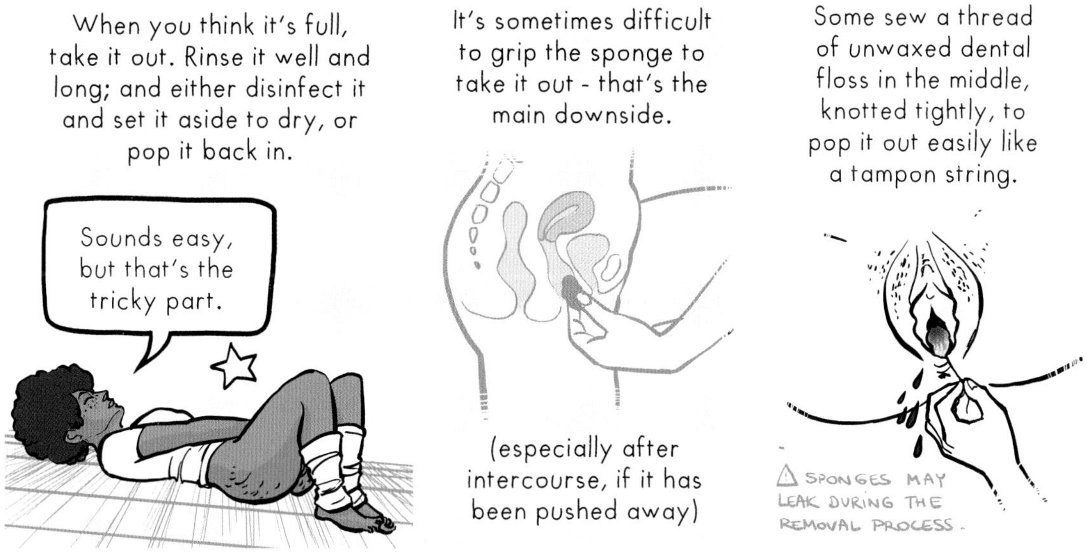
When you think it's full, take it out. Rinse it well and long; and either disinfect it and set it aside to dry, or pop it back in.
Sounds easy, but that's the tricky part.
It's sometimes difficult to grip the sponge to take it out - that's the main downside.
(especially after intercourse, if it has been pushed away)
Some sew a thread of unwaxed dental floss in the middle, knotted tightly, to pop it out easily like a tampon string.
⚠ SPONGES MAY LEAK DURING THE REMOVAL PROCESS.

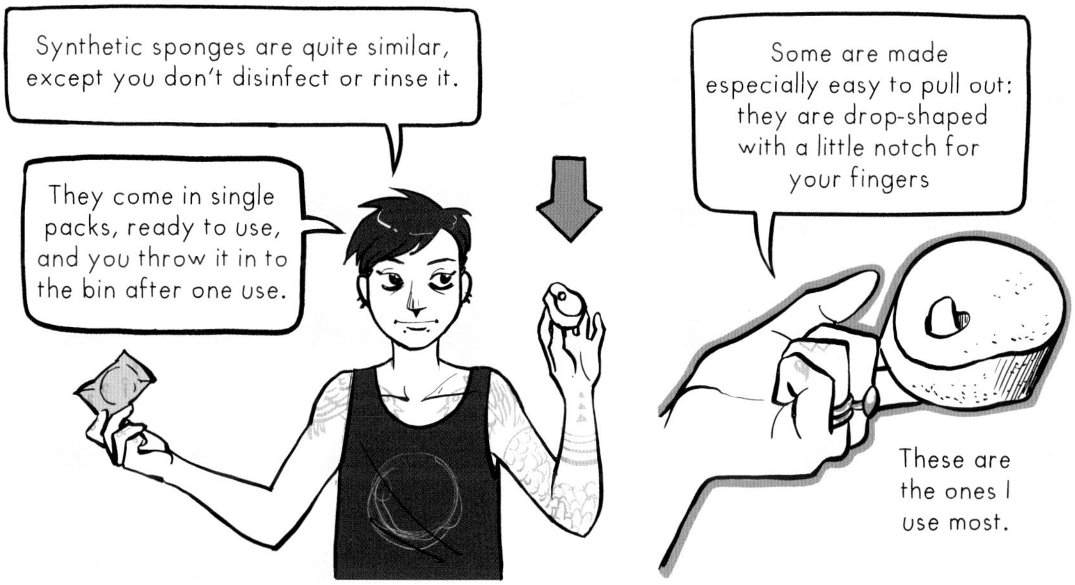
Synthetic sponges are quite similar, except you don't disinfect or rinse it.
They come in single packs, ready to use, and you throw it in to the bin after one use.
Some are made especially easy to pull out: they are drop-shaped with a little notch for your fingers
These are the ones I use most.

	NATURAL SEA SPONGE	SYNTHETIC SPONGE
PROS	- no chemicals - reusable - cheap	- easy to use - comes in single pack
CONS	- not vegan! - washing it can be very awkward in public restrooms	- expensive - single use

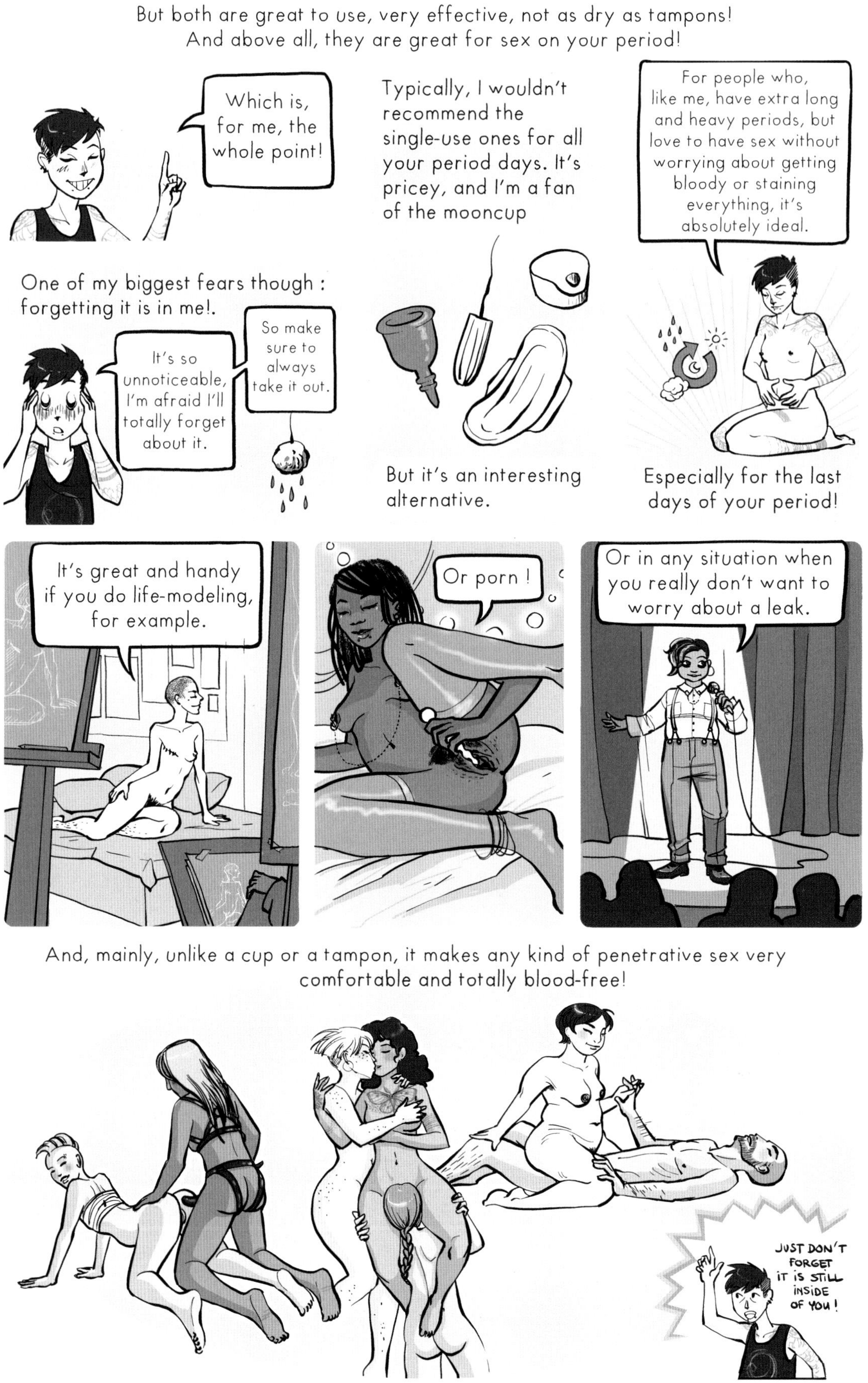
But both are great to use, very effective, not as dry as tampons!
And above all, they are great for sex on your period!
Which is, for me, the whole point!
Typically, I wouldn't recommend the single-use ones for all your period days. It's pricey, and I'm a fan of the mooncup
For people who, like me, have extra long and heavy periods, but love to have sex without worrying about getting bloody or staining everything, it's absolutely ideal.
One of my biggest fears though : forgetting it is in me!.
It's so unnoticeable, I'm afraid I'll totally forget about it.
So make sure to always take it out.
But it's an interesting alternative.
Especially for the last days of your period!
It's great and handy if you do life-modeling, for example.
Or porn !
Or in any situation when you really don't want to worry about a leak.
And, mainly, unlike a cup or a tampon, it makes any kind of penetrative sex very comfortable and totally blood-free!
JUST DON'T FORGET IT IS STILL INSIDE OF YOU!

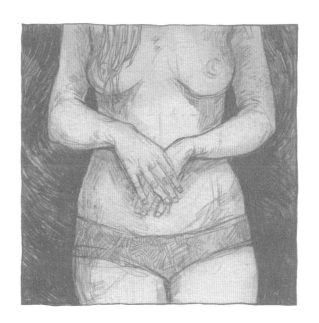

BODY IMAGE
by Thomke Meyer

Thomkemeyer.tumblr.com

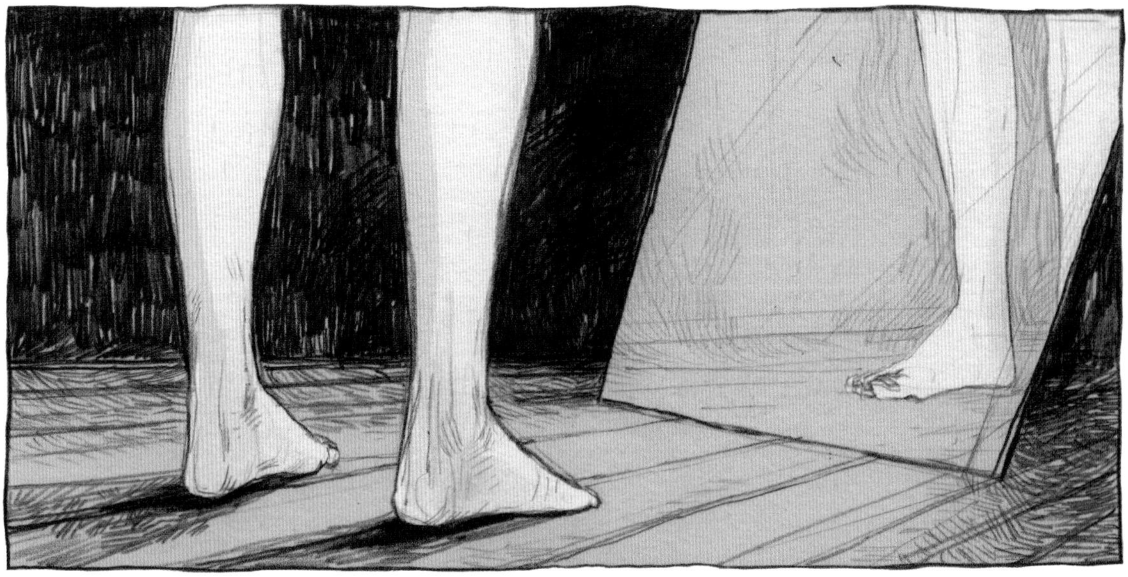

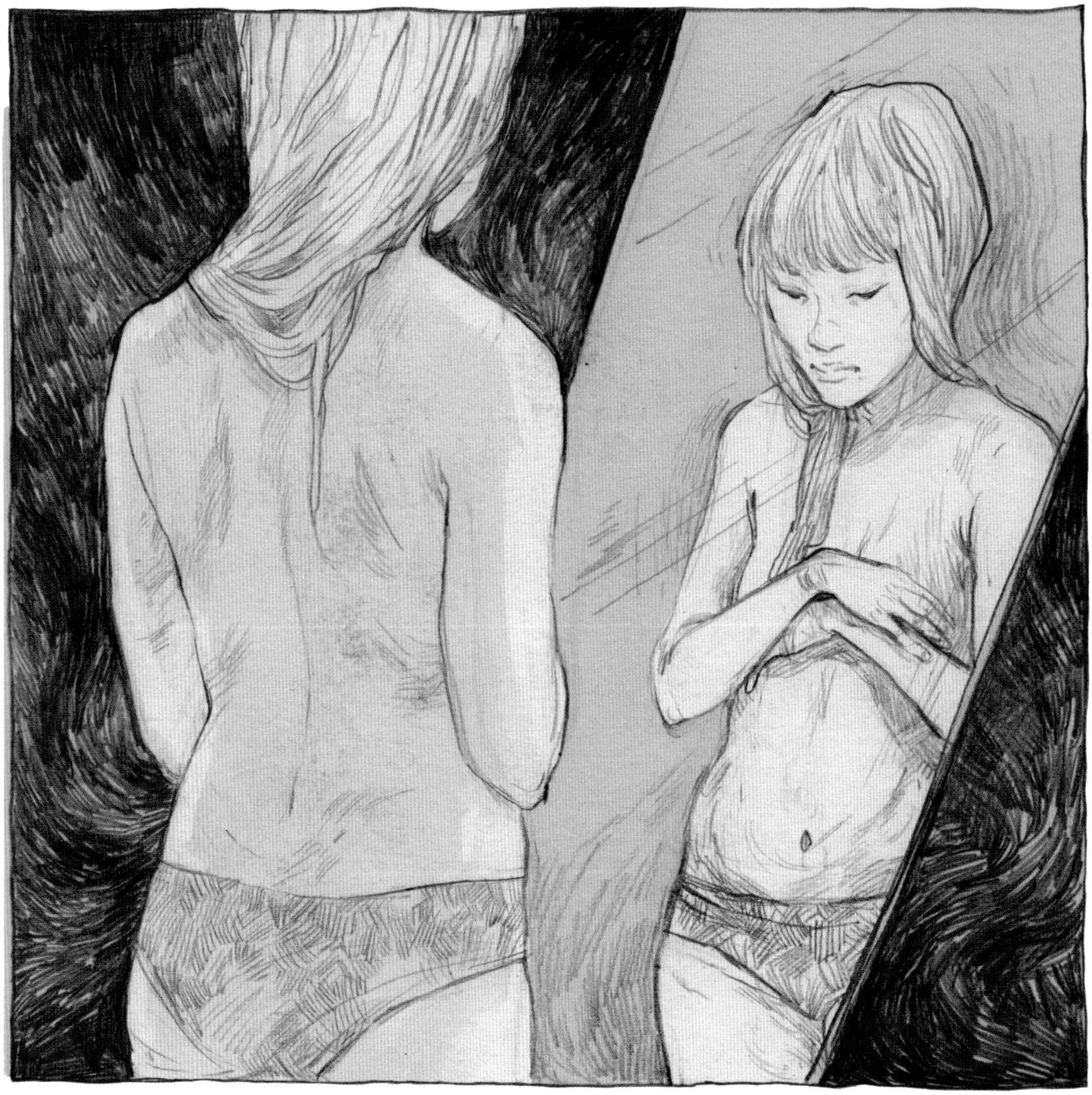

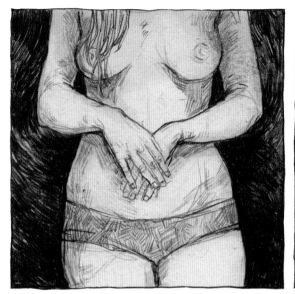
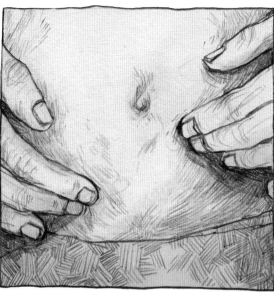
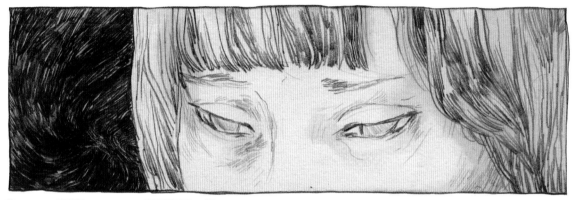
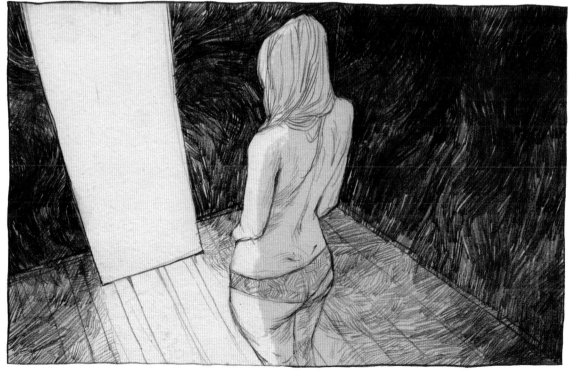

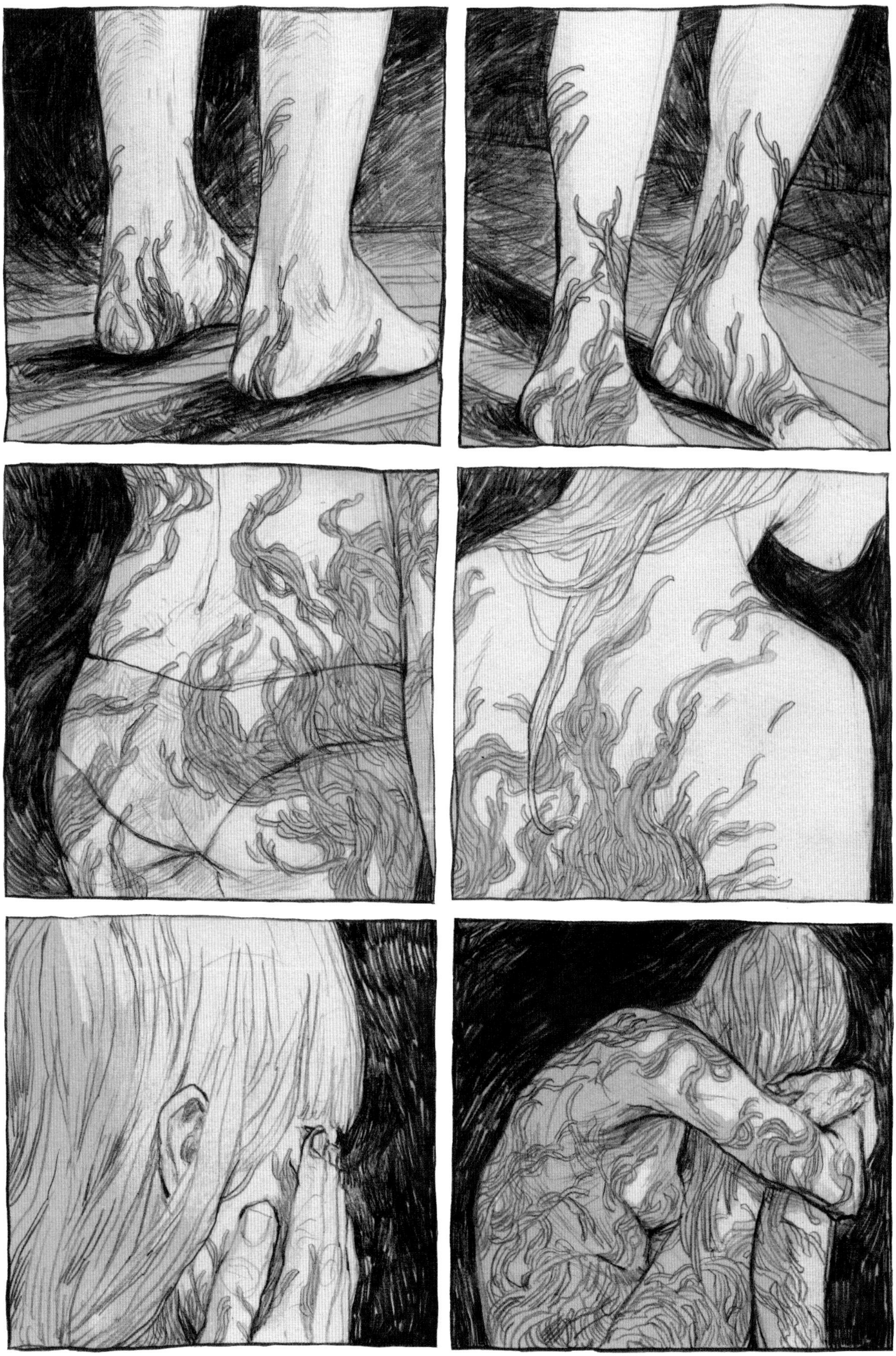

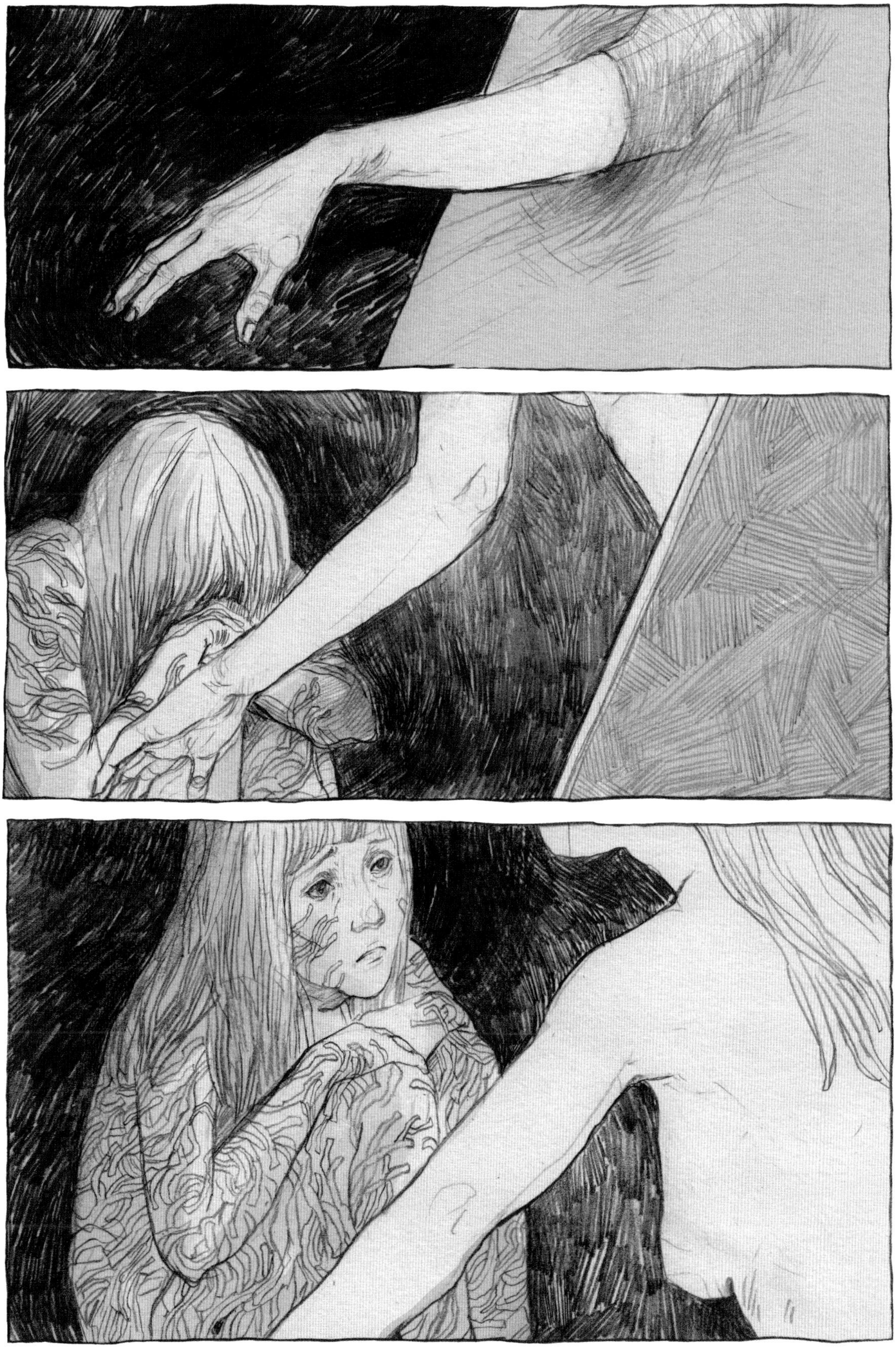

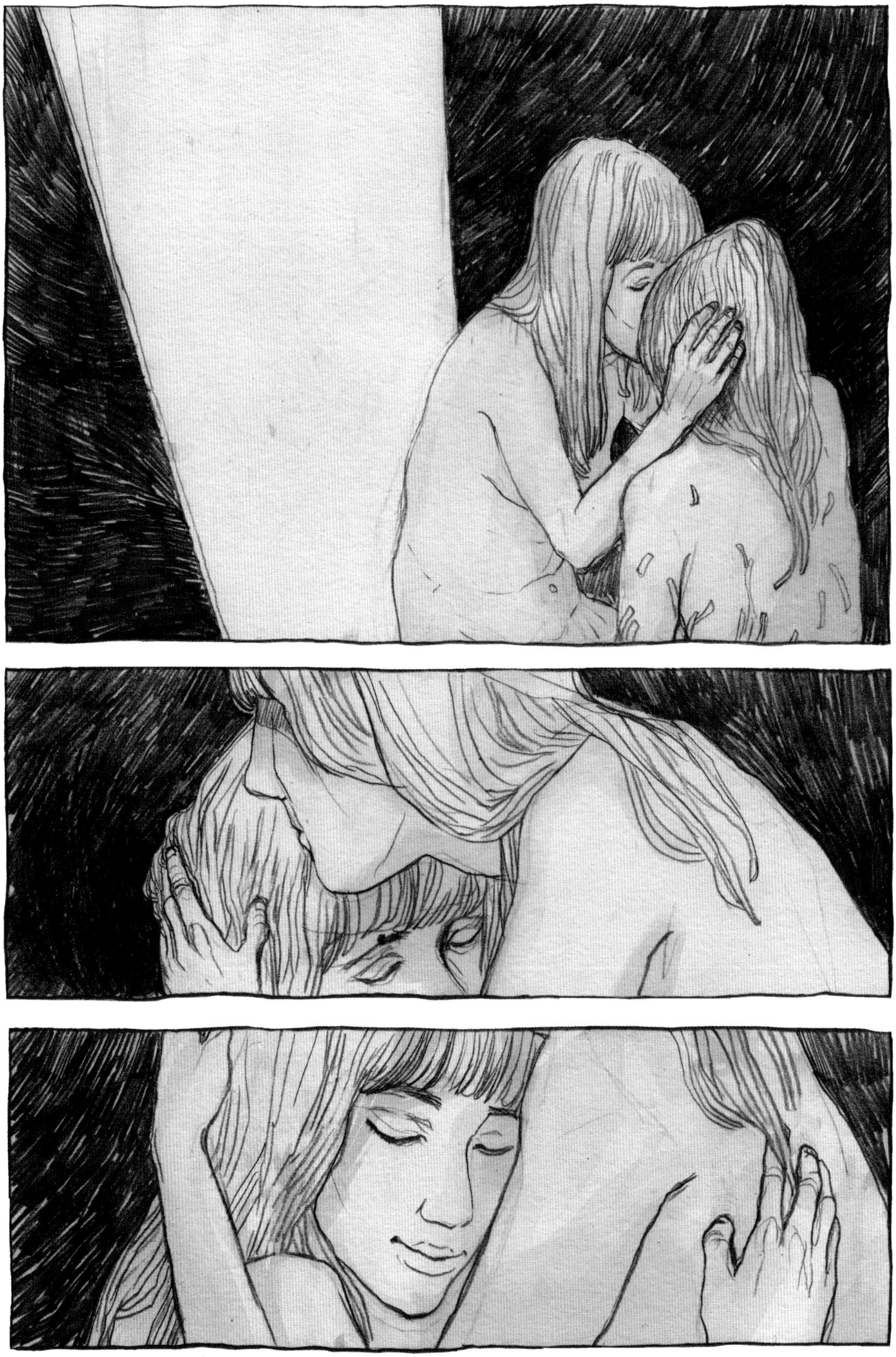

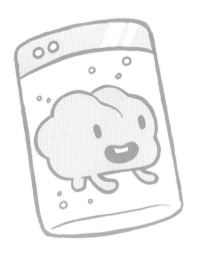

BRAIN ORGASM SCIENCE

by Tait Howard

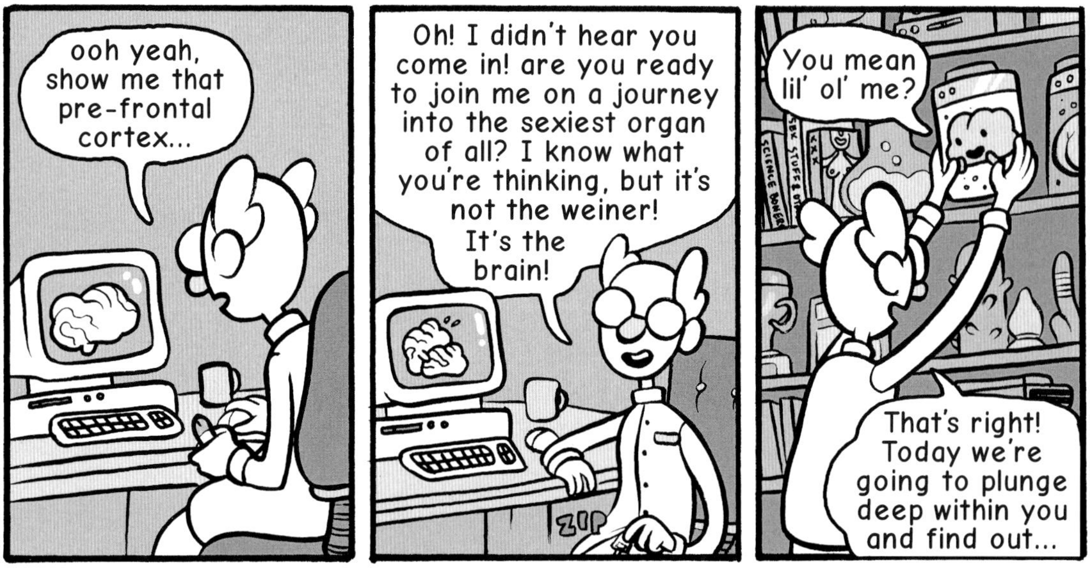
ooh yeah, show me that pre-frontal cortex...
Oh! I didn't hear you come in! are you ready to join me on a journey into the sexiest organ of all? I know what you're thinking, but it's not the weiner!
It's the brain!
ZIP
You mean lil' ol' me?
That's right! Today we're going to plunge deep within you and find out...

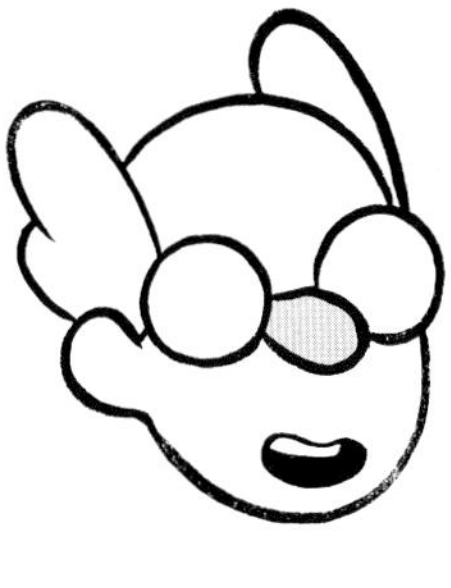

WHAT HAPPENS IN THE BRAIN DURING AN ORGASM

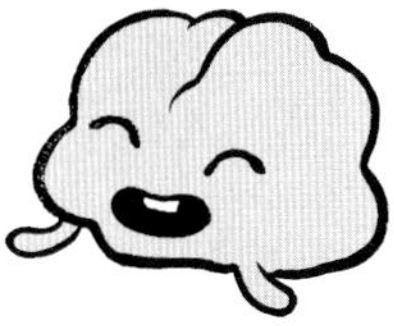

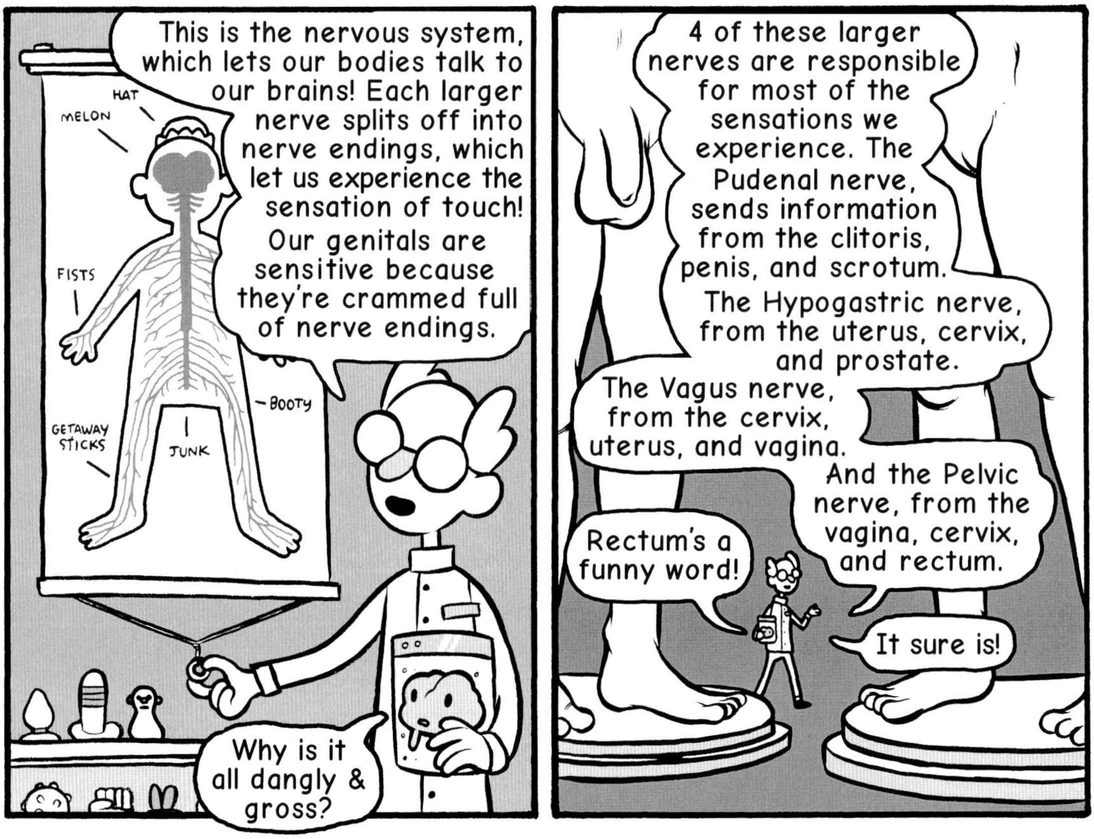
This is the nervous system, which lets our bodies talk to our brains! Each larger nerve splits off into nerve endings, which let us experience the sensation of touch!
Our genitals are sensitive because they're crammed full of nerve endings.
HAT
MELON
FISTS
BOOTY
GETAWAY STICKS
JUNK
Why is it all dangly & gross?
4 of these larger nerves are responsible for most of the sensations we experience. The Pudenal nerve, sends information from the clitoris, penis, and scrotum.
The Hypogastric nerve, from the uterus, cervix, and prostate.
The Vagus nerve, from the cervix, uterus, and vagina.
And the Pelvic nerve, from the vagina, cervix, and rectum.
Rectum's a funny word!
It sure is!

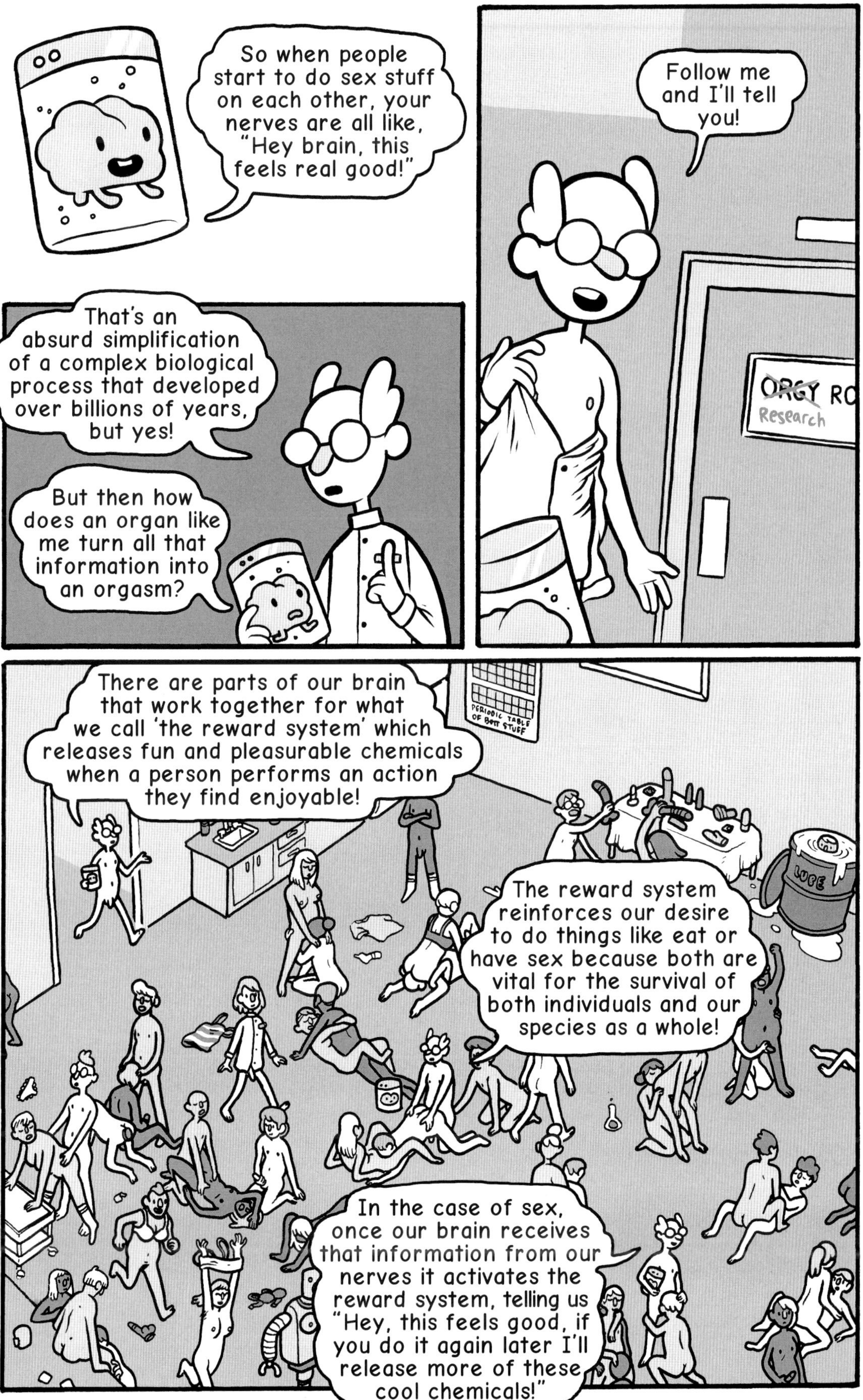
So when people start to do sex stuff on each other, your nerves are all like, "Hey brain, this feels real good!"
Follow me and I'll tell you!
ORGY RO
Research
That's an absurd simplification of a complex biological process that developed over billions of years, but yes!
But then how does an organ like me turn all that information into an orgasm?
There are parts of our brain that work together for what we call 'the reward system' which releases fun and pleasurable chemicals when a person performs an action they find enjoyable!
PERIODIC TABLE OF BUTT STUFF
LUBE
The reward system reinforces our desire to do things like eat or have sex because both are vital for the survival of both individuals and our species as a whole!
In the case of sex, once our brain receives that information from our nerves it activates the reward system, telling us "Hey, this feels good, if you do it again later I'll release more of these cool chemicals!"

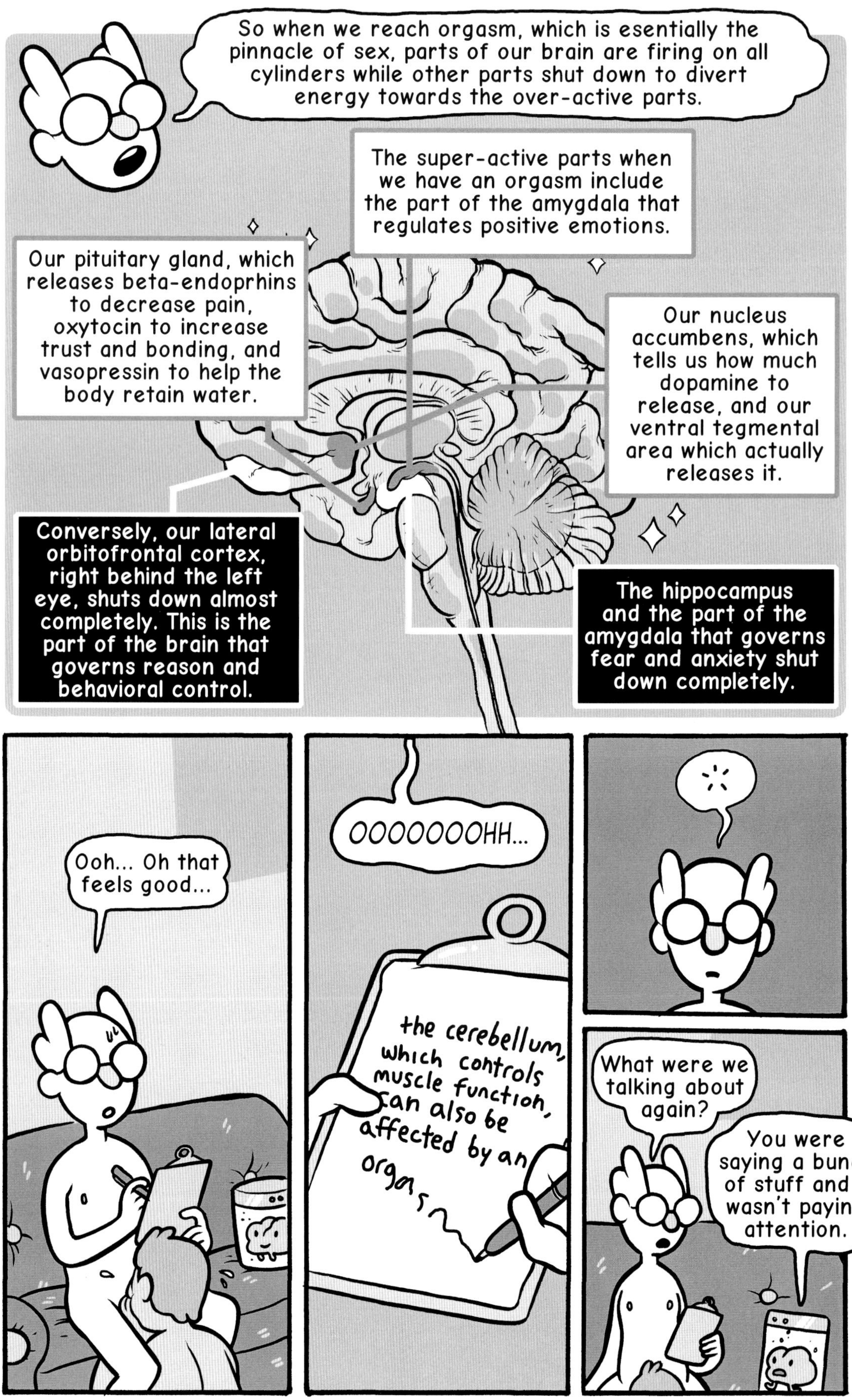

So when we reach orgasm, which is esentially the pinnacle of sex, parts of our brain are firing on all cylinders while other parts shut down to divert energy towards the over-active parts.
The super-active parts when we have an orgasm include the part of the amygdala that regulates positive emotions.
Our pituitary gland, which releases beta-endoprhins to decrease pain, oxytocin to increase trust and bonding, and vasopressin to help the body retain water.
Our nucleus accumbens, which tells us how much dopamine to release, and our ventral tegmental area which actually releases it.
Conversely, our lateral orbitofrontal cortex, right behind the left eye, shuts down almost completely. This is the part of the brain that governs reason and behavioral control.
The hippocampus and the part of the amygdala that governs fear and anxiety shut down completely.
Ooh... Oh that feels good...
OOOOOOOHH...
the cerebellum, which controls muscle function, can also be affected by an orgasm
What were we talking about again?
You were saying a bunch of stuff and I wasn't paying attention.

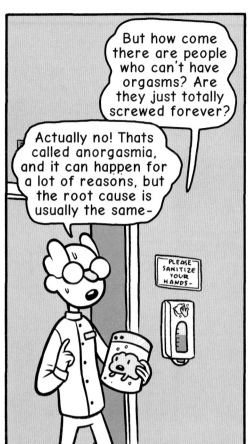

But how come there are people who can't have orgasms? Are they just totally screwed forever?

Actually no! Thats called anorgasmia, and it can happen for a lot of reasons, but the root cause is usually the same—

PLEASE SANITIZE YOUR HANDS—

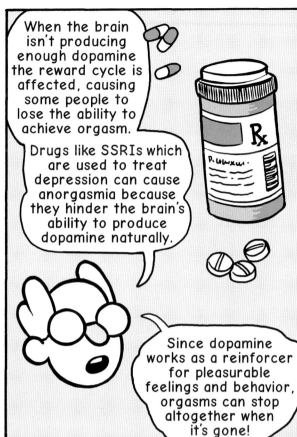

When the brain isn't producing enough dopamine the reward cycle is affected, causing some people to lose the ability to achieve orgasm.

Drugs like SSRIs which are used to treat depression can cause anorgasmia because they hinder the brain's ability to produce dopamine naturally.

Rx

Since dopamine works as a reinforcer for pleasurable feelings and behavior, orgasms can stop altogether when it's gone!

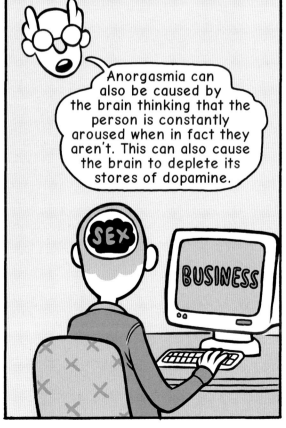

Anorgasmia can also be caused by the brain thinking that the person is constantly aroused when in fact they aren't. This can also cause the brain to deplete its stores of dopamine.

SEX

BUSINESS

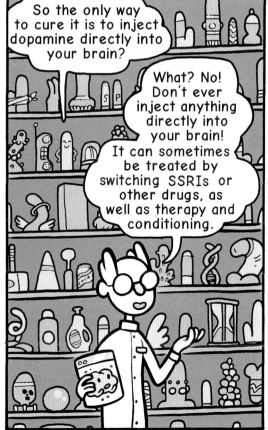

So the only way to cure it is to inject dopamine directly into your brain?

What? No! Don't ever inject anything directly into your brain!

It can sometimes be treated by switching SSRIs or other drugs, as well as therapy and conditioning.

Some people can feel orgasms in other parts of their bodies too! such as:

Nipples

Hands

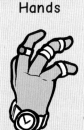

Feet

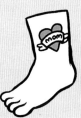

Scalps, and more!

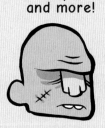

Researchers think that this is caused by the nerves that lead from the body part in question going to the same part of the brain that the genitals do!

People with missing limbs have also reported feeling orgasms in their absent parts! This happens when the cortical homunculus, which maps our brain to corresponding body parts, will sometimes repurpose the part of the brain that used to control the missing limb to the genitals instead!

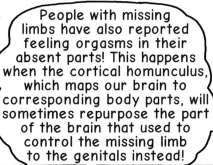

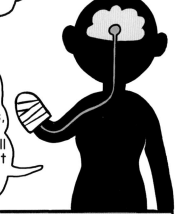

So next time you explode your load, climax, cum, shoot your wad, pop your top, shoot, squirt, ejaculate, blow your roof off, pull the trigger on your love gun, or take the tickle-train to tingle-town, be sure to thank all of that gooey grey matter for making it possible!

Thanks, me!

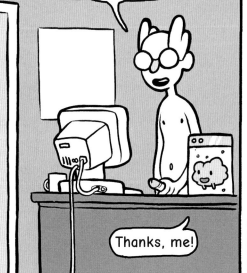

Hey what the-

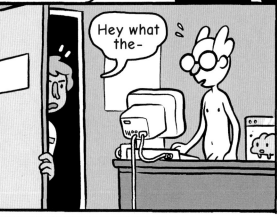

If you're going to masturbate do it in your own office!

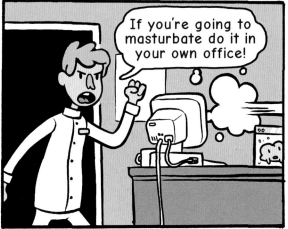

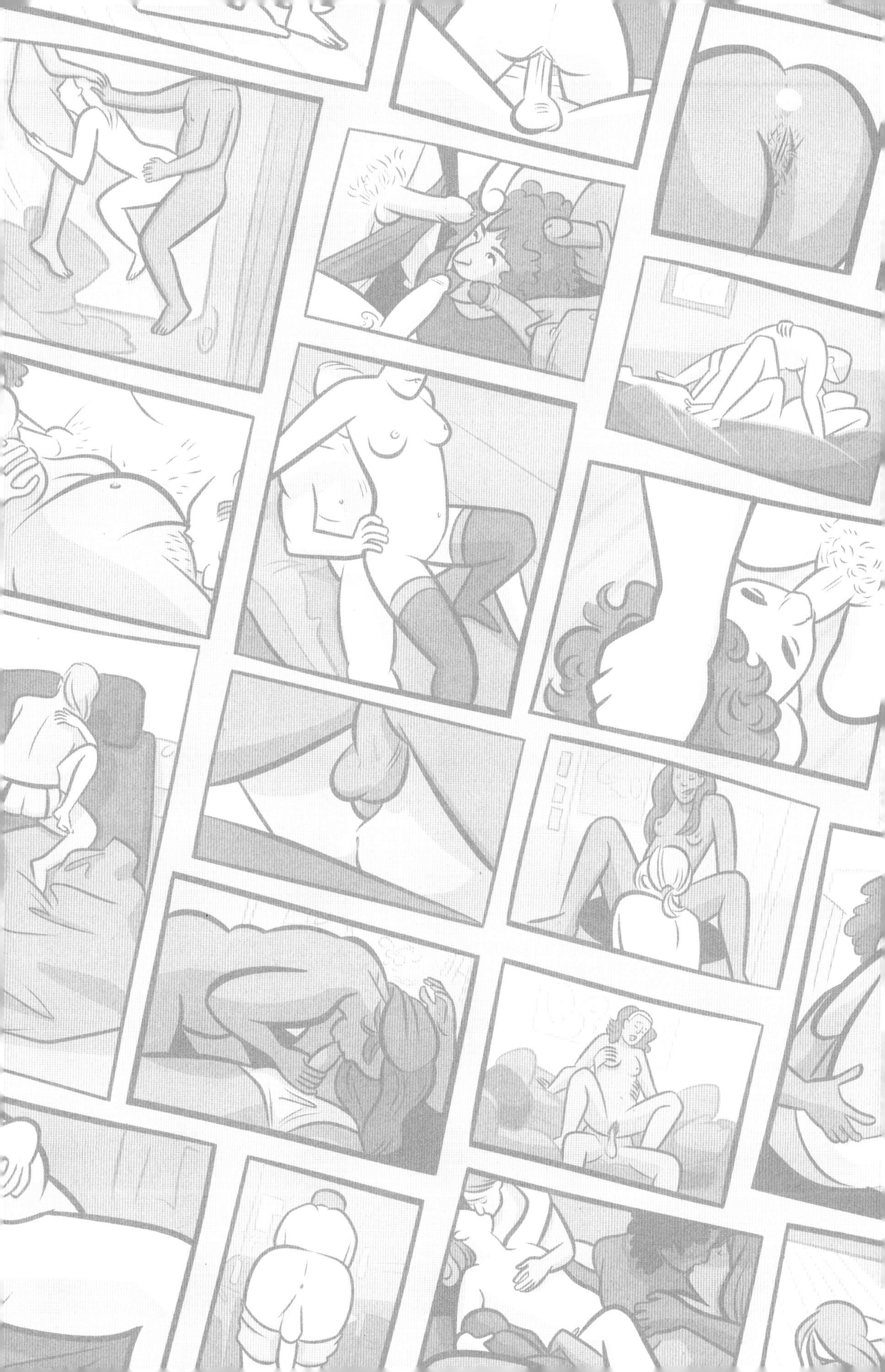

Oh Joy Sex Toy

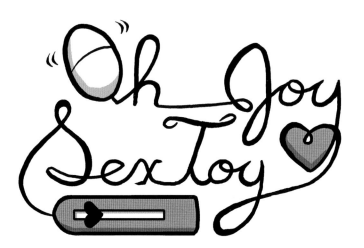